DAY-CASE ANAESTHESIA
AND SEDATION

Day-Case Anaesthesia and Sedation

EDITED BY J. G. WHITWAM
MB, ChB, PhD, FRCP, FRCA
Professor and Director, Department of Anaesthesia
Royal Postgraduate Medical School
Hammersmith Hospital, London

FOREWORD BY A. A. SPENCE
CBE, MD, MB, ChB, FRCA, FRCP (Glas),
FRCS (Ed), FRCP (Ed)
Professor of Anaesthetics
University of Edinburgh

OXFORD
Blackwell Scientific Publications
LONDON EDINBURGH BOSTON
MELBOURNE PARIS BERLIN VIENNA

Editorial Offices:
Osney Mead, Oxford OX2 0EL
25 John Street, London WC1N 2BL
23 Ainslie Place, Edinburgh EH3 6AJ
238 Main Street, Cambridge
Massachusetts 02142, USA
54 University Street, Carlton
Victoria 3053, Australia

Other Editorial Offices:
Librairie Arnette SA
1, rue de Lille
75007 Paris
France

Blackwell Wissenschafts-Verlag GmbH
Düsseldorfer Str. 38
D-10707 Berlin
Germany

Blackwell MZV
Feldgasse 13
A-1238 Wien
Austria

First published 1994

Set, printed and bound in Great Britain at the University Press, Cambridge

DISTRIBUTORS

Marston Book Services Ltd
PO Box 87
Oxford OX2 0DT
(*Orders*: Tel: 0865 791155
Fax: 0865 791927
Telex: 837515)

USA
Blackwell Scientific Publications, Inc.
238 Main Street
Cambridge, MA 02142
(*Orders*: Tel: 800 759-6102
617 876-7000)

Canada
Times Mirror Professional Publishing, Ltd
130 Flaska Drive
Markham, Ontario L6G 1B8
(*Orders*: Tel: 800 268-4178
416 470-6739)

Australia
Blackwell Scientific Publications Pty Ltd
54 University Street
Carlton, Victoria 3053
(*Orders*: Tel: 03 347-5552)

A catalogue record for this title is available from the British Library

ISBN 0-632-03704-0

Library of Congress
Cataloging-in-Publication Data

Day-case anaesthesia and sedation: anaesthesia and sedation for day-case procedures and ambulatory surgery / edited by J.G. Whitwam.
p. cm.
Includes bibliographical references and index.
ISBN 0-632-03704-0
1. Anesthesia. 2. Ambulatory surgery. 3. Analgesia.
I. Whitwam, J. G. (James G.)
[DNLM: 1. Ambulatory Surgery. 2. Ambulatory Care. 3. Anesthesia—methods. 4. Analgesia—methods. WO 200 D2725 1994]
RD82.D39 1994
617.9′6—dc20
DNLM/DLC
for Library of Congress

Contents

Contributors, viii

Foreword, xi
A. A. Spence

Preface, xiii

Part 1: General Principles of Pharmacology and Subjects Relevant to the Practice of Day-Case Anaesthesia

1 History and Scope of Day-Case Anaesthesia: Past, Present and Future, 3
I. Smith and P. F. White

2 Pharmacology and Day-Case Anaesthesia, 20
D. P. Dob and J. G. Whitwam

3 Pharmacological Principles in Paediatric Patients, 58
N. S. Morton and D. Lord

4 Anaphylactic and Anaphylactoid Reactions, 69
J. Pepys and M. M. Fisher

5 Cardiopulmonary Resuscitation, 87
D. A. Zideman and W. F. Dick

6 Methods for Assessment of Recovery, 104
G. G. Lockwood

7 Safe Endoscopy, 118
E. B. Keeffe

8 Management of Diabetic Day-Case Patients, 133
K. Shotliff and E. M. Kohner

9 Pain Treatment in the Day-Care Unit, 138
W. W. A. Zuurmond

10 The Future: the Effect of Minimally Invasive Therapy on Day-Case Anaesthesia, 151
J. G. Whitwam

Part 2: Anaesthesia, Analgesia, Sedation

ADULT ANAESTHESIA

11 Adult Day-Case Anaesthesia, 165
A. P. Fisher and E. K. Krzeminska

12 Laparoscopy and its Complications, 202
A. M. Skelly and J. G. Whitwam

13 Ophthalmic Day-Case Anaesthesia, 212
C. Carr

14 General Anaesthesia for Outpatient Dentistry, 226
A. Padfield

15 Local Anaesthesia in Day-Case Surgery, 238
W. W. A. Zuurmond and J. J. de Gange

16 Sedation and Sedoanalgesia, 262
J. G. Whitwam and Chen Wang

17 Patient Controlled Sedation, 275
L. B. Cook and J. G. Whitwam

18 Anaesthetic Circuits and Ventilation Systems, 289
M. K. Chakrabarti, P. Ravussin and J. G. Whitwam

PAEDIATRIC ANAESTHESIA

19 General Principles of Paediatric Day-Case Anaesthesia, 303
N. S. Morton and D. Lord

20 General Anaesthesia for Paediatric Day-Case Surgery, 313
D. Lord

21 Local Anaesthesia for Paediatric Day-Case Surgery, 332
N. S. Morton

Part 3: Procedural Safety

22 Issues Involved in Safe Practice, 347
D. M. Nolan

23 Nursing and Unit Organization, 369
S. Penn

Part 4: Legal Issues

24 Legal Aspects of Day-Case Surgery, 383
N. Davies

25 The Practitioner, the Anaesthetist and the Law, 389
D. Poswillo

Appendices

1 Criteria for Day-Cases and Outpatients, 399
2 Malignant Hyperpyrexia, 400
3 High Frequency Ventilation/High Frequency Oscillation, 404
4 Semantics of Day-Case Anaesthesia, Analgesia and Sedation, 405
5 Bleeding Disorders and Day-Case Surgery, 406
6 Sickle Disease, 410
7 Summary of Patient Assessment and Process, 412

Index, 416

Contributors

C. Carr MA, MBBS, FRCA, *Consultant Anaesthetist, Moorfields Eye Hospital, City Road, London EC1V 2PD*

M. K. Chakrabarti BSc, MPhil, MBE, *Senior Chief Technician, Department of Anaesthesia, Royal Postgraduate Medical School, Hammersmith Hospital, Du Cane Road, London W12 0NN*

L. B. Cook MBBS, FRCA, *Senior Registrar, Department of Anaesthetics, Hammersmith Hospital, Du Cane Road, London W12 0NN*

N. Davies QC, *3 Serjeants' Inn, London EC4 1BQ*

J. J. de Gange MD, PhD, *Professor of Anaesthesiology, Department of Anaesthesiology, Academic Hospital, Vrije Universiteit, Amsterdam, The Netherlands*

W. F. Dick, *Klinik für Anästhesiologie, Johannes Gutenberg Universität, Langenbeck Strasse 1, D-6500 Mainz 1, Germany*

D. P. Dob BSc (Hons), MBBS, FRCA, *MRC Research Fellow, Department of Anaesthetics, Hammersmith Hospital, Du Cane Road, London W12 0NN*

A. P. Fisher FRCA, *Consultant Anaesthetist, King's College Hospital, Denmark Hill, London SE5 9RS*

M. M. Fisher MB, ChB, MD, FFARACS, FANZCA, *Head, Intensive Therapy Unit, Royal North Shore Hospital, St Leonards, New South Wales 2065, Australia*

E. B. Keeffe MD, *Clinical Professor of Medicine, University of California, San Francisco; Chief, Division of Gastroenterology and Hepatology; Director, Gastroenterology Laboratory; Medical Director, Liver Transplant Program, California Pacific Medical Center; Secretary to the American Society for Gastrointestinal Endoscopy*

E. M. Kohner MD, FRCP, FCOphth, *Professor of Medical Ophthalmology, Diabetic Retinopathy Unit, Royal Postgraduate Medical School, Hammersmith Hospital, Du Cane Road, London W12 0NN*

E. K. Krzeminska FRCA, *Senior Registrar, Department of Anaesthetics, King's College Hospital, Denmark Hill, London SE5 9RS*

G. G. Lockwood FRCA, *Senior Lecturer, Department of Anaesthetics, Royal Postgraduate Medical School, Hammersmith Hospital, Du Cane Road, London W12 0NN*

D. Lord, *Consultant Anaesthetist, Booth Hall Children's Hospital, Charlestown Road, Blackley, Manchester M9 2AA*

N. S. Morton MB, ChB, FRCA, FFARCS(Ire), *Consultant in Paediatric Anaesthesia and Intensive Care, Department of Anaesthetics, The Royal Hospital for Sick Children, Yorkhill NHS Trust, Glasgow G3 8SJ*

D. M. Nolan, *Consultant Anaesthetist, Withington Hospital, Nell Lane, West Didsbury, Manchester M20 8LE*

A. Padfield MB, FRCAnaesth, DA, *Consultant Anaesthetist and Honorary Clinical Lecturer, Royal Hallamshire and Charles Clifford Dental Hospitals, University of Sheffield*

S. Penn RGN, *Manager, Day Surgery Unit, Addenbrooke's Hospital, Hills Road, Cambridge CB2 2QQ*

J. Pepys MD, FRCP, FRCPath, FFOM, *Honorary Consultant, Immunological Medicine Unit, Royal Postgraduate Medical School, Hammersmith Hospital, Du Cane Road, London W12 0NN*

D. Poswillo CBE, DDS, MD, DSc, FRCPath, *Emeritus Professor, Department of Oral and Maxillofacial Surgery, Guy's Hospital, St Thomas Street, London SE1 9RT*

P. Ravussin, *Royal Postgraduate Medical School, Hammersmith Hospital, Du Cane Road, London W12 0NN*

K. Shotliff MRCP, *Research Fellow, Diabetic Retinopathy Unit, Royal Postgraduate Medical School, Hammersmith Hospital, Du Cane Road, London W12 0NN*

A. M. Skelly, *Royal Postgraduate Medical School, Hammersmith Hospital, Du Cane Road, London W12 0NN*

I. Smith BSc, MBBS, FRCA, *Senior Registrar, Midlands Anaesthetic Training Scheme, Birmingham*

Chen Wang, *Royal Postgraduate Medical School, Hammersmith Hospital, Du Cane Road, London W12 0NN*

P. F. White PhD, MD, FFARACS, *Professor and Holder of the McDermott Chair in Anesthesiology, Department of Anesthesiology and Pain Management, University of Texas Southwestern Medical Center, Dallas TX 75235–9068, USA*

J. G. Whitwam MB, ChB, PhD, FRCP, FRCA, *Professor and Director, Department of Anaesthetics, Royal Postgraduate Medical School, Hammersmith Hospital, Du Cane Road, London W12 0NN*

D. A. Zideman QHP(c), BSc, MBBS, FRCA, *Consultant Anaesthetist, Royal Postgraduate Medical School, Hammersmith Hospital, Du Cane Road, London W12 0NN*

W. W. A. Zuurmond MD, PhD, *Department of Anaesthesia, Academic Hospital, Vrije Universiteit, Amsterdam, The Netherlands*

Foreword

The growth of day surgery, at least in the United Kingdom, is a product of a wider revolution in health care delivery, in which the major factor is cost containment. In addition, however, doctors, managers and politicians have come to realize that there are considerable social and consumer benefits. Although the scope of surgery must be limited, the range of procedures has grown as confidence develops. Changes in operating methods also are having an impact, with endoscopic surgery as the biggest single factor for further change, although its scope remains to be defined reliably. Finally, the development of therapeutic procedures from other disciplines (radiology, dentistry, pain management) fits comfortably with the day surgery ethos, stimulating and benefiting from this whole area of change.

To those whose basic specialist education preceded these changes, and to others, it is obvious that day and short-stay procedures with invasion and danger to the tissues, including anaesthesia or sedation, have major implications for risk management. Thus day care is not simply to be added to the established repertoires; it is a definable practice on its own, depending, as does all sound therapy, on good science. Sadly, at the moment, many doctors have not heeded, let alone led, that process within the clinical team. Indeed, apart from the efforts of a few enthusiasts, much of the body of knowledge has been put together by drug and equipment salesmen and by lay administrators, none of whom have the correct background. Now, as this book testifies, it is time for systematic study and intensive audit of activity. We need to know the real health 'gain' and also to define and minimize deficit. There is a need for clinical guidelines, and some appear within this text, but there is also a need to be critical of guidelines through audit and experimentation. Nothing should be regarded as set in concrete.

Professor Joe Whitwam has recognized all these problems and the need for a book to deal with them. But that is a very inadequate curtain-raiser for what is here. This work is highly original in its planning, extends far beyond an elementary guide to its subject, yet identifies the main messages so well that there is a wide potential readership from a variety of backgrounds and levels of understanding. The mainly scientific chapters are up-to-date and very readable. They are essential for those on the steep learning curve of anaesthesia and sedation. I would also urge established practitioners to look closely. At least, they will find an up-to-date view, and perhaps, as in my case, they will learn one or two things that they did not know before.

The clinical practice chapters will stand as an essential and authoritative source, while the editor's linking text not only serves to orientate, but informs and challenges as well. I should add that there are some chapter titles which struck me initially as having arrived in the wrong book, but I assure the reader that they have quite central relevance to the purpose of this volume.

It has been my privilege to know Professor Whitwam for some 30 years and to share with others the knowledge that he is one of the best anaesthetists of our generation. He is also—and I say this affectionately—reliably idiosyncratic. All these qualities have come together here uniquely and delightfully.

ALASTAIR A. SPENCE
November 1993

Preface

This book is concerned with sedation, analgesia and anaesthesia suitable not only for conventional day-case surgery as currently practised in day-care units, but also for use during endoscopic and interventional therapeutic procedures, for example in departments of radiology, gastroenterology and cardiology. In addition to discussions of adult and paediatric anaesthesia, both local and general, there is a long section concerned with sedation. This provides clear, unequivocal guidelines and descriptions of how to perform sedation techniques, including the methods currently in use for patient controlled sedation and requirements for safe practice. Chapters on demand sedation and also assessment of recovery provide information which practitioners wishing to set up their own demand systems and undertake research may find useful.

In addition to core material, a series of carefully selected topics describe practical aspects of subjects important to the safe management of patients undergoing anaesthesia and sedation, for example drug reactions, cardiopulmonary resuscitation, diabetes and relevant haematological disorders, anaesthesia and gas delivery circuits, together with aspects of jet and cuirass ventilation, problems of endoscopy and a current review of the complications of laparoscopy. It is the first general book to contain a description of the new European and North American guidelines on cardiopulmonary resuscitation. Finally there is a section on the medicolegal principles of sound practice.

The book draws on the experience and views of a group of carefully chosen specialists with a wide range of clinical interests and seniority to give a balanced perspective of current practice and also those developments which can be anticipated to have increasing application in the future. It includes an overview of the impact of minimally invasive therapy on anaesthesia and it is intended to be of interest not only to anaesthesiologists, but also of practical use to specialists concerned with interventional procedures. At present there is an insufficient supply of trained anaesthetists to meet the future requirements of sedation practice and the specialists in charge of minimally invasive therapy are increasingly having to provide or organize the practice of safe sedation and analgesia for themselves.

It should be of interest to all such clinicians, including gastroenterologists, rheumatologists and cardiologists, interventional radiologists and endoscopic surgeons.

Much endoscopic surgery, particularly laparoscopic procedures, requires general anaesthesia and hence surgeons are more directly involved with anaesthesiologists who are therefore readily available to them.

It has been assumed that well-trained, experienced anaesthesiologists can administer safe anaesthesia with rapid recovery and turnover of patients and are familiar with the best drugs and monitoring systems currently available for this purpose. The book has been prepared with this consideration in mind. Thus whereas the practical aspects of sedation techniques are described for those with little or no formal training in anaesthesia, no attempt has been made to provide instructions of how to provide general anaesthesia, since this would not only be patronizing to anaesthesiologists, but also it was felt that the main thrust should be concerned with currently accepted principles and the organization of care and safety. However, the more general anaesthetist should find the specialist chapters including demand sedation, local anaesthesia and day-case pain therapy of considerable interest. Emphasis has also been given to those areas of major concern to anaesthesiologists about which even the most experienced senior staff may have insecurities in relation to the present state of the art, for example new views on resuscitation, drug reactions, new drugs, management of diabetes and haemorrhagic disorders, complications of laparoscopy, sedation techniques, laser surgery of the airway, jet and cuirass ventilation and not least sound legal principles.

In addition there are guidelines for procedural safety in nuclear magnetic resonance imaging units, radiology departments and during laser surgery.

Day-case surgery started with dental anaesthesia and world-wide the bulk of dental procedures are still carried out in privately owned facilities, principally using local anaesthesia with or without sedation, with recourse to general anaesthesia only when necessary. However, such patients are, strictly speaking, outpatients (see Appendix 1) since a day case has been defined as a patient who is admitted for a planned procedure on a non-resident basis, who requires facilities for recovery and a period of postprocedural observation. In normal day-care arrangements, recovery facilities are available if required; for a whole day stay usually only up to approximately 10 h, it is accepted that a small percentage of patients may require to be formally admitted to the supporting hospital for a minimum of overnight stay, i.e. approximately 24 h. Technically this definition excludes minor procedures undertaken in dental clinics, outpatient, and accident and emergency departments (see Appendix 1).

Whenever patients are returned home to a professionally unmonitored environment after increasingly major therapeutic interventions, anaesthetists, surgeons, interventionalists and increasingly hospital managers, are taking a calculated risk that there will be no complications requiring immediate treatment which could threaten life or induce long-term morbidity. Moreover, the flexibility and extent of therapy for pain, nausea and vomiting, may be limited and apart from humanitarian considerations such problems can be the subject of serious litigation.

A whole variety of questions can be posed: How should patients be assessed preoperatively? Should there be any age limitation? Why are 65 years and 100 kg the maximum age and weight allowed in some units? What should be the minimum period of fluid deprivation and starvation, if any, before anaesthesia, whether local or general, and sedation? Should intravenous fluid loading be practised during the procedure to delay the need for oral fluids postoperatively? Should trasylol (aprotinin) be used to protect clot formation in patients treated with salicylates and non-steroidal anti-inflammatory drugs (NSAIDs) in selected patients now that laparoscopic cholecystectomy is on the day-case agenda? Should the use of the new prepacked disposable patient controlled analgesia (PCA) systems, which can be mounted on the forearm, be considered for use in the home environment? Is it possible that cases of acid aspiration syndrome have occurred at home after gastroscopy in patients whose laryngeal reflexes were depressed by sedative drugs immediately after removal of the endoscope without the causal link being made? When does rapid eye movement (REM) sleep with its associated nocturnal episodes of hypoxaemia return after day-case anaesthesia? Are there special issues of consent? There is little hard data from well-controlled studies and audits on these issues, some of which are fundamental to the organization of day-case units.

At the heart of all the discussion and debate is procedural and hence public safety, and there is little doubt that the seniority, experience and knowledge of the staff undertaking the work is paramount. However, their work requires good organization and management.

Arguably one of the worst fates that can befall a human being, particularly when young, is the recurrence of a carcinoma of the face with bone involvement, or a melanoma, due to inadequate initial surgery, and such patients on the one hand should be referred to experienced specialists and on the other should not be delegated to the 'lumps and bumps' list to be performed by inexperienced junior surgeons.

There are two major factors driving the move to undertake more surgery on an ambulatory or outpatient basis: costs and the introduction of new technology. The second factor is arguably the more important in the long term since it is allowing the treatment of an increasing range of pathology in a less invasive way. The key is visualization of structures, without the need for exposure by surgical access, so far principally using the fibreoptic endoscope, digital subtraction angiography and ultrasound, and this has allowed the development of minimally invasive therapy.

There are two principal results. First, much conventional surgery is now being undertaken less invasively using endoscopes, and has spawned a proliferation of new societies and journals concerned with endoscopic surgery. Second, and again in the long term probably of greater import, is the entry of a great many specialists, who were formerly concerned largely with diagnosis, into the therapeutic arena, notably radiologists, gastroenterologists and cardiologists. Nowhere is this seen more dramatically than in the development of angioplasty, and the introduction of stents into both the vascular system and ducts and conduits of all types. The interventional radiologist has converted some of the treatment of obstruction of the blood supply to the lower limbs from a conventional abdominal vascular surgical procedure, often requiring high dependency or intensive care facilities, to a closed procedure requiring only counselling and local infiltration of the groin with or without sedation, and which can be performed in large numbers of selected patients on a day-care basis.

Thus the terms 'anaesthesia' and 'surgery' are too narrow to encompass the ever wider range and increasing number of interventional day-case procedures for which the practice of safe sedation and analgesia, alone or in combination, is becoming increasingly important, and which are conducted in departments away from not only the main operating theatres but also the new day surgery units.

From an anaesthetic point of view the whole emphasis is on speed of recovery of the patients and minimizing risk and morbidity with the introduction of local anaesthesia and anxiolytic drugs whenever possible, since sedation can be an unnecessarily deep state. The technique is described as sedoanalgesia in the UK and monitored anaesthetic care in the USA. As in surgery, for procedural safety it is vital that experienced staff anaesthesiologists are involved in the whole process of the management of ambulatory surgery in day-case units. Others involved, particularly the nursing staff, radiographers, receptionists and operating theatre assistants require leadership and clear guidelines, for example in the assessment for admission, discharge criteria and consent of patients. Each unit will develop its own ambience and, within a core of activity common to all such units, its own procedural arrangements.

Although it is often assumed that surgery and other interventional procedures are being introduced, particularly by health-care managers, to obtain more work from existing facilities and budgets, i.e. purely on the basis of cost, it must be remembered that there are real positive benefits for patients. These include, for example, reduced personal costs, in an insured fee for service health-care environment, particularly with the removal of the need for the hotel facility, convenience for the family, and reduced loss of earnings due to the more rapid recovery time following minimally invasive procedures, although the latter is only indirectly a day-care issue.

JAMES G. WHITWAM
July 1993

Part 1:
General Principles of Pharmacology and Subjects Relevant to the Practice of Day-Case Anaesthesia

This part starts with Chapter 1 which reviews the history and current scope of day-case surgery.

The second chapter on pharmacological principles pays attention to some of the newer drugs, notably mivacurium, and considerable discussion is given to the new inhalational agents, which are currently undergoing trials, that is desflurane and sevoflurane. These latter two agents have considerable potential in the field of day-case anaesthesia, since recovery from desflurane as the sole anaesthetic is quicker than from propofol. However, desflurane presents problems from the point of view of its boiling point and administration, the etherish smell of the agent and the postoperative recovery period where some nausea may occur. Sevoflurane on the other hand is a pleasanter agent for the patient and provides faster recovery than isoflurane.

This chapter also deals not only with the pharmacology of the benzodiazepines and the central role of midazolam in sedation, but also with some of the newer concepts of synergism and the exploitation of synergism to induce anaesthesia for which co-induction is used. By this is meant the administration of small amounts of one drug to reduce the amount required of the main agent. For example, by the administration of small doses of alfentanil and midazolam it is possible to reduce the induction dose of propofol by 86%. The application of co-induction should ensure faster recovery since smaller doses of two drugs are used. Thus, whereas synergism between analgesic and sedative drugs can present a serious hazard in the practice of sedation by the unknowledgeable, the professional anaesthetist can exploit the same phenomenon to advantage.

Propofol is now commonly used for the induction of anaesthesia of short duration, as in the day-case setting. The saturation by propofol infusions of the cytochrome system which is involved in the metabolism of alfentanil increases the duration of action of the latter drug and it seems that such interactions are likely to become increasingly important in the study of drugs in the future. This part also includes an outline of newer additional drugs, for example $5HT_3$ antagonists and non-steroidal anti-inflammatory drugs (NSAIDs). However, the principal discussion of local anaesthesia and the pharmacology for example of the benzodiazepines and sedo-analgesia occurs in Part 2.

Chapter 4 on anaphylactoid reactions to drugs, written by Professor J. Pepys, currently at Hammersmith Hospital, and Dr Malcolm Fisher from the Royal North

Shore Hospital, Sydney, is authoritative and in terms of reported incidents this part is up to date at the time of writing.

Similarly resuscitation (Chapter 5) written by Dr Zideman and Professor Dick is written on the basis of the new European and American standards and this is the first publication of its type containing this new material.

Chapter 6 on methods of assessment of recovery is extremely important from two points of view. The first is in terms of audit and the clinical management of patients, and the second in the development of new drugs and protocols in the future, since objective methods of assessing recovery will become increasingly important. Dr Lockwood has produced a comprehensive review of the subject as it stands at the moment and it is a first class source for anyone working in this field.

Gastrointestinal endoscopy (Chapter 7) has a significant share of day-case and outpatient procedures and Professor Keeffe, who is a gastroenterologist, has comprehensively reviewed the issues surrounding endoscopic procedures. It is in this chapter that the philosophy of producing recommendations for training in new technologies becomes apparent. Professor Keeffe has produced a view of this subject which is relevant to anyone practising in this field anywhere in the world. Many of his comments on training and other issues are apposite in other areas of day-case surgery and anaesthesia.

Diabetes is a common and potentially dangerous disease which complicates the management of many types of patient. Dr Shotliff and Professor Kohner practise laser therapy on patients with diabetic retinopathy. They use periorbital block and sedation for many of their procedures. In a succinct account of the subject they provide an authoritative short practical protocol for the management of mild, moderate and severe diabetics in the day-case setting.

Anaesthesiologists practise a wide variety of techniques in the management of patients with both acute and chronic pain including for example nerve blocks, tractotomy, guanethidine Bier blocks and the introduction of epidural catheters for the prolonged administration of analgesic drugs in ambulatory patients. Dr Zuurmond gives a comprehensive description of this type of work in day-case patients. Since this is within the remit of anaesthesiologists and hence anaesthesia, but is not part of mainstream anaesthesia *per se*, it is included in this section of the book.

Finally, Chapter 10 concludes this part with a review of some of the present and potential future developments in minimally invasive therapy, their impact on clinical treatment and some of their implications for the practice of anaesthesia, particularly the expansion of day-case procedures and sedation.

Chapter 1
History and Scope of Day-Case Anaesthesia: Past, Present and Future

I. Smith and P. F. White

Modern anaesthetic practices have evolved from the efforts of early dental surgeons to persuade patients to accept their services, and thus to safeguard their income, by means of rendering their trade painless. Although dental anaesthesia is now generally regarded as a highly specialized form of day-case anaesthesia, it is interesting to observe that the first recipients of 'modern anaesthesia' would have been day-case patients. The first anaesthetic administered for a surgical procedure was probably given by Crawford W. Long, who excised two small tumours from the neck of James Venable on 30 March 1842. Long charged $2 for the surgery and 25 cents for the anaesthetic. Unfortunately, Long did not publish his results until 1849, and the 'discovery' of anaesthesia is usually attributed to William Thomas Morton, a dentist. Morton publicly demonstrated ether anaesthesia in the Bullfinch amphitheatre of the Massachusetts General Hospital, on Friday 16 October 1846 [1]. Despite the apparent magnitude of these events and the rapid dissemination of knowledge of the technique, anaesthesia was slow to become universally accepted. As a result, the number of surgical operations performed did not increase dramatically until the turn of the century.

The beginnings of day-case surgery, as it is currently defined, can be traced to the early 1900s, when Nicoll reported operating on a series of 8988 children as day-cases at the Glasgow Royal Hospital for Sick Children over a 10-year period [2]. Then in 1916, Ralph M. Waters opened his 'Downtown Anesthesia Clinic' in Sioux City, Iowa [3]. This facility, which provided care for dental and minor surgery cases, is generally regarded as the prototype for the modern free-standing day-case unit. The clinic evolved over the subsequent years and underwent expansion, in 1925, when Waters moved to Kansas City. More recent practitioners also reported favourable results with day-case surgery [4, 5].

Hospital-based day-case surgery in the USA was first established with the development of a formal outpatient surgical programme at the University of California at Los Angeles in 1962, and the opening of similar facilities at George Washington University in 1966 and in Providence, Rhode Island, in 1968. Further development of day-case anaesthesia as a subspecialty occurred with the establishment of the Society of Freestanding Ambulatory Surgical Centers—now called the Federated Ambulatory Surgery Association (FASA)—in 1974, and the Society for Ambulatory Anesthesia (SAMBA) in 1984. By 1985, 7.3 million operations in the USA (representing 34% of all elective surgical procedures) were performed as day-cases. In addition, a further three-quarters of a million day-case procedures were performed in free-standing units. In 1993, over 16.5 million day-case operations (60% of all elective operations) are performed yearly in the USA.

In the UK, the growth in day-case surgery has occurred at a slower pace than in the USA, where much of the expansion was fuelled by the desire of the medical insurance companies to contain rising health-care costs. In Britain, tradition has favoured the retention of an overnight stay following many types of surgical procedures. However, in recent years growth has occurred in day-case surgery, and is likely to accelerate with the move towards a purchaser–provider system under the recent health-care reforms [6]. At present, day-case surgery accounts for only 15% of operations in the UK, but the Royal College of Surgeons [7] has recommended that this should rapidly be increased towards 50–60%. In 1988, a multidisciplinary organization consisting of surgeons, radiologists and anaesthetists, called the Society for Minimally Invasive Therapy, held its first meeting in London. The growth of this international organization has been stimulated by the rapid development of endoscopic surgical techniques. The list of procedures which are considered suitable to be performed as day-cases is changing rapidly and varies considerably between different countries, and even within different regions of a country [8, 9].

Benefits of day-case surgery

Day-case surgery offers a number of advantages for both the patients and the health-care system. Patients like day-case surgery [10] because it decreases their separation time from the home and family environment and decreases their likelihood of contracting hospital-acquired infections and complications. Compared to a traditional hospital admission, there is also a reduction in the demand for postoperative medications and a more rapid recovery [11]. Unlike inpatient surgery, day-case surgery does not depend upon the availability of a hospital bed. This may permit the patient greater flexibility in selecting the time of surgery. Furthermore, the cost (per case) of day-case surgery may be 25–75% lower than that of similar inpatient care and the 'throughput' of patients can be considerably increased [12–14].

In a publicly funded health-care system, the increased use of day-case surgery can significantly decrease waiting times [15]. However, the ability to treat more patients in a given time period may cause total costs to rise, the so-called 'efficiency trap' [9]. In addition, the hospital beds that are made available by a move to day-case surgery do not usually remain empty, but instead are occupied by other needy patients [9, 16], which will also tend to increase overall costs. Furthermore, a move from inpatient to day-case surgery may have implications for the workload and work patterns of hospital and community-based nursing staff [17]. Despite these drawbacks, increased day surgery should improve the overall value for money of health care.

Patient selection

In order for day-case surgery to be safe, efficient and successful, careful selection of patients and procedures is crucial. A selection of procedures that are typically performed as day-cases are shown in Table 1.1. Procedures must be chosen that can be performed in a reasonable period of time (e.g. less than 90 min), are not associated with excessive blood loss or fluid shifts, do not require highly specialized equipment (e.g. lasers and microscopes) [18], or excessive postoperative care, and which are not associated with postoperative pain that is more severe than can be easily managed by patients in their own homes. Even in otherwise suitable cases (e.g. inguinal hernia repair), there are subpopulations of patients who are at increased risk of surgical complications or the need for more extensive surgery, and greater requirements for postoperative analgesics, immobilization and/or special nursing care [19]. Even laparoscopic surgery may result in a surprisingly high incidence of unanticipated hospital admission as a result of visceral perforation or the need for more extensive surgery than originally planned [20]. Furthermore, laparoscopy is frequently associated with postoperative morbidity, including nausea, vomiting and myalgia, in addition to abdominal and shoulder pain [21]. Of patients having this procedure, 40–50% require analgesic therapy after leaving the hospital [22, 23]. Other studies indicate that only 33–57% of patients undergoing laparoscopy are able to resume normal activities within 48 h, and the majority require 2–5 days to recover completely [23–25].

Once a range of procedures has been identified as being suitable for day surgery, the intended patients must also be assessed to ensure their acceptability for day surgery. Patients with serious coexisting diseases should be in a stable condition at the time of their operation to avoid an adverse response to surgery and anaesthesia. All day-case patients should be capable of understanding instructions for pre- and postoperative

Table 1.1 Surgical procedures commonly performed as day-cases. Modified from Urquhart and White [93] with permission

Dental	Extractions, conservation
Dermatology	Excision of skin lesions
Ear/nose/throat	Tonsillectomy, adenoidectomy, myringotomy, laryngoscopy, polypectomy
Eye	Tonometry, cataracts, strabismus surgery
General surgery	Biopsy and small lesion excision, varicose veins, herniorrhaphy, haemorrhoidectomy
Gynaecology	Dilatation and curettage, Bartholin's cyst, laparoscopies
Orthopaedic	Manipulation under anaesthesia, carpal tunnel, extremity surgery
Urology	Cystoscopy, orchidopexy, vasectomy
Paediatric	Circumcision, herniorrhaphy, examination under anaesthetic
Endoscopy	Endoscopy, colonoscopy, bronchoscopy
Plastic surgery	Cosmetic repairs, septorhinoplasty
Pain management	Chemicalsympathectomy, epidural injection

care and, following surgery, they should be accompanied home by a responsible escort. Someone should also be available to care for them during the first night after surgery and be able to assist them in obtaining emergency medical care, if needed. Once a patient is accepted for day-case surgery, they should be properly prepared for an anaesthetic technique which provides optimum intraoperative conditions, while at the same time ensuring rapid return of consciousness and protective reflexes at the completion of surgery, minimal residual effects on the central nervous system (so-called hangover), little impairment of postoperative cognitive function, minimal side effects, and, ideally, a degree of residual analgesia during the early recovery period. Postoperatively, pain and nausea must be effectively treated to permit early discharge of patients and to ensure their continuing comfort at home.

Traditionally in the USA, day-case surgery has been restricted to healthy patients who meet the American Society of Anesthesiologists (ASA) physical classification I or II. This follows from the finding that the incidence of perioperative complications is considerably increased in the presence of pre-existing disease, especially if the disease process involves the cardiovascular system (Table 1.2). However, providing that their disease has been stable and well controlled for 3 months or longer, patients of ASA physical status III may also safely undergo day-case surgery [26].

Table 1.2 Factors influencing the incidence of perioperative complications associated with day-case surgery. Modified from White [42] with permission

Factors	Incidence
Pre-existing disease	
None	1 in 156
Diabetes	1 in 149
Asthma	1 in 139
Chronic lung disease	1 in 112
Hypertension	1 in 87
Cardiovascular disease	1 in 74
Type of anaesthesia	
Local	1 in 268
Regional	1 in 277
Local/regional with sedation	1 in 106
General	1 in 120
Duration of surgery (h)	
< 1	1 in 155
1–2	1 in 84
2–3	1 in 54
> 3	1 in 35

Age of patients

In general, there is no correlation between the patient's age and their outcome following day-case surgery [27]. However, elderly patients are probably more likely to have social factors which render them less suitable for this type of surgery. Furthermore, recovery of fine motor skills and cognitive function is slowed with increasing age [28–30], therefore older patients may require a greater degree of post-discharge supervision than younger ones, which may place a greater burden on family members. At the opposite extreme of age, ex-preterm infants have an increased incidence of postoperative apnoeic episodes [31], which persists until they have exceeded approximately 46 weeks postconceptual age [32]. These infants should probably be admitted to hospital for overnight respiratory monitoring following even minor operations under general anaesthesia.

For older children, day-case surgery is generally advantageous, compared to inpatient care. Separation from parents is a major cause of anxiety for most children, and is especially common in those aged 1–4 years. While such separation can never be completely avoided when surgery is required, day-case surgery can reduce this to a minimum and avoid the need for the child to spend a night away from their familiar home environment.

Preoperative assessment

Since successful day-case surgery is dependent upon appropriate patient selection, there needs to be a reliable and accurate mechanism for assessment of patients scheduled for day-case surgery. Given that surgical, medical and social factors are all involved in the selection process, surgeons, anaesthetists and family practitioners should participate in the decision making. Although patients are not seen by an anaesthetist until the day of surgery in many day-surgery units, a thorough medical assessment is required well in advance of the planned surgery date if delays and cancellations are to be minimized. This will then allow time for the completion of any special investigations, and may also permit time for assessment and treatment of any pre-existing medical conditions. The preoperative assessment may be conducted by referring the patient to an 'anaesthetic clinic' immediately following their referral for day surgery. However, such a system may present logistical problems for both hospitals and patients. For this reason, alternative forms of assessment are currently under investigation. Better communication with surgical colleagues will result in fewer unsuitable patients being referred for day-case surgery. It is also possible to collect information from patients by way of a postal questionnaire or a telephone enquiry [33]. However, response rates to postal surveys are frequently disappointingly low, and not all patients may be easily reached by telephone.

Recently, interest has been shown in computerized information gathering systems. One such system (HealthQuiz) is now commercially available. This laptop computer device displays a series of screening questions, followed up by more specific enquiries, depending on the answers received. Patients respond using three buttons, clearly labelled 'yes', 'no' or 'don't know'. At the end of the screening session, a summary is produced which includes suggestions for further questioning and provides recommendations regarding appropriate laboratory tests. Patients have found this device simple to use, and a recent clinical trial demonstrated that patients gave similar answers 97% of the time when asked identical questions either by the computer or in a traditional interview format [34]. Furthermore, patients appear to give more accurate answers to personal and sensitive questions posed by a machine rather than during an interview. A further significant advantage of such systems is that patients may be guided in their use by non-medically qualified personnel. Future developments will see the combination of information-gathering systems with patient education packages. Preliminary results suggest that preoperative education of patients by computerized devices using interactive video technology results in stricter compliance with preoperative instructions than following a traditional interview [35].

Patient preparation

Appropriate preoperative preparation of patients will make day-case surgery both safer and more acceptable to patients. Preparation should be aimed at reducing the risks inherent in general anaesthesia, and in making the experience a pleasant one for the patient and their family. Preoperative preparation should be aimed at reducing patient anxiety by pharmacological and non-pharmacological means, where appropriate. Finally, preventative measures may be taken to reduce postoperative side effects (e.g. nausea and pain).

When general anaesthesia is employed, protective airway reflexes are obtunded, and there is a risk of aspiration. By avoiding the intake of solid food before surgery, the stomach may be allowed to empty naturally. However, in the absence of oral intake, gastric secretions continue to be produced, which will increase gastric volume. Traditionally, patients preparing for general anaesthesia have been asked to fast for at least 6 h, and frequently from midnight of the day before surgery. However, it is known that liquids are cleared much more rapidly than solids. Recent work has shown that clear liquids may safely be ingested up to 2 h before surgery, without increasing residual gastric volume [36–38]. Furthermore, the intake of oral fluids may actually dilute gastric secretions and stimulate gastric emptying, thereby lowering residual gastric volumes and acidity [36]. A further advantage is that patients find preoperative fluid restriction particularly unpleasant, and permitting oral fluids results in reduced anxiety, as well as decreased feelings of thirst and hunger [39]. For patients at risk of pulmonary aspiration, H_2 antagonists can reduce residual gastric acidity. Given the remarkably low incidence of clinically significant aspiration following day-case surgery (e.g. 1 in 2000 anaesthetics with a mortality rate close to 1 in 50000 [40]), routine prophylaxis with an H_2 blocker is not justified. The necessarily clinical trials to demonstrate the possible benefit from routine use of these expensive drugs have not been performed to date.

Patients scheduled to undergo elective surgery are typically anxious. In the days before modern anaesthetics and analgesics, perioperative pain and the (not insignificant) risk of death were the main concerns. At the present time, postoperative pain, perioperative 'awareness' and failure to recover from anaesthesia are more common concerns. Despite an almost universal utilization of premedication for inpatients over many years, day-case patients have customarily been denied pharmacological anxiolysis in the belief that the available agents would significantly delay their return to 'street fitness'. With the availability of short-acting benzodiazepines (e.g. midazolam), it is now possible to provide reliable sedation and anxiolysis without a clinically significant delay in recovery times or discharge ('home readiness'). Oral administration of temazepam and midazolam may be highly effective. Temazepam, 20 mg, and midazolam, 10 mg, (using the parenteral solution) were found to be equally effective for sedation and anxiolysis compared to placebo [41]. Patients preferred the active premedicant to the placebo, and were equally satisfied with either anxiolytic drug; neither of which had any adverse effect on recovery times. Unfortunately, many day-case patients are denied the benefits of premedicant drugs, simply because there is insufficient time for these drugs to act between the arrival of the patient and the induction of anaesthesia. For this reason, non-pharmacological factors (e.g. improved preoperative education) that can reduce anxiety are to be encouraged.

Choice of anaesthetic technique

Day-case surgery may potentially be conducted under general, regional or local anaesthesia. The choice of technique depends upon both surgical and patient factors. In addition, sedation may be added to local anaesthetic-based techniques (called monitored anesthesia care in the USA). General anaesthesia remains the most popular technique with both patients and hospital staff. However, an increasing percentage of cases are being performed with sedation techniques in the USA [42]. The increasing availability of drugs with short and highly predictable durations of effect, lack of accumulation, and minimal side effects, have made brief surgical procedures safer and more pleasant for patients, and are currently permitting longer and more complex surgery to be performed on a day-case basis.

Intravenous agents are now routinely used for induction of anaesthesia. Thiopentone has long been the standard agent for this purpose, however, it can impair fine motor skills for several hours and is less suitable for short day-case procedures. The first significant advance over thiopentone was methohexitone, a barbiturate with a shorter elimination half-life, which permitted significantly faster awakening and recovery [43]. Nevertheless, its use was still associated with a significant 'hangover' and it also produces a variety of undesirable excitatory side effects [44]. Etomidate has also been used for induction and maintenance of general anaesthesia for short outpatient

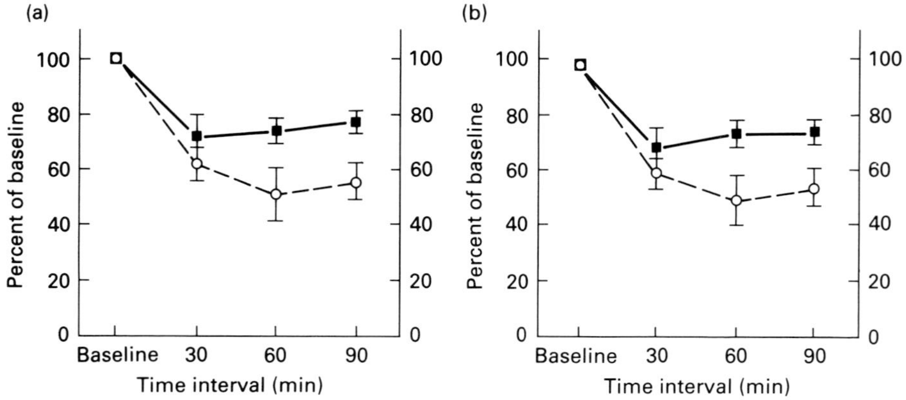

Fig. 1.1 Recovery of cognitive function, as assessed by digit-symbol substitution test (mean ± SEM values) in patients receiving either isoflurane (○— —○) or desflurane (■——■). (a) Number of pairs completed; (b) number of pairs corrected. $^*P < 0{\cdot}05$, from isoflurane. Redrawn from Ghouri *et al.* [60] with permission.

procedures [45]. However, recovery was not found to differ greatly from that with methohexitone [46, 47]. Furthermore, etomidate is associated with myoclonic movements, pain on injection and postoperative nausea and vomiting.

Propofol has recently become the induction agent of choice in day-case anaesthesia. It is associated with very rapid emergence as a result of its early redistribution and short elimination half-life. Recovery following propofol induction is faster than that with methohexitone, thiopentone or etomidate [48–51]. In addition, propofol is associated with a degree of euphoria on emergence and a reduced incidence of postoperative nausea [52–55]. Although the search for improved intravenous anaesthetics is continuing (e.g. pregnanolone), no experimental agent appears to have as favourable an early recovery profile as propofol. However, the term co-induction is increasingly being used to indicate the exploitation of synergism for the induction of anaesthesia. For example the administration of a small dose of midazolam at the start of anaesthesia can cause a major reduction in the amount of induction agent required, whether thiopentone, methohexitone or propofol, and hence improve the haemodynamic profile during the induction process without compromising recovery (Chapter 2).

For maintenance of anaesthesia, volatile agents have always been popular. The increasing series of halogenated ether compounds are generally associated with low blood : gas solubilities, permitting rapid onset and offset of effect, combined with greater haemodynamic stability. For day-case anaesthesia, many investigators have found few differences between halothane, enflurane and isoflurane [56, 57], while other workers have found enflurane to produce the most rapid recovery [58, 59]. Desflurane has recently become available in the USA and is likely to become extremely popular for maintenance of day-case anaesthesia. This agent possesses the lowest blood : gas solubility of any volatile anaesthetic, and is associated with more rapid awakening and decreased postoperative impairment of cognitive function than isoflurane (Fig. 1.1)

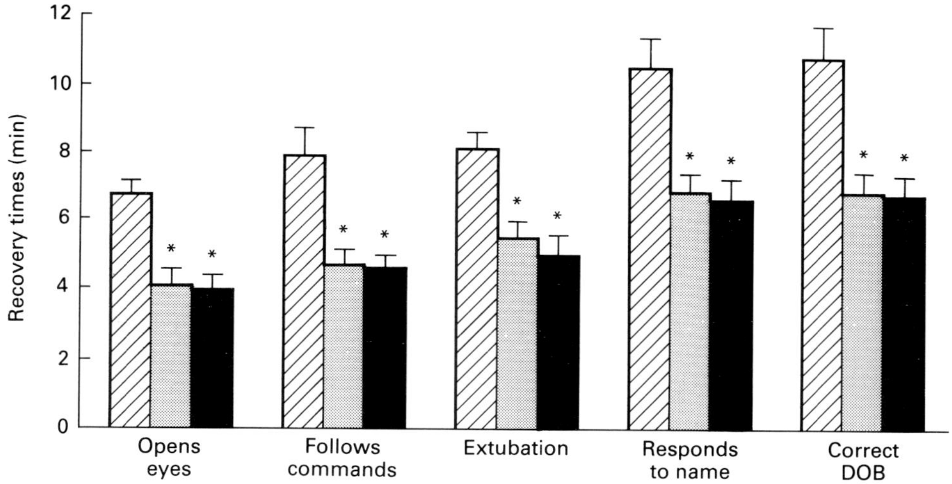

Fig. 1.2 Time (mean ± SEM) from discontinuation of anaesthesia until patients were able to open their eyes; obey commands; have their tracheal tube removed; and state their name and date of birth (DOB). (▨) Propofol induction, isoflurane maintenance; (▩) propofol induction, sevoflurane maintenance; and (■) sevoflurane induction and maintenance. $^*P < 0{\cdot}05$, from isoflurane. Redrawn from Smith *et al* [61] with permission.

[60]. Sevoflurane is also under widespread clinical investigation. This agent has also demonstrated faster awakening times than isoflurane (Fig. 1.2) [61], and may be especially useful as an induction agent, because it is non-irritating to the airway. Increasingly, propofol infusions are being used during the maintenance period to improve the quality of recovery from general anaesthesia. However, for brief day-case procedures, this technique has not been shown to permit faster recovery and discharge than either desflurane [62] or enflurane [63].

Face masks and oral airways are frequently employed for brief day-case procedures. However, more recently, endotracheal intubation has become more widespread in the day-surgery setting. Although all types of day-case anaesthesia may be managed successfully with one or other of these techniques, both have disadvantages. The laryngeal mask airway (LMA) is now employed in many situations where either a face mask or endotracheal tube would otherwise have been used. Advantages of the LMA include a clearer, hands-free airway compared to a face mask [64] and reduced requirement for anaesthetic agents, a lowered incidence of postoperative sore throat, decreased acute haemodynamic responses and avoidance of muscle relaxants and laryngoscopy compared to an endotracheal tube, Unfortunately, the laryngeal mask does not protect the airway against aspiration, and additional research is needed to determine whether the risk of regurgitation differs from that with a face mask technique.

The flexibility of day-case surgery can be greatly enhanced by the use of a wide variety of local and regional anaesthetic techniques. Common side effects of general

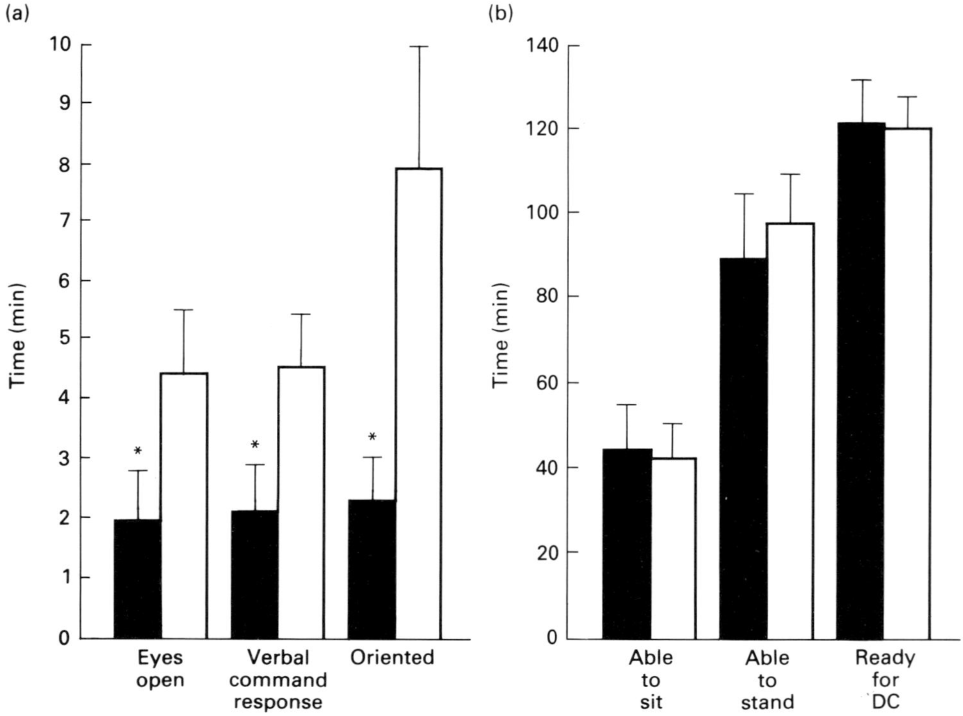

Fig. 1.3 Recovery times (mean ± SEM) from discontinuation of sedative infusion until patients were able to (a) open their eyes, obey commands or were orientated to time and place; (b) were able to sit and stand unassisted, and were judged to be fit for discharge. (□) Midazolam; (■) propofol. $^*P < 0{\cdot}05$, from midazolam. Redrawn from White and Negus [68] with permission.

anaesthesia (e.g. nausea, vomiting, dizziness, lethargy) are avoided, the risks of aspiration pneumonitis are minimized, postanaesthesia nursing care may be decreased, and residual analgesia is provided in the early postoperative period [65, 66]. Simple surgical procedures can be performed with local infiltration, whereas more extensive operations may be undertaken using field blocks and intravenous regional anaesthesia. For lower body procedures, spinal and epidural techniques may be utilized. Spinal anaesthesia is preferable to an epidural, since it is more readily performed and produces more rapid and consistent effects. Leakage of cerebrospinal fluid (CSF) may result in a severe, postural headache, which has limited the popularity of this technique. Modern technology permits the production of very fine (e.g. 27 gauge), pencil-pointed (e.g. Whitacre) needles, which produce an almost negligible incidence of postdural puncture headache. The greatest limiting factor to the use of spinal anaesthesia is now probably the persistence of sympathetic block into the recovery period (even when short-acting local anaesthetics are used).

Many patients would find the use of local and regional anaesthetic techniques intolerable were it not for the ability to provide adequate sedation and anxiolysis with adjuvant drugs. Once again, newer intravenous agents with a brief duration of action

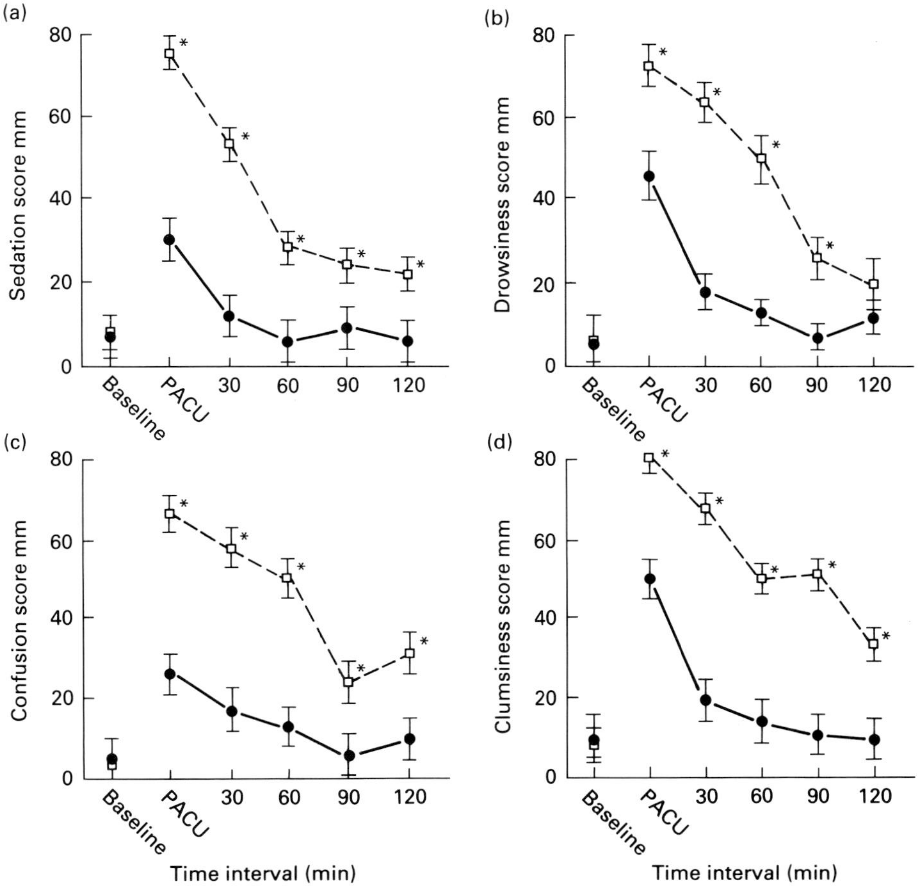

Fig. 1.4 Postoperative visual analogue scales for (a) sedation; (b) drowsiness; (c) confusion; and (d) clumsiness as assessed by patients who received either midazolam (□— —□) or propofol (●——●) by infusion during procedures performed under local or regional analgesia. Values are median (±SEM). $*P < 0{\cdot}05$, from propofol. Redrawn from White and Negus [68] with permission.

are now commonly used. Midazolam, 2 mg i.v., has been shown to increase significantly sedation, amnesia and anxiolysis during procedures performed under local anaesthesia, without delaying recovery [67]. Low-dose infusions of propofol permit satisfactory levels of sedation, which are rapidly adjustable and which permit a rapid recovery (Figs 1.3 & 1.4) [68]. The intraoperative use of patient-controlled analgesia with alfentanil during minor diagnostic and investigative procedures was equally satisfactory compared to physician-controlled alfentanil administration [69]. More recently, Ghouri and colleagues [70] have described patient-controlled administration of midazolam and propofol during day-case surgery performed under local anaesthesia.

Postoperative analgesia

The ability to control postoperative pain satisfactorily may make the difference between performing a given procedure on an inpatient or day-case basis. Following day-case surgery, pain should be controllable with conventional oral analgesics (e.g. paracetamol and codeine) before patients are discharged. However, potent, rapid-acting opioid analgesics (e.g. fentanyl, alfentanil, sufentanil) are very useful in treating early postoperative pain. While opioid analgesics have long been used to treat postoperative pain, their use may be associated with an increased incidence of postoperative nausea and vomiting, which reduces their desirability for day cases. Recently there has been greatly increased use of potent non-steroidal anti-inflammatory agents (e.g., diclofenac, ketorolac), which are effective in reducing the requirements for opioid analgesics [71–73]. For example, 6-hourly ketorolac (30 mg) after minor orthopaedic surgery markedly decreased the need for morphine and significantly improved pain scores [74]. Other (less expensive) non-steroidal agents can be administered orally in the preoperative period. For example, oral ibuprofen was found to provide prolonged postoperative analgesia with less nausea compared to parenteral fentanyl following laparoscopic surgery [75].

The use of local anaesthetic techniques, either for intraoperative analgesia or as an adjunct to general anaesthesia, can provide useful supplemental analgesia during the early postoperative period. Simple wound infiltration has been shown to improve postoperative analgesia following a variety of lower abdominal, extremity and laparoscopic procedures [76–79]. Following diagnostic laparoscopy, abdominal pain may be prevented by the use of a rectus sheath block [80], while the addition of a mesosalpinx block may reduce the deep pelvic pain from tubal ligation [80]. Shoulder pain is also common following laparoscopic surgery, and this has recently been reported to be effectively treated with subdiaphragmatic infiltration of local anaesthetic solution [81]. Following arthroscopic knee surgery, instillation of 30 ml of 0·5% bupivacaine into the joint space significantly reduced postoperative opiate requirements and permitted earlier ambulation and discharge but had no effect on the patient's assessment of pain [82]. Stein *et al.* [83] have reported low-dose intra-articular morphine can reduce delayed postoperative pain, and this interesting finding has recently been confirmed by other investigators [84].

Supplemental sedation, anxiolysis and analgesia may also be provided with the α_2 agonist agents, dexmedetomidine and clonidine. Dexmedetomidine has been shown to provide significant pain relief and reduced opioid analgesic requirements in women recovering from day-case laparoscopic sterilization [85]. However, the usefulness of these agents may be limited by an unacceptably high incidence of postoperative sedation and bradycardia.

Future expansion of day-case surgery will probably require further improvements in our ability to provide effective postoperative pain relief. One method which may be applicable is subcutaneous patient-controlled analgesia [86], which has already been shown to be practical outside the hospital [87].

Postoperative side effects

Side effects which might be regarded as minor in other situations may contribute to delays and unanticipated hospital admissions when they occur in day-case patients. Newer drugs tend to be pharmacodynamically 'cleaner' compared with earlier agents, and appear to be associated with a decrease in postoperative side effects. For example, residual lethargy and psychomotor impairment is less with propofol than with other available intravenous anaesthetics. Similarly, the non-depolarizing muscle relaxants do not produce the myalgias and neck stiffness which may be troublesome for ambulatory patients receiving suxamethonium [24, 88]. Even more recent ultra short-acting agents such as mivacurium may avoid the need to use reversal agents.

Of all the anaesthetic side effects after day surgery, nausea and vomiting remain the most troublesome. Although nausea is unpleasant at any time, it is a common cause of unanticipated hospital admission following day-case surgery [89]. A variety of anti-emetic preparations have been utilized both prophylactically and to treat intractable postoperative nausea. However, until recently, all of the available agents have undesirable psychotropic side effects. Recently, ondansetron, a 5HT antagonist, has become available for the treatment of postoperative nausea and vomiting [90]. It is effective in countering chemotherapy-induced nausea, and early comparative trials would suggest that it is superior to droperidol and metoclopramide in preventing postoperative vomiting [91]. Furthermore, ondansetron appears to be free of the side effects commonly associated with other anti-emetic agents [90]. However, the high cost of this agent may limit its more widespread use. Further studies evaluating its cost-effectiveness (e.g. in preventing unnecessary hospital admission) are clearly needed.

Summary

Day-case anaesthesia is now a recognized anaesthetic subspecialty, with its own unique set of problems. As experience helps to determine which patients and procedures are most suitable for day surgery, further expansion of day-case surgery is likely. The rate of expansion of day-case surgery in the future will probably vary from country to country, dependent upon local needs and the level of ancillary home health-care services. Many recently developed drugs have pharmacological profiles which are ideally suited to day-case anaesthesia. Nevertheless, troublesome side effects remain all too common. Finally, while many of the newer drugs are ideal for day-case use, the cost of these agents is usually many times higher than the drugs that they replace. If a move towards greater use of day-case surgery also requires a move towards more expensive drugs, then the potential for financial savings will be greatly reduced.

Future studies on new day-case drugs and techniques need to focus not only on subjective improvements for the patient, but also on overall cost-effectiveness [92]. These studies must compare the increased cost of newer treatments with the financial savings resulting from earlier hospital discharge, reduced consumption of supplemental drugs and earlier return to normal activities. Unfortunately, many of the exciting new drugs currently being investigated may not offer a significant advantage over the more traditional agents when subjected to rigorous cost-effectiveness testing.

References

1 Calverley RK. Anesthesia as a specialty: past, present, and future. In: Barash PG, Cullen BF, Stoelting RK, eds. *Clinical Anesthesia*. Philadelphia: JB Lippincott, 1989: 3–33.
2 Nicoll JH. The surgery of infancy. *Br Med J* 1909; ii: 753–4.
3 Waters RM. The down-town anesthesia clinic. *Am J Surg* 1919; 33 (suppl): 71–3.
4 Herzfeld G. Hernia in infancy. *Am J Surg* 1938; 39: 422–8.
5 Webb E, Graves H. *Anesthesia for the Ambulant Patient*. Philadelphia: JB Lippincott, 1966.
6 Partridge AD, Brennan MF, Gray NH. *Day Surgery: Making it Happen. A study conducted by the NHS management executive value for money unit*. London: HMSO, 1991.
7 Royal College of Surgeons of England, Commission on the Provision of Surgical Services. *Guidelines for Day Case Surgery*. London: HMSO, 1985.
8 Henderson J, Goldacre MJ, Griffith M, Simmons HM. Day case surgery: geographical variation, trends and readmission rates. *J Epidemiol Comm Health* 1989; 43: 301–5.
9 Morgan M, Beech R. Variations in lengths of stay and rates of day case surgery: implications for the efficiency of surgical management. *J Epidemiol Comm Health* 1990; 44: 90–105.
10 Audit Commission. *Measuring Quality: the patient's view of day surgery*. London: HMSO, 1991.
11 Lahti PT. Early postoperative discharge of patients from the hospital. *Surgery* 1968; 63: 410–15.
12 Caldamone AA, Rabinowitz R. Outpatient orchidopexy. *J Urol* 1982; 127: 286–8.
13 Kaye KW, Clayman RV, Lange PH. Outpatient hydrocele and spermatocele repair under local anesthesia. *J Urol* 1983; 130: 269–71.
14 Pineault R, Contandriopoulos A-P. Randomized clinical trial of one-day surgery-patient satisfaction, clinical outcomes, and costs. *Med Care* 1985; 23: 171–82.
15 Haworth EA, Balarajan R. Day surgery—does it add to or replace inpatient surgery? *Br Med J* 1987; 294: 133–5.
16 Hatch LR. Day care surgery: do we and our patients need it? *Canad Anaesth Soc J* 1983; 30: 542–3.
17 Stott NCH. Day case surgery generates no increased workload for community based staff. True or false? *Br Med J* 1992; 304: 825–6.
18 Kallar SK, Everett LL. Controversies in ambulatory anesthesia: preoperative evaluation. *Anesth Rev* 1992; 19: 27–32.
19 Pritchard TJ, Bloom AD, Zollinger RM Jr. Pitfalls in ambulatory treatment of inguinal hernias in adults. *Surg Clin N Am* 1991; 71: 1353–62.
20 Biswas TK, Leary C. Postoperative hospital admission from a day surgery unit: a seven-year retrospective survey. *Anaesth Intens Care* 1992; 20: 147–50.
21 Smith I, Ding Y, White PF. Muscle pain after outpatient laparoscopy—influence of propofol versus thiopental and enflurane. *Anesth Anal* 1993; 76: 1881–4.
22 Brash JH. Outpatient laparoscopic sterilization. *Br Med J* 1976; i: 1376–7.
23 Collins KM, Docherty PW, Plantevin OM. Postoperative morbidity following gynaecological outpatient laparoscopy. A reappraisal of the service. *Anaesthesia* 1984; 39: 819–22.
24 Brindle GF, Soliman MG. Anaesthetic complications in surgical out-patients. *Canad Anaesth Soc J* 1975; 22: 613–19.
25 Fraser RA, Hotz SB, Hurtig JB, Hodges SN, Moher D. The prevalence and impact of pain after day-case tubal ligation surgery. *Pain* 1989; 39: 189–201.
26 *FASA Special Study 1*. 700 N. Fairfax Street, No. 520, Alexandria, Virginia 22314, 1986.
27 Meridy HW. Criteria for selection of ambulatory surgical patients and guidelines for anesthetic management. *Anesth Analg* 1982; 61: 921–6.

28 Kortilla K, Saarnivaara L, Takkanen J *et al.* Effect of age on amnesia and sedation induced by flunitrazepam during local anaesthesia for bronchoscopy. *Br J Anaesth* 1978; 50: 1211–18.
29 Sear JW, Cooper GM, Kumar V. The effect of age on recovery. A comparison of the kinetics of thiopentone and althesin. *Anaesthesia* 1983; 38: 1158–61.
30 Chung F, Lavelle PA, McDonald S, Chung A, McDonald N. MMS: a screening test for elderly outpatients. *Anesthesiology* 1989; 69: A900.
31 Steward DJ. Preterm infants are more prone to complications following minor surgery than term infants. *Anesthesiology* 1982; 56: 304–6.
32 Liu LMP, Coté CJ, Goudsouzian NG *et al.* Life-threatening apnea in infants recovering from anesthesia. *Anesthesiology* 1983; 59: 506–10.
33 Philip BK. Patient's assessment of ambulatory anaesthesia and surgery. *J Clin Anaeth* 1992; 4: 355–8.
34 Lutner RE, Roizen MF, Stocking CB *et al.* The automated interview vs. the personal interview. *Anesthesiology* 1991; 75: 394–400.
35 Foster WE, Griffith KE, Beck PM, Newson CD, White PF. Computer-assisted preoperative assessment for ambulatory anesthesia (Abstract). 1993; 79: A45.
36 Maltby JR, Sutherland AD, Sale JP, Shaffer EA. Preoperative oral fluids: is a five-hour fast justified prior to elective surgery? *Anesth Analg* 1986; 65: 1112–16.
37 Goodwin APL, Rowe WL, Ogg TW, Samaan A. Oral fluids prior to day surgery. *Anaesthesia* 1991; 46: 1066–8.
38 Read MS, Vaughan RS. Allowing pre-operative patients to drink: effects on patient's safety and comfort of unlimited oral water until 2 hours before anaesthesia. *Acta Anaesth Scand* 1991; 35: 591–5.
39 Splinter WM, Stewart JA, Muir JG. The effect of preoperative apple juice on gastric contents, thirst, and hunger in children. *Can J Anaesth* 1989; 36: 55–8.
40 Olsson GL, Hallen B, Hambraeus-Jonzon K. Aspiration during anaesthesia. *Acta Anaesth Scand* 1986; 30: 84–92.
41 Turner GA, Paech M. A comparison of oral midazolam solution with temazepam as a day case premedicant. *Anaesth Intens Care* 1991; 19: 365–8.
42 White PF. Outpatient anesthesia—an overview. In White PF, ed. *Outpatient Anesthesia*. New York: Churchill Livingstone, 1990: 1–48.
43 Cooper GM. Recovery from anaesthesia. *Clin Anaesth* 1984; 2: 145–62.
44 Whitwam JG, Manners JM. Clinical comparison of thiopentone and methohexitone. *Br Med J* 1962; i: 1663–5.
45 White PF. Continuous infusions of thiopental, methohexital or etomidate as adjuvants to nitrous oxide for outpatient anesthesia. *Anesth Analg* 1984; 63: 282.
46 Miller BM, Hendry JGB, Lees NW. Etomidate and methohexitone. A comparative clinical study in out-patient anaesthesia. *Anaesthesia* 1978; 33: 450–3.
47 Craig J, Cooper GM, Sear JW. Recovery from day-case anaesthesia. *Br J Anaesth* 1982; 54: 447–50.
48 O'Toole DP, Milligan KR, Howe JP, McCollum JSC, Dundee JW. A comparison of propofol and methohexitone as induction agents for day case isoflurane anaesthesia. *Anaesthesia* 1987; 42: 373–6.
49 Ræder JC, Misvær G. Comparison of propofol induction with thiopentone or methohexitone in short outpatient general anaesthesia. *Acta Anaesth Scand* 1988; 32: 607–13.
50 Heath PJ, Ogg TW, Gilks WR. Recovery after day-case anaesthesia. A 24-hour comparison of recovery after thiopentone or propofol anaesthesia. *Anaesthesia* 1990; 45: 911–15.
51 Servin F, Pommereau R, Rowan C, Nimier M, Desmonts JM. Comparison of intraoperative course

and recovery following anesthesia with etomidate or propofol in patients over 80 years. *Anesthesiology* 1990; 73: A318.
52 Doze VA, Westphal LM, White PF. Comparison of propofol with methohexital for outpatient anesthesia. *Anesth Analg* 1986; 65: 1189–95.
53 Borgeat A, Wilder-Smith OHG, Saiah M, Rifat K. Subhypnotic doses of propofol possess direct antiemetic properties. *Anesth Analg* 1992; 74: 539–41.
54 Marshall CA, Jones RM, Bajorek PK, Cashman JN. Recovery characteristics using isoflurane or propofol for maintenance of anaesthesia: a double-blind controlled trial. *Anaesthesia* 1992; 47: 461–6.
55 Raftery S, Sherry E. Total intravenous anaesthesia with propofol and alfentanil protects against postoperative nausea and vomiting. *Can J Anaesth* 1992; 39: 37–40.
56 Tracey JA, Holland AJC, Unger L. Morbidity in minor gynaecological surgery: a comparison of halothane, enflurane and isoflurane. *Br J Anaesth* 1982; 54: 1213–15.
57 Carter JA, Dye AM, Cooper GM. Recovery from day-case anaesthesia. *Anaesthesia* 1985; 40: 545–8.
58 Azar I, Karambelkar DJ, Lear E. Neurologic state and psychomotor function following anesthesia for ambulatory surgery. *Anesthesiology* 1984; 60: 347–9.
59 Fisher DM, Robinson S, Brett CM, Perin G, Gregory A. Comparison of enflurane, halothane and isoflurane for diagnostic and therapeutic procedures in children with malignancies. *Anesthesiology* 1985; 63: 647–50.
60 Ghouri AF, Bodner M, White PF. Recovery profile after desflurane-nitrous oxide versus isoflurane-nitrous oxide in outpatients. *Anesthesiology* 1991; 74: 419–24.
61 Smith I, Ding Y, White PF. Comparison of induction, maintenance and recovery characteristics of sevoflurane-N_2O and propofol-sevoflurane-N_2O with propofol-isoflurane-N_2O. *Anesth Analg* 1992; 74: 253–9.
62 Van Hemelrijck J, Smith I, White PF. Use of desflurane or outpatient anesthesia: a comparison with propofol and nitrous oxide. *Anesthesiology* 1991; 75: 197–203.
63 Ding Y, Fredman B, White PF. Recovery following outpatient anesthesia: use of enflurane versus propofol. *J Clin Anesth* 1993; in press.
64 Smith I, White PF. Use of the laryngeal mask airway as an alternative to a face mask during outpatient arthroscopy. *Anesthesiology* 1992; 77: 843–6.
65 Bridenbaugh LD. Regional anaesthesia for outpatient surgery. *Canad Anaesth Soc J* 1983; 30: 548–52.
66 Philip BK, Covino BG. Local and regional anesthesia. In: Wetchler BV, ed. *Anesthesia for Ambulatory Surgery*. Philadelphia: JB Lippincott, 1985; 309–74.
67 Taylor E, Ghouri AF, White PF. Midazolam in combination with propofol for sedation during local anesthesia. *J Clin Anesth* 1992; 4: 213–16.
68 White PF, Negus JB. Sedative infusions during local or regional anesthesia—a comparison of midazolam and propofol. *J Clin Anesth* 1991; 3: 32–9.
69 Zelcer J, White PF, Chester S, Paull JD, Molnar R. Intraoperative patient-controlled analgesia: an alternative to physician administration during outpatient monitored anesthesia care. *Anesth Analg* 1992; 75: 41–4.
70 Ghouri AF, TerKonda R, Taylor E, White PF. Patient-controlled sedation: a comparison of three techniques during local anesthesia. *Anesth Analg* 1992; 74: S110.
71 Gillies GWA, Kenny GNC, Bullingham RES, McArdle CS. The morphine sparing effect of ketorolac tromethamine. *Anaesthesia* 1987; 42: 727–31.
72 Campbell WI. Analgesic side effects and minor surgery: which analgesic for minor and day-case surgery? *Br J Anaesth* 1990; 64: 617–20.

73 McLoughlin C, McKinney MS, Fee JPH, Boules Z. Diclofenac for day-care arthroscopy surgery: comparison with a standard opioid therapy. *Br J Anaesth* 1990; 65: 620–3.

74 Kinsella J, Moffat AC, Patrick JA *et al.* Ketorolac trometamol for postoperative analgesia after orthopaedic surgery. *Br J Anaesth* 1992; 69: 19–22.

75 Rosenblum M, Weller RS, Conard PL, Falvey EA, Gross JB. Ibuprofen provides longer lasting analgesia than fentanyl after laparoscopic surgery. *Anesth Analg* 1991; 73: 255–9.

76 Bourne MH, Johnson KA. Postoperative pain relief using local anesthetic instillation. *Foot Ankle* 1988; 8: 350–1.

77 McKenzie R, Phitayakorn P, Uy NTL *et al.* Topical bupivacaine and etidocaine analgesia following fallopian tube banding. *Can J Anaesth* 1989; 36: 510–14.

78 Kaplan P, Freund R, Squires J, Herz M. Control of immediate postoperative pain with topical bupivacaine hydrochloride for laparoscopic falope ring tubal ligation. *Obstet Gynaecol* 1990; 76: 798–802.

79 Partridge BL, Stabile BE. The effects of incisional bupivacaine on postoperative narcotic requirements, oxygen saturation and length of stay in the post-anesthesia care unit. *Acta Anaesth Scand* 1990; 34: 486–91.

80 Smith BE, MacPherson GH, deJonge M, Griffiths JM. Rectus sheath and mesosalpinx block for laparoscopic sterilization. *Anaesthesia* 1991; 46: 875–7.

81 Narchi P, Benhamou D, Fernandez H. Intraperitoneal local anaesthetic for shoulder pain after day-case laparoscopy. *Lancet* 1991; 338: 1569–70.

82 Smith I, Van Hemelrijck J, White PF, Shively R. Effects of local anesthesia on recovery after outpatient arthroscopy. *Anesth Analg* 1991; 73: 536–9.

83 Stein C, Comisel K, Haimeri E *et al.* Analgesic effect of intraarticular morphine after arthroscopic knee surgery. *New Engl J Med* 1991; 325: 1123–6.

84 Joshi GP, McCarroll SM, O'Brien TM, Lenane P. Intraarticular analgesia following knee arthroscopy. *Anesth Analg* 1993; 76: 333–6.

85 Aho MS, Erkola OA, Scheinin H, Lehtinen A, Korttila K. Effect of intravenously administered dexmedetomidine on pain after laparoscopic tubal ligation. *Anesth Analg* 1991; 73: 112–18.

86 White PF. Subcutaneous PCA: an alternative to i.v.-PCA for postoperative pain management. *J Clin Pain* 1990; 6: 297–300.

87 Chandler LH, White PF. Ambulatory PCA—a new approach to postoperative pain management. *Anesth Analg* 1991; 72: S33.

88 Urbach GM, Edelist G. An evaluation of the anaesthetic techniques used in an outpatient unit. *Canad Anaesth Soc J* 1977; 24: 401–7.

89 Kapur PA. The big 'little' problem. *Anesth Analg* 1991; 73: 243–5.

90 Bodner M, White PF. Antiemetic efficacy of ondansetron after outpatient laparoscopy. *Anesth Analg* 1991; 73: 250–4.

91 Alon E, Himmelseher S. Ondansetron in the treatment of postoperative vomiting: a randomized, double-blind comparison with droperidol and metoclopramide. *Anesth Analg* 1992; 75: 561–5.

92 White PF, Watcha MF. Are new drugs cost-effective for patients undergoing ambulatory surgery? *Anesthesiology* 1993; 78: 2–5.

93 Urquhart M, White PF. Outpatient anaesthesia. In: Nimmo WS, Smith G, eds. *Anaesthesia*. Oxford: Blackwell Scientific Publications, 1989: 665–86.

Chapter 2
Pharmacology and Day-Case Anaesthesia

D. P. Dob and J. G. Whitwam

When a drug is administered in anaesthesia it is often used for a single primary effect such as the induction of sleep, analgesia, reflex depression or muscle relaxation. Single inhalational anaesthetic agents can achieve all these effects but in varying relative degree due to the varying concentration response curves for different modalities of effect so that to achieve, for example, muscle relaxation the level of 'anaesthesia' may be unnecessarily deep. Hence balanced anaesthesia using a combination of intravenous or local anaesthesia drugs is preferred albeit against a background of light inhalational anaesthesia. Each drug may have unwanted side effects, e.g. cardiovascular or respiratory depression, excitatory phenomena or nausea and vomiting (Table 2.1).

The duration of action of a drug depends on its bioavailability and processing by the body, i.e. pharmacokinetics. The effect of the drug on the patient is referred to as pharmacodynamics. A thorough knowledge of the pharmacokinetic characteristics of drugs indicate those which may allow a rapid return of the patient to 'street fitness' and hence which are suitable for day-case procedures. Arguably one of the clearest expositions of basic pharmacology, particularly pharmacokinetics, is by Calvey and Williams [1].

Day-case anaesthesia should include: (a) rapid smooth onset of action particularly in the absence of premedication; (b) rapid recovery without residual side effects, and active metabolites; and (c) absence of adverse effects, such as nausea and vomiting which is extremely important for ambulatory surgery. Emetic symptoms not only affect the recovery times but also the incidence of an unanticipated hospital admission.

Intravenous anaesthetics

These drugs all have a common purpose, the removal of consciousness [2]. However, some, although short acting and otherwise suitable for day-case anaesthesia, may have serious side effects which limit their use. Hence, apart from duration of action a comparison of anaesthetic drugs is based largely on their adverse side effects, i.e. pharmacodynamics. Postoperative morbidity affects between 20 and 30% of patients. Problems encountered include respiratory and cardiovascular depression, nausea and vomiting, and central nervous system complications, e.g. psychic phenomena which may be due to, or exacerbated by, the anaesthetic technique [3, 4]. It is generally accepted that most anaesthetic drugs impair psychomotor performance for some time

Table 2.1 Adverse reactions to agents used for the induction of anaesthesia. From Whitwam [2]

Type A. Dose dependent; incidence high; mortality low
Induction complications
Excitatory phenomena, e.g. involuntary muscle movement such as tremors
Respiratory upset (cough, hiccup, laryngospasm)
Respiratory depression
Cardiovascular effects
Recovery
Psychic phenomena—dreaming, hallucinations, dissociative phenomena, delirium and agitation, emotional reactions
Motor phenomena—changes in muscle tone, involuntary muscle movement (e.g. tremors and convulsions)
Effects on pain
Nausea and vomiting
Duration of action and cumulation
Placental transmission and foetal effects
Tissue irritation and damage (drug and solvent)
Pain on injection, venous complications, effect of intra-arterial injection
Effect on endocrine function (etomidate)
Type B. Incidence low; morbidity and mortality high
Anaphylactic responses (anaphylactoid)
Interaction with inherited abnormalities
Malignant hyperpyrexia
Myotonic syndromes
Cholinesterase phenomena
Halothane hepatitis (familial disposition)

after their administration [5]. Pharmacokinetic properties which predict a rapid recovery time are a short distribution phase, high clearance and short elimination half-life. These characteristics are also important for drugs used to provide total intravenous anaesthesia (TIVA).

Drugs commonly used to induce anaesthesia by the intravenous route include propofol, thiopentone, methohexitone, etomidate, ketamine and midazolam. Currently the most important group of drugs used for sedation is the benzodiazepines, and the drug of choice is midazolam [6].

Benzodiazepines

History

The first BZD, chlordiazepoxide was synthesized in 1956 and introduced to clinical

Table 2.2 Benzodiazepines for which parenteral preparations for intravenous use are available

Agonists	Antagonists
Midazolam	Flumazenil
Diazepam	
Flunitrazepam	
Lorazepam	

practice in 1960 as an orally administered anxiolytic. In 1977 specific BZD receptors were described in the central nervous system (CNS) [7, 8] associated with receptors for γ-amino butyric acid (GABA) to form a protein complex containing a chloride ion channel referred to as the GABA-BZD-Cl^- channel complex [9–14]. Similar receptors are now known to be widely distributed throughout the body [15] including the myocardium [16]. In the early 1980s midazolam Ro21-3965 (Dormicum, Versed, Hypnovel, Doricum, Dormonid, Flormidal) was introduced. It is the first water soluble BZD and has the shortest duration of action of all BZD agonists so far developed for clinical use. The first specific BZD antagonist flumazenil, Ro15-1788 (Anexate, Lanexate), which is also water soluble, was synthesized in 1979, characterized in 1981, and introduced into clinical practice from the mid-1980s onwards. It introduced an agonist–antagonist technique whereby BZD-induced sedation, or anaesthesia, can be terminated at will [17]. The BZDs for which formulations for intravenous use are available are summarized in Table 2.2.

Pharmacology

Receptors. Conventional BZDs have full agonist effects at their receptors, causing, in increasing dose and receptor occupancy, anxiolysis through sedation, amnesia and muscle relaxation to anaesthesia (Table 2.3) although clearly there is considerable overlap of the various behavioural changes.

Ligands which bind to these receptors with the opposite effect to the BZDs, to cause anxiety, arousal and convulsions are called inverse agonists (e.g. methyl β-carboline carboxylate, βCCM, [18–20] anxiety peptides [21–25] while those which in themselves are not convulsive, but which kindle the system for other convulsive agents are referred to as partial inverse agonists (e.g. FG7142, CGS-8216, ethyl β-carboline carboxylate—βCCE, Ro15-4513) [26]. In addition there are partial agonists (e.g. Ro16-6028, Ro17-1812, ZK91296, CGS-9896) [26] and antagonists (flumazenil, Ro15-3505, ZK93426).

Thus there are five groups of ligands for BZD receptors [27] and flumazenil antagonizes the other four groups. It reverses all the effects of conventional BZD without affecting their bioavailability or kinetics [28, 29]. At very high doses (e.g. 75–100 mg kg^{-1}), flumazenil shows some agonist activity in animal models.

Table 2.3 Reciprocal dose effect of benzodiazepine (BZD) agonist and flumazenil

BZD agonist	Effect	Flumazenil
Low dose	Anxiolysis	High dose
	Anticonvulsive effect	
	Slight sedation	
	Reduced attention	
	Amnesia	
	Intense sedation	
	Muscle relaxation	
High dose	Hypnosis (anaesthesia)	Low dose

The postulated receptor occupancies of BZD receptors for different effects are anticonvulsive 20–25%, anxiolytic 20–30%, sedative 25–50% and hypnotic 60–90% [30].

After midazolam, the reaction time, a measure of mental concentration, recovers at plasma concentrations between 100 and 25 ng ml^{-1} [31], while sedation persists until the plasma concentration is below 75 ng ml^{-1}. Amnesia is total above 100 ng ml^{-1} [32] and anaesthesia occurs above 250 ng ml^{-1} [33–35].

Myocardial BZD receptors. The GABA-BZD-Cl^- channel system has been demonstrated in myocardial papillary muscle of the guinea pig. It has the effect of decreasing myocardial contractility and shortening the duration of the action potential [16]. BZDs have been used in the treatment of arrhythmias associated with chloroquine poisoning [36].

General pharmacology. There are over 30 BZDs on the market principally for oral administration. In general in suitable formulation they are absorbed by all routes, oral, sublingual, nasal, rectal, intramuscular and intravenous. The bioavailability after oral administration depends on first pass extraction by the liver and is around only 44% for midazolam and 16% for flumazenil which are the most rapidly metabolized BZDs.

Metabolism is by hydroxylation or decarboxylation, desalkylation (e.g. desmethyl, desethyl) followed by glucuronidation with both biliary and urinary excretion. The metabolites are often active and longer lasting than the parent drug so that the administered drug is a 'pro-drug'. Three, oxazepam, temazepam, lorazepam, are not metabolized, but merely glucuronated before excretion, and before the introduction of triazolam and midazolam were regarded as short acting (e.g. half-life β for lorazepam $\approx$ 12 h).

In a sense BZDs do not have primary effects but act through the GABA system. There is a ceiling to the effect they can produce which is dependent on receptor occupancy and ongoing GABA activity. They have a much higher therapeutic index

Table 2.4 Therapeutic Index (ThI) = MT (maximum tolerated, i.e. highest non-lethal dose i.v. in rodents)/CD (clinical anaesthetic doses in man)

Drug	Mean MT mg kg^{-1}	CD mg kg^{-1}	ThI (man)
Midazolam	53·5	0·07–0·3	177+
Flumazenil	64·3	0·005–0·15	428+
Thiopentone	37·5	3·0–3·5	10·7+
Propofol	25	2·0–2·5	10+

Table 2.5 Principal differences between midazolam and diazepam

	Midazolam	Diazepam
Water solubility	+	—
Pain on injection	< 2%	Diazepam emulsion < 1% Diazepam ≈ 40%
Metabolites	Hydroxy (4α-dihydro)	Desmethyl
Half-life β drug (h)	2·5–3·5	30
Half-life β metabolites (h)	< 1·5	100
Enterohepatic circulation	—	+
Amnesia	++	+

than conventional intravenous induction agents, e.g. thiopentone, propofol (Table 2.4). In normal clinical doses their effects on the cardiovascular and respiratory systems are relatively small.

Until relatively recently no anaphylactic reactions to BZDs have been reported, apart from those in the early 1980s in Sweden due to a cremophor preparation of diazepam, which is no longer available. However a reaction of this type has now been related to the administration of midazolam in which a patient developed angioedema after its administration on two separate occasions [37].

BZDs can be used to induce anaesthesia in the presence of malignant hyperthermia and porphyria.

Midazolam versus diazepam. The principal differences between midazolam and diazepam which can affect their clinical use are summarized in Table 2.5. These are primarily the pharmacokinetics where significant plasma concentrations of diazepam and its desmethyl derivative may persist for days with the potential for enterohepatic circulation, and hence midazolam is associated with earlier complete recovery and fewer longer term side effects than diazepam [38]. Midazolam also has the advantage of being water soluble and providing a greater degree of amnesia.

An equipotency ratio of 0·07 mg kg^{-1} of midazolam to 0·15 mg kg^{-1} of diazepam was proposed in the early 1980s [39]. It is now recognized that midazolam is more potent and that a relative dose of 0·05 mg kg^{-1} or lower is more appropriate. Although the onset time of midazolam [39] is faster than diazepam the time to peak effect can be up to 5 min [40]. These two factors have probably combined so that in previous comparative studies [40] the dose of midazolam has been high relative to diazepam.

Bolus dose versus titration. Because of the slow onset times of the BZDs it is possible for even the most patient clinician to overdose with both drugs. By using a bolus injection of the BZD the sedative dose should be reduced by approximately one-third for both midazolam [41] and diazepam [42] and some authorities use only approximately one-half of the normal dose of midazolam and work in a dose range of 2–3 mg intravenously.

PCA. Several methods of providing PCA have now been described. These will be discussed under practice procedures and theoretical considerations are discussed in Chapter 17.

Genetic polymorphism. In 1986, Dundee and his associates [46] suggested, on the basis of retrospective data from studies conducted during the previous 5–6 years, that in about 6% of the population the terminal half-life of midazolam was in the range 8–22 h compared with the majority where the mean half-life is about 2·4 h. This would indicate polymorphism in the cytochrome P450 system for the metabolism of BZDs and would have implications for the use of flumazenil. However Kassai in a prospective study on 168 hospitalized patients with normal hepatic and renal function found no evidence for this [43]. The mean plasma half-lives for men and women were 2·6 and 3·1 h respectively and in patients under and over 60 years 2·8 and 3·0 h respectively [44]. Other factors which may prolong its half-life are hypovolaemia [45], critical illness [46] and there may also be ethnic differences [47].

Drug interactions (Table 2.6)

Opioids and barbiturates

Cook *et al.* [48] described the use of intramuscular pethidine as a premedication 30–40 min before the induction of sedation for gastroscopy with intravenous diazepam [48]. Since then many gastroenterologists use not only pethidine but also a variety of other opioids intravenously combined with BZDs for sedation.

In addition to analgesia the opioids cause respiratory depression, bradycardia and hypotension due to baroreflex sensitization [49], muscle rigidity and nausea and vomiting [50].

Ben-Shlomo *et al.* [51] determined 50% of the effective dose (ED_{50}) for the induction of hypnosis with fentanyl and midazolam. They found that the administration of only

Table 2.6 Midazolam drug interactions in man. ED_{50} of equi-effective doses for the induction of sleep or light anaesthesia as indicated by failure to open eyes on command. ED_{50} for each drug alone = 100%. Numbers in table = percentage of the doses of each drug which when used in combination produce the same ED_{50} as each drug when used alone

	Drug combination to produce ED_{50} of 100%			
Synergism	Second drug	Second drug ED_{50}%	Midazolam ED_{50}%	Reference
Opioid	Fentanyl	25	23	[51]
	Alfentanil	33	21	[52]
Barbiturate	Thiopentone	25	25	[53]
	Methohexitone	33	27	[54]
Propofol		41	35	[55]

25% of the ED_{50} of fentanyl i.v. reduced the ED_{50} dose of midazolam by 77%, i.e. to 23% of its value when administered alone, showing genuine synergism between the two drugs.

Synergism of a similar order of magnitude has been shown to exist between midazolam and alfentanil [52], thiopentone [53], methohexitone [54], propofol [55] and morphine [56]. Tucker *et al.* [57] found that fentanyl caused a greater degree of respiratory depression with a significant reduction in oxygen saturation (SaO_2) when combined with both midazolam and diazepam.

The precise interaction between nalbuphine and the BZDs has not been evaluated. Suffice it to say that nalbuphine prolongs the recovery time and the incidence of side effects of diazepam-induced sedation [58]. In one study two patients who received nalbuphine in addition to midazolam developed obstructive apnoea [59] in spite of the ceiling effect of nalbuphine on respiratory depression when administered alone [60].

The conclusion is that once a patient has received either midazolam or any other BZD, great care should be exercised in the administration of an opioid, e.g. fentanyl, sulfentanil, alfentanil, nalbuphine, morphine and pethidine, a barbiturate or propofol and vice versa. A major reduction in the dose of the second drug should be anticipated if the induction of anaesthesia with potentially dangerous side effects are to be avoided such as apnoea and loss of the airway, with subsequent hypoxaemia, and also a fall in arterial pressure. These remarks will also probably apply to a combination of many psychosedative drugs with the BZDs.

Recently Vinik and Kissin [61] discussed triple synergism whereby following small doses of midazolam and alfentanil the anaesthetic induction dose of propofol could be reduced by 86%.

H_2 receptor antagonists

The cytochrome P450 enzyme system is involved in the metabolism of the benzodiazepines in the liver and hence drugs such as cimetidine but possibly not ranitidine could be expected to prolong their action. However the position is not clear cut because in volunteer studies the concurrent administration of either oral cimetidine or ranitidine increased the bioavailability of oral midazolam by approximately 30% [62, 63]. Oral cimetidine caused a relatively small increase in the rate of fall in plasma levels of a sedative dose (5 mg i.v.) of this drug [64].

Ketorolac

Ketoralac [65] is a non-steroidal anti-inflammatory drug (NSAID) with analgesic properties equivalent to 10 mg morphine. However, it causes no cardiovascular or respiratory depression and an extremely small incidence of nausea. Its interactions with BZDs should not be clinically significant in terms of respiratory depression. However, one of the side effects of ketorolac is a small degree of somnolence but as yet no serious interactions have been reported.

Flumazenil

Flumazenil is a water-soluble BZD [30, 66–68]. It is a competitive antagonist at the BZD receptor and antagonizes all other ligands for this receptor. It reverses all the modalities of effect of the BZDs without affecting their bioavailability or kinetics and has minimal effects on the normal CNS with slight agonist and some anticonvulsive properties. Incremental doses up to 0·5–1·0 mg i.v. are effective clinically while doses of 600 mg orally and 100 mg i.v. are well tolerated in normal volunteers.

It is rapidly absorbed orally, with a high hepatic clearance and bioavailability averages only 16%. The mean volume of distribution (VD_{SS}) is $0{\cdot}95 \pm 0{\cdot}16$ l kg^{-1} (mean $\pm$ SD), clearance (Cl_pd) is 920 ± 216 ml min^{-1} and half-life β is $0{\cdot}9 \pm 0{\cdot}2$ h. Only 40% is bound to plasma proteins. It rapidly enters and subsequently clears the CNS. Less than 0·2% is excreted unchanged. Hydroxylation and desmethylation occur.

Its duration of action following a single intravenous injection has varied from 15–140 min depending on the dose but its mean duration of action in normal subjects is about 58 min.

In endoscopy clinics where conscious BZD sedation is used, flumazenil allows immediate reduction of sedation if verbal contact is lost or apnoea occurs. Because of its relatively short duration of action, to minimize the risk of resedation, long-acting agonist drugs should be avoided, and midazolam is the drug of choice. Flumazenil has been used to reverse midazolam-supplemented anaesthesia [68–71].

Flumazenil in clinical doses has similar side effects to a placebo. Sixty-seven out of 301 normal volunteers variously exhibited extremely transient episodes of dizziness, headache, flushing and anxiety following bolus intravenous doses in excess of 5 mg and as high as 60 mg (Data on file, F. Hoffman-La Roche Ltd).

Flumazenil reversal of sedation. There are now many studies reporting the use of flumazenil in reversing midazolam [72–75] and diazepam [72, 74, 76, 77] sedation particularly following endoscopy and minor surgery [74–78].

The potential indications for flumazenil in sedation are:

1 Medical (i.e. safety): (a) as an emergency drug, e.g. in case verbal communication is lost and/or the breathing becomes obstructed and laboured or absent; or (b) to deliberately reverse patients of poor physical status as soon as the procedure is complete.

2 Health economics—to speed up the flow of patients and to minimize dependence on fully staffed expensive conventional recovery facilities.

Although flumazenil reverses the prospective amnesic effects of BZDs that for the procedure is retained. Anxiety has been reported following its administration. Most such reactions are due to the rapid reversal of heavily sedated amnesic patients in an unfamiliar environment [76]. However, it can produce panic attacks in patients subject to such attacks [79].

Paradoxical reactions to the effects of midazolam in elderly patients, with anxiety and restlessness rather than sedation, have been successfully treated with flumazenil [72].

One of the major advantages of reversal of BZDs with flumazenil, compared for example with the use of naloxone to reverse opioids, is that there is no cardiovascular rebound with hypertension [69, 80].

Previous areas of critical debate

These are resedation, the use of flumazenil in chronic BZD users and ventilatory responsiveness to changes in blood gas tensions.

Resedation. In the past the desirability of the very existence of flumazenil has been challenged [81].

As the effects of flumazenil decline, i.e. about 45–60 min after its administration, the patient returns to the level of sedation which would have existed at that time if flumazenil had not been administered. Normally without flumazenil, given a correct dose of midazolam, a patient would be ready for discharge about 1 h after completion of the procedure with no danger of resedation due to enterohepatic circulation, as is the case with diazepam, since the elimination of midazolam and its metabolites is complete within 5–8 h in the type of patient undergoing outpatient or day-care procedures. Thus the administration of flumazenil on completion of the procedure after sedation with midazolam provides immediate clinical recovery since the patients can walk and sit in a chair, rather than recover on a trolley or bed, are no longer amnesic and are therefore capable of receiving instructions. After about 1 h they can be accompanied home in the normal way without the need of a conventional day ward. Midazolam is a highly potent drug and recent criticisms of the use of flumazenil to reverse its effects are due to a lack of understanding of the low dose of midazolam which is required to induce adequate clinical anxiolysis. There also appears to be in some cases an ignorance of the pharmacology of the newer BZDs since many clinicians still regard midazolam as equivalent to diazepam in all respects. The current use of the original formulation of diazepam with its propensity to cause pain on injection and permanent venous thrombosis in countries where a diazepam emulsion preparation is available, would support the view that its continued use is more to do with long-standing prescribing habits. Arguably the continued use of either in preference to midazolam is sometimes based on similar considerations rather than on currently accepted pharmacological data.

Chronic BZD users. Concern has also been expressed that flumazenil could precipitate an acute withdrawal syndrome [82] in patients receiving prolonged BZD medication comparable to that induced by naloxone in chronic opioid users. Withdrawal symptoms, never prolonged or severe, have followed the administration of flumazenil in several species of BZD-treated animals [83]. However, a recent paper suggests that far from being a problem, flumazenil may be useful in the treatment of BZD tolerance [84]. This was an investigation using positron emission tomography (PET scanning) to study receptor occupancy in patients with temporal lobe epilepsy who had become tolerant to clonazepam. A single dose of flumazenil (1·5 mg i.v.) restored the effectiveness of clonazepam such that the patients were seizure-free for 6–21 days. They attributed the absence of withdrawal seizures to three possible factors:

1 Anticonvulsive effects of flumazenil.

2 The fact that 1·5 mg of flumazenil only occupies 45–55% of the BZD receptors and clonazepam 2–5 mg only 30%.

3 Configurational 'resetting' of the receptors by flumazenil.

An intriguing concept which could follow from this work is that patients on long-term BZD administration, who could have become tolerant to their effects and hence have an unpredictable response for example to midazolam, should receive 2–3 mg of flumazenil to reset say over 60% of the receptors. Approximately 2 h later, when the antagonistic effect of the flumazenil has disappeared, the patient may then show a normal response to midazolam which could subsequently be reversed by flumazenil in the normal way.

Ventilatory response to hypoxaemia and hypercarbia. It has been suggested that whereas the effect of flumazenil in reversing sedation is immediate, full recovery of chemoreflexes is delayed [85, 86]. However, there are several problems in this interpretation of studies on the effect of midazolam on the ventilatory responses to hypoxaemia and carbon dioxide (CO_2).

1 Normal subjects show a large random variation in responsiveness over time and on different days [87]. Power *et al.* [87] in controlled studies each lasting over 6 h, where a placebo was administered, found spontaneous variations of the standard deviation of responses in normal volunteers in excess of 50% of the mean values for the slope of the carbon dioxide response curves and over 25% for the intercept. Thus changes less than this in response to a drug, even if statistically significant, would not have any practical significance. Thus when using carbon dioxide response curves as a method of evaluating respiratory depression, it is not enough to undertake a control readings. Rather, the normal variation in the group over time or on different days, must be investigated before any conclusions can be drawn about the depressant effect of psychosedative drugs unless these are obvious or verge on apnoea as can be the case, for example, with the opioids and barbiturates.

2 Responses to hypoxaemia are non-linear.

3 During a period of sustained hypoxaemia, as can happen during gastroscopy, central adaptations occur so that the initial vigorous response, which is not affected by small doses of midazolam, declines [88] which could be falsely interpreted as due to the depressant effect of the sedative drug.

4 Earlier studies on the effects of midazolam and diazepam showed that neither had any great effect on carbon dioxide responsiveness. For example, Forster *et al.* [89] found that although 0·15 mg kg^{-1} of midazolam and 0·3 mg kg^{-1} of diazepam caused a reduction in the slope of the carbon dioxide response curve by 4 min there was no change in the intercept. Moreover Power *et al.* [90] showed that neither midazolam 0·075 mg kg^{-1} nor diazepam 0·15 mg kg^{-1} caused any significant changes in carbon dioxide responsiveness. In general BZDs cause minimal respiratory depression [91].

5 It has also been suggested that during prolonged sedation with diazepam, mean duration 145 min (dose 1 mg min^{-1} i.v.) that the recovery of ventilatory depression is due to the onset of tolerance to diazepam [86], a phenomenon which has been described previously for midazolam in animals [92]. At the doses used these workers claimed that flumazenil did not reverse diazepam induced depression of the hypoxic ventilatory response [86].

6 Recent evidence suggests that 15 mg flumazenil may be required in humans for full receptor occupancy [84]. Thus the suggested failure of up to 2·0 mg of flumazenil to reverse completely all the effects of the BZDs may be simply a question of inadequate dosage. Moreover, if an element of acute tolerance, for example to midazolam, has been induced by prolonged sedation which can occur within 2 h in animals [92], and has been postulated by Mora *et al.* for diazepam in humans [86], then it has been shown in humans that flumazenil could reverse such tolerance, e.g. to clonazepam [84]. This would restore the effectiveness of the agonist which would then require more flumazenil to block the renewed activity.

7 A more recent paper has finally resolved the debate on the effect of flumazenil on the midazolam induced ventilatory response to hypoxia. Blouin *et al.* [93] have clearly shown that in human volunteers during isohypercarbia flumazenil restores the hypoxic ventilatory drive previously depressed by midazolam [93].

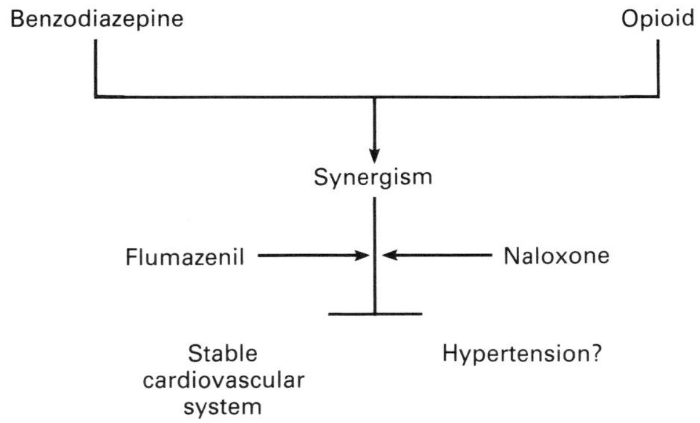

Fig. 2.1 Principle of use of naloxone and flumazenil. Each is specific for its drug type. For example if inadvertent overdose due to synergism occurs leading to anaesthesia, reversal of the benzodiazepine with flumazenil will cause arousal while retaining the benefit of the opioid analgesia and without 'rebound' hypertension. If consciousness is not reversed immediately, e.g. within 60 s, then naloxone should also be administered.

Flumazenil is specific for the BZD component of sedation. The effect of a second type of drug, e.g. an opioid, will persist (Fig. 2.1) [94].

Propofol

Propofol (2,6-diisopropylphenol) is a chemically inert phenol derivative, which is a short-acting anaesthetic agent with a rapid onset of action. It produces unconsciousness within 30 s, i.e. approximately one arm–brain circulation time. It may be used to induce and/or maintain general anaesthesia [95, 96] and for sedation of patients undergoing day-case anaesthesia. It has also been used for patient controlled sedation in patients undergoing day-case procedures [97].

Induction of anaesthesia

Presented in intralipid (1% suspension) propofol has an onset of action comparable to other intravenous induction agents, with features similar to thiopentone since both cause cardiovascular [98, 99] and respiratory depression [100, 101], and a smooth induction of anaesthesia [102]. It causes a lower incidence of excitatory phenomena (see Table 2.1) when compared with methohexitone and etomidate [103] although approximately 14% of patients receiving propofol show some excitatory phenomena and there is debate about whether it can cause convulsions [104]. It also depresses perilaryngeal sensitivity which facilitates the insertion of a tracheal tube or a laryngeal mask [105].

Pharmacokinetics

Propofol is rapidly metabolized and is only suitable for intravenous administration. The decline in propofol concentrations after a single bolus dose or following the termination of an infusion can be described by a three compartment model, with a fast initial distribution (half-life α of 2–4 min) followed by rapid metabolic elimination (half-life β of 30–60 min), with a slower final phase (half-life 184–502 min) which is due to return of propofol from poorly perfused tissues. It has a clearance of 1·5–2 l min^{-1}.

Metabolism

Propofol is extensively metabolized in the liver, principally by conjugation. Within 5 days 88% of a dose is excreted in the urine and less than 0·3% is excreted unchanged in the urine; less than 2% is eliminated in the faeces. The major metabolites are the glucuronic acid conjugate of propofol (40%) and the 1- and 4-glucuronides and 4-sulphate of its derivative 2,6-diisopropyl, 4-quinol [106–109].

It is metabolized during the anhepatic phase of liver transplantation [109] and extrahepatic metabolism also has been demonstrated in humans after cardiopulmonary bypass [110]. The site of this metabolism may be the gastrointestinal tract with a capacity equivalent to 10% of the liver [111, 112]. It may be reformed from its metabolites in the kidney, since it has been found to have a higher concentration in sheep renal veins than their renal arteries. This has not been confirmed in humans, but it may offer a further possible explanation of its relatively long terminal half-life in spite of a high hepatic clearance [113].

Recovery characteristics

It is clear that propofol provides a short recovery time which makes it suitable for day-case anaesthesia. Is this true under all circumstances?

Propofol as an induction agent. In early day-case studies anaesthesia was induced with propofol and maintained with inhalational agents for up to 15 min. Patients were able to open their eyes between 5 and 8 min after the end of the procedure and to recall their date of birth correctly 1 min later [113] and a number of studies have found that propofol was followed by faster emergence than, for example, thiopentone, methohexitone and etomidate [114–118].

In a recent study [119] it has been suggested that propofol has a postoperative anti-anxiety effect compared with thiopentone when they are used as induction agents for day-case anaesthesia. However, although this was a double-blind study, there were variations in anxiety levels dependent on gender, for example male patients were reluctant to admit to anxiety when compared to females. Further studies are required to confirm these findings.

Thus it is well established that the induction of general anaesthesia with propofol is associated with a more rapid return to the conscious and orientated state in the immediate postoperative period compared with thiopentone. However, the practical importance of this difference could be of limited clinical significance when the agent is only restricted to use as an induction agent. For example Valanne and Kortilla [120] suggest it offers little advantage when compared with induction of anaesthesia with methohexitone when it is continued with an enflurane and nitrous oxide combination.

However, recently reported studies continue to show an advantage for propofol. For example, Chittleborough *et al.* [121] found that the mean recovery times required to meet discharge criteria were significantly shorter in a group anaesthetized with propofol and maintained with nitrous oxide and enflurane, than a similar group induced with thiopentone. Gupta *et al.* [122] compared thiopentone and propofol for induction of anaesthesia maintained by isoflurane and nitrous oxide. Measurements of a perception accuracy test, showed a significantly faster return to normal values in the propofol group.

The current balance of opinion would suggest that the choice of intravenous induction agents does influence recovery times when anaesthesia is maintained for relatively short periods with volatile agents, as in day-case anaesthesia, and in this respect propofol is the induction agent of choice.

Propofol for TIVA. Propofol infusions are used for the maintenance of anaesthesia wholly or in part for TIVA or sedation. Are they advantageous in day-case surgery?

For short outpatient procedures, lasting less than 60 min, maintained with a variable infusion of propofol combined with nitrous oxide, early recovery times compared favourably with methohexitone infusions supplemented with nitrous oxide [123]. Also compared with thiopentone–enflurane anaesthesia, intravenous anaesthesia with propofol provided good surgical conditions and a faster recovery, with earlier discharge and less postoperative morbidity [124]. Doze *et al.* [125] also found that propofol combined with nitrous oxide compared favourably with a thiopentone–isoflurane nitrous oxide sequence for the maintenance of anaesthesia during short outpatient procedures. Nightingale and Lewis [126, 127] found that recovery occurred significantly earlier in the TIVA group when measured by critical flicker fusion testing and simple reaction times. Valanne [128] also found that patients anaesthetized with propofol could be discharged significantly faster than those where anaesthesia was maintained with nitrous oxide isoflurane for medium duration oral surgery.

In contrast Zuurmond *et al.* [129] studied patients undergoing arthroscopy and found no difference between a group anaesthetized with a propofol infusion and a group induced with propofol and maintained with nitrous oxide and isoflurane. Milligan *et al.* [130] found initial recovery more rapid with incremental doses of propofol for TIVA, compared with induction with propofol followed by and maintained with isoflurane but the difference disappeared by 1 h.

Marshall *et al.* [131] found no difference between two techniques comparing propofol alone and in combination with isoflurane. There was a lower incidence of emesis in the propofol group but this was reversed when an alfentanil infusion was added.

In summary, it seems that the differences in recovery from TIVA with propofol combined with other agents and patients induced with propofol and maintained with isoflurane may be small and not easily detected and some authors have not found them to be significant. However, when propofol is used as the sole agent, in the absence of all other agents, whether inhalational (e.g. nitrous oxide) or intravenous (e.g. alfentanil) there will be a relatively rapid 'clear headed' recovery without nausea compared with other techniques.

Other side effects of propofol

Propofol has anti-emetic properties [131, 132]. When it is used as the sole agent in short procedures nausea and vomiting are very rare, and this could have an impact on one of the major causes of overnight admission to hospital after day-case anaesthesia; however, the use of opioids with propofol may negate this effect [131]. Several authors have reported a lower incidence of nausea and vomiting when propofol is part of the anaesthetic technique [133–135].

Propofol causes both cardiovascular and respiratory depression. The hypotensive response is usually not associated with the baroreflex-mediated tachycardia which occurs with other intravenous induction agents such as methohexitone or thiopentone. Often the effect of propofol on heart rate is neutral or a limited bradycardia and it has 'vagotonic' properties [136]. Fentanyl, sufentanil and alfentanil all cause baroreflex sensitization, manifested by hypotension with bradycardia [137]. Combinations of vagotonic drugs can cause severe bradycardia which may be life-threatening requiring the administration of vagolytic drugs such as atropine or glycopyrrolate. In an extreme case a combination of fentanyl and propofol caused asystole [138].

Propofol is associated with pain on injection. The reported incidence varies from 28% when injected into the small veins on the dorsum of the hand to only 6% for the larger veins in the antecubital fossa [133]. The pain on injection may be reduced by the addition of 10 mg lignocaine to the formulation or the preadministration of lignocaine into the same vein immediately before injection.

Drug interactions with propofol

Metabolic. Propofol is broken down by the cytochrome system (P450) and therefore propofol infusions which saturate these systems can increase the duration of action of other drugs. For example, studies in both humans and pigs have shown that propofol inhibits the degradation of alfentanil and sufentanil [139].

Synergism. Pharmacodynamic interaction of drugs, for example in terms of their sedative and hypnotic effects in the central nervous system can occur at cellular level where two drugs act at the same or different receptors. Alternatively, if their distribution in the brain is different, they can affect different neural networks which overlap. Propofol has been shown to act synergistically with midazolam [140] and alfentanil [141]. Such synergism can be exploited, where a small dose of one drug (e.g. midazolam) is administered to reduce the dose of the induction agent. More recently

Vinik and Kissin [61] have used the term 'triple synergism' to refer to the use of appropriate combinations of midazolam, alfentanil and propofol, whereby the induction dose of propofol has been reduced by 86%. Such techniques are referred to as 'co-induction'.

Thiopentone and methohexitone

Thiopentone and methohexitone are barbiturates used for the induction of anaesthesia by the intravenous route.

Thiopentone is a thiobarbiturate which induces anaesthesia in one arm–brain circulation time. It has a pK_a of 7·6 indicating that 61% is un-ionized at pH 7·4. This partially explains its rapid peak concentration in the brain and its extensive distribution to all body tissues.

Recovery from such anaesthesia is primarily due to a rapid redistribution. The decay can be described by a triexponential equation interpreted as a three compartment model. Two distribution phases, a rapid (half-life of 2–7 min) and a slower one (half-life of 42–60 min) are followed by a terminal elimination phase with a much longer half-life, with a normal range from 300 to 720 min. This long elimination half-life and its large volume of distribution contribute to the relatively slow longer term recovery. For example a single dose of thiopentone of 6 mg kg^{-1} can impair simulated driving skills for up to 8 h after anaesthesia [142].

After repetitive injections or continuous infusions of thiopentone, marked cumulative effects are observed and it is not suitable for maintenance of anaesthesia by infusion.

Despite its disadvantages however, the ease of administration and low incidence of side effects makes thiopentone easy to use. Indeed since its introduction in 1934 it still is the 'gold standard' by which other agents of similar purpose are judged.

Methohexitone is an oxybarbiturate which has pharmacokinetic properties which are much more suitable than thiopentone for day-case anaesthesia. It has a much smaller volume of distribution (60–80 l) and a far higher clearance (700–900 ml min^{-1}) which gives an elimination half-life which is significantly shorter than thiopentone [143]. This difference in elimination half-life values contributes to the more prolonged recovery after thiopentone infusions compared to methohexitone [143]. When administered by repeated bolus doses, methohexitone offers a more rapid recovery than thiopentone [144].

Like propofol, methohexitone causes a relatively high incidence of pain on injection but this is much less than for propofol, and can be reduced by preinjection with lignocaine. Involuntary myoclonic movements and hiccuping can be minimized by using an optimal dose and pretreatment with a narcotic analgesic [145]. However, a smooth induction may not be guaranteed and premedication with hyoscine, phenothiazines and H_1 antagonists, particularly for example promethazine, should be avoided [2].

Methohexitone is generally considered to be superior for day-case anaesthesia to thiopentone and etomidate because of its low incidence of side effects and faster recovery times [146].

Methohexitone may also be used by infusion with fairly rapid emergence if the infusion lasts less than 1 h [147]. However, Steegers and Foster [148] found that 96% of patients were responding well to questions 20 min after propofol infusion compared with only 46% after methohexitone.

Alkaline barbiturate solutions can cause tissue irritation and pain if injected intravenously and serious sequelae if injected intra-arterially. They produce a dose-dependent cardiovascular and respiratory depression, in common with the other intravenous induction agents with the exception of ketamine.

In summary, although these two barbiturates have been used for outpatient surgery, their pharmacokinetic properties make them less suitable than propofol if rapid recovery and not cost is the issue.

Etomidate

Etomidate is an imidazole compound which causes rapid induction of anaesthesia within 30 s. It has a pK_a of 4·24 and is largely un-ionized at plasma pH, so that it crosses the blood–brain barrier readily. It is metabolized mainly by the liver to pharmacologically inactive compounds.

Although it has a very high clearance rate it also has a substantial volume of distribution, which means that prolonged infusions can cause drug accumulation. This, coupled with the fact that it is thought to cause transient depression of adrenal steroidogenesis after single doses or infusions [149–151], means that it is not used for the intravenous maintenance of anaesthesia by infusion.

Recovery of psychomotor function with etomidate is intermediate between thiopentone and methohexitone since it has a relatively short elimination half-life of about 2–5 h. It has been observed that patients, undergoing laparoscopy, in whom anaesthesia was induced with etomidate took longer to waken than those who received propofol [152].

However, etomidate does have significant disadvantages for day-case anaesthesia. It is associated with involuntary movements, and myoclonus on induction with pain on injection [114]. It is also associated with significantly inferior recovery when compared to thiopentone, methohexitone and propofol [114], and a particular problem, relevant to outpatient anaesthesia, is the relatively high incidence of nausea and vomiting associated with its use [2, 153].

Although the involuntary movements may be effectively eliminated when a benzodiazepine [154] precedes the induction dose, and the incidence of nausea and vomiting may be reduced by prior administration of droperidol, on balance etomidate is an unattractive choice for induction or maintenance of anaesthesia in day cases.

Ketamine

Ketamine is an arylcyclohexylamine, structurally related to phencyclidine. It is administered as a racemic mixture of two enantiomers: the (+) enantiomer is 3·4 times as potent as the (−) enantiomer [155].

It produces a 'dissociative' state of anaesthesia. It has a high hepatic clearance rate, with a large volume of distribution and an elimination half-life of 3 h. Norketamine is the principal metabolite and this is less active than ketamine itself. It causes sympathetic stimulation with tachycardia, an increase in cardiac output and blood pressure, and bronchodilatation. The airway reflexes are relatively well preserved. Its use in day-case anaesthesia is limited, however, because of a high incidence of psychomimetic sequelae (see Table 2.1) and the relatively slow recovery. Ketamine has been studied in day surgery [156] but was associated with a high incidence of delayed discharge and visual disturbances with confusion. There is evidence that benzodiazepines, especially midazolam, are effective in attenuating these emergence phenomena [157].

Low-dose intramuscular ketamine premedication has been shown to improve acceptance of a halothane gaseous induction in paediatric patients. Although the immediate recovery time was not prolonged in the ketamine group, there was an increase in the time to discharge [158].

Ketamine is used throughout the world, and is arguably the most widely used anaesthetic drug, particularly in emergency or difficult situations, but its use in routine day-case anaesthesia is limited because of emergence phenomena and its relatively long duration of action.

Midazolam

Midazolam is an imidazo benzodiazepine derivative which may be used for sedation, premedication or intravenous induction of anaesthesia. It is water soluble and is associated with a low incidence of pain on injection, e.g. 1–2% which is only slightly higher than diazepam in intralipid form (diazemuls).

It is not used commonly as an induction agent because of concerns regarding delayed recovery and residual amnesia [159], although it may be used as a premedicant intramuscularly [160]. There is considerable variation in the response to midazolam and with the recommended dose of 0·3 mg kg^{-1} induction of anaesthesia may not be achieved in 3 min in unpremedicated healthy patients [161]. Flumazenil has been used to reverse sedation following midazolam induced anaesthesia in ambulatory surgery patients [162].

Norton and Dundas [163] compared midazolam subsequently reversed with flumazenil, with propofol for induction of anaesthesia maintained with isoflurane. They found that although flumazenil improved recovery and indices of psychomotor impairment, propofol was associated with more rapid medium-term recovery and less impairment of memory. There appears to be no great advantage for a midazolam/flumazenil technique in day-case anaesthesia.

Co-induction

In recent years the administration of a small dose of midazolam, e.g. up to 2.5 mg, has been found to confer significant advantages for the induction of anaesthesia without compromising recovery. This technique exploits synergism between the benzodiazepine and the common induction agents, e.g. propofol. The principal advantages are amnesia for the induction process, a major reduction in the requirement of the induction agent and a more stable haemodynamic profile, in relation to the effect of the induction agent on the cardiovascular system and in obtunding the response to laryngoscopy [164–167]. The term triple synergism has been used when a combination of midazolam, alfentanil and propofol are used for the induction of anaesthesia. This technique, exploiting the synergistic effects of different drugs to advantage, is finding increasing application for the induction of anaesthesia [61].

Inhalation agents

Inhalation agents currently in common use for day-case anaesthesia are halothane, enflurane, isoflurane and nitrous oxide. The new agents desflurane and sevoflurane may become important in the near future, because of their favourable pharmacokinetic properties.

Table 2.7 shows some of the important characteristics of the inhalation agents which affect their use in day-case anaesthesia. In general, the lower the lipid solubility and the higher the minimal alveolar concentration (MAC) value, the better the agent will be for the rapid induction of anaesthesia and recovery and hence for day-case anaesthesia. This assumes that the vapour pressure at room temperature allows its use, it is not flammable or irritant, has only minimal side effects (e.g. hypotension, respiratory depression, nausea and vomiting), and preferably a low total metabolism in humans.

Desflurane

Desflurane is a new methyl ether derivative which has great potential for day-case anaesthesia. Its physical properties distinguish it as an agent with a rapid onset and offset of action, with minimal metabolism (0·02%) compared to other inhalation agents.

The MAC of desflurane is 6–7·2% and is less potent than halothane, enflurane, isoflurane and sevoflurane. This relative lack of potency is ascribed to its lower lipid gas solubility (see Table 2.1). However, its very low blood: gas solubility (0·4) ensures rapid equilibration of the alveolar partial pressure of desflurane with the partial pressure in the brain.

Desflurane is also less soluble in human tissue than either sevoflurane, halothane or isoflurane [168], therefore less is absorbed into the tissue compartment. These

Table 2.7 Characteristics of the inhalational agents

	Desflurane	Sevoflurane	Isoflurane	Enflurane	Halothane	Nitrous oxide
Partition coefficients						
Blood : gas	0·4	0·6	1·4	1·9	2·3	0·5
Olive oil : gas	19·0	53·0	41·0	96·0	224·0	1·4
Boiling point (°C)	23·5	58·5	48·5	56·5	50·2	−89·0
Vapour pressure at 20°C (kP_a)	88·53	21·3	31·86	22·93	32·5	44×10^2
MAC in oxygen (%)	6·0/7·2	1·7/2·0	1·2	1·6	0·7	105
Stability in soda–lime	Stable	?Unstable	Stable	Stable	Stable	Stable
Etherality	Pungent	Pleasant	Pungent	Pungent	Pleasant	Pleasant
Metabolism	0·02%	2–3%	0·2%	2–3%	20%	≈ 0

MAC, minimal alveolar concentration.

characteristics suggest that rapid awakening after desflurane anaesthesia is very likely. However, desflurane has disadvantages. It is pungent and causes coughing, laryngospasm and excitation when used for gaseous induction [169]. This problem may be avoided in day-case anaesthesia by induction with propofol followed by maintenance with desflurane. The boiling point of 23·5°C means that it cannot be delivered using standard vaporizers and pressurized vaporizers are now being used. It is also expensive.

Arguably however, in terms of speed of recovery, an anaesthetic technique based on propofol and desflurane would have major advantages for day-case anaesthesia. For example Ghouri *et al.* [170] found that 76% of patients who received desflurane nitrous oxide anaesthesia were able to complete a digit symbol substitution test 0·5 h post anaesthesia compared to only 46% of patients who received isoflurane nitrous oxide. The induction and maintenance of anaesthesia using desflurane and propofol as principal agents has been compared [171] and emergence was found to be significantly faster in the desflurane group. Wrigley *et al.* [172] also found that early recovery of psychomotor performance was significantly better in the desflurane compared with the propofol group. Equivocal results have been found in another study by Graham and Aitkenhead [173] on 57 female patients undergoing laparoscopic surgery. Although recovery of consciousness and orientation were more rapid in patients maintained with desflurane, there were no significant differences in digit substitution tests and p-deletion tests between the desflurane and propofol groups.

The balance of opinion would suggest that desflurane offers advantages of very rapid reawakening and could have a major role in day-case anaesthesia in the future. It has cardiovascular effects similar to those of isoflurane [174]. In humans it is less likely than halothane to cause arrhythmias [175], and does not cause a coronary steal phenomenon in animal models [176].

Although there are no studies concerning the effects of desflurane on the airways, it is probably a bronchodilator, as are halothane, enflurane and isoflurane. It is a central respiratory depressant, but less so than isoflurane and enflurane. It causes a dose-related increase in cerebral blood flow and intracranial pressure, and in common with the other inhalational agents potentiates neuromuscular blocking drugs. Its effects on postoperative nausea and vomiting require further study particularly when it is used with propofol. For example, compared with isoflurane Ghouri *et al* [170] found a higher incidence (52%) following desflurane whereas Wrigley *et al.* [172] found no difference.

In summary desflurane is a very important prospect for day-case anaesthesia with a rapid onset of action and short recovery time. Its known disadvantages are irritation of the airway and etherish odour, the need for specialized delivery systems and cost.

Sevoflurane

Sevoflurane is a methyl propyl ether in clinical use in Japan. It has a low blood:gas solubility coefficient of 0·6 and an MAC of 1·7–2. Sevoflurane, although not eliminated as quickly as desflurane, is eliminated much faster than halothane and isoflurane which would predict that its onset and offset of action is slower than desflurane and more rapid than halothane, which has proved to be the case. Its vapour pressure of 21·3 kP_a at 20°C and its boiling point of 58·5°C mean that it can be used with conventional vaporizers.

It does not cause irritation of the upper airway, and is 'pleasant' to inhale. A comparison of the induction and emergence times of sevoflurane with enflurane found the emergence times were significantly shorter with sevoflurane [177].

The characteristics above suggest sevoflurane might be useful in day-case anaesthesia. However, there are serious problems with this agent. Firstly, the plasma concentrations of fluoride ions have been reported as increasing markedly after sevoflurane administration. Although there was no evidence of gross changes in renal function in the patients so far studied [178] this could conceivably, as with methoxyflurane, compromise its use. Secondly, sevoflurane may not be stable in the presence of soda–lime [169].

In humans, sevoflurane decreases systemic blood pressure, with little effect on the heart rate [169] and is less likely to cause arrhythmias than halothane. It appears to have similar effects on cerebral blood flow and intracranial pressure to desflurane and isoflurane.

In summary, hitherto sevoflurane has not been as extensively investigated as desflurane in humans. It is certainly easier to use and does not need any specialized vaporizing equipment. However, its stability and toxicity *in vivo* are in doubt, and there are questions about its reactivity with soda–lime. These must be resolved before it is more widely introduced.

Isoflurane and enflurane

Isoflurane and enflurane are both extensively used in day-case surgery. The blood : gas solubilities of isoflurane and enflurane are 1·4 and 1·9 respectively.

They have effectively replaced halothane in the day-case area because of the higher solubility of halothane in lipid associated with its lower MAC value and slower recovery. However, the relationship between isoflurane and enflurane is not so simple, since although isoflurane is less soluble in lipid than enflurane, it has a lower MAC value of 1·2 compared with 1·6 when theoretically it should lie between enflurane and sevoflurane. It is possible that the dissociation of solubility in olive oil and MAC values for isoflurane is caused by stereoscopic receptor interactions based on chirality [179]. Thus the question could arise as to whether its potency follows the MAC, where correlations may not be direct for the blood : gas and olive oil : gas partition coefficients and hence clinical induction and recovery studies are required to answer these questions.

However, several studies have been performed which show no significant difference in recovery times between halothane, enflurane and isoflurane [180, 181].

Isoflurane causes upper airway irritation and is difficult to use for gaseous induction. In children it has been associated with significant disadvantages of coughing and laryngospasm [182]. Isoflurane offers very few advantages when compared to enflurane. It is, however, less metabolized than enflurane (only $\approx$ 0·2% compared to enflurane $\approx$ 2% and halothane $\approx$ 20%). Given that the emergence times are similar with isoflurane and enflurane, the indications for using it in day-case anaesthesia are not clear cut.

Enflurane has a fairly rapid onset and offset time, only slightly longer than isoflurane which may not be clinically significant. It is metabolized more than isoflurane, however, to free fluoride ions but this has not prevented its general use and sevoflurane shows the same phenomena. Free fluoride ions may rise to particularly high levels in patients taking enzyme-inducing medicines such as isoniazid. Arguably neither enflurane nor sevoflurane should be administered under these circumstances.

However, it remains a relatively cheap, rapidly acting and safe alternative to the other inhalational agents, and from the overall point of view of costs and side effects, is a very good choice in day-case anaesthesia.

Halothane is still the most useful drug for inhalational induction in children, because it is pleasant to breathe and does not cause airway irritation. However, sevoflurane may eventually supplant it for this purpose.

The potential for hepatic necrosis with halothane presents a serious problem in developed countries, where alternatives are available. As many as 25–30% of patients given halothane show evidence of minor hepatic dysfunction, and hepatic necrosis may occur with an incidence of 1 in 3700, depending on the number of previous exposures [183]. Its sudden unexpected occurrence precludes the continued use of halothane in day-case anaesthesia since arguably a predictable law suit will eventually overtake any cost advantage.

The possibility of hepatic necrosis on repeated exposure to halothane presents the anaesthetist with a difficult choice. The Committee on Safety of Medicines [184] have issued guidelines on the use of halothane. They recommended a period of at least 3 months should elapse before repeated exposure to halothane, but halothane hepatitis may occur sporadically up to several years after previous exposure. Therefore, this recommendation may not be completely safe.

Nitrous oxide has been in clinical use for many years. Its low blood:gas solubility ensures rapid changes in the partial pressure of the agent in the brain. It is generally used as a vehicle adding to the anaesthetic effects of the volatile agents.

Its main disadvantage is a tendency to cause nausea and vomiting postoperatively. Although some workers suggest there is an association between nitrous oxide and nausea, others question the importance of the gas in this respect [185]. However, when nitrous oxide is combined with opioid analgesia, the incidence of nausea and vomiting may be significantly higher [186].

In summary inhalational agents have a great part to play on the maintenance of anaesthesia for day-case surgery.

Desflurane may become the rapidly acting drug and sevoflurane the most pleasant while also providing rapid recovery [187]. However, if there is little to choose between the duration of action of halothane, enflurane and isoflurane, enflurane may well be the best choice in terms of cost-effectiveness since for procedures of short duration the potential advantages of low flow circuits are not fully exploited.

Analgesic agents

Opioids

Opioid analgesics are frequently administered during day-case anaesthesia as part of a 'balanced technique'. The ideal opioid has fast onset and offset times with minimal 'hangover' and side effects. Particularly, nausea and vomiting should be minimal. Table 2.8 shows data for some of the commonly used opioids.

Although the use of opioids perioperatively reduces the incidence of complications at induction and provides for smoother anaesthesia [188], it also increases the incidence of postoperative nausea and vomiting [189].

The older drugs such as morphine and pethidine are still used but the newer drugs fentanyl, alfentanil and sufentanil have faster onset and more rapid redistribution times giving them a better action profile.

Fentanyl is very widely used in day-case anaesthesia. It has a rapid onset and an elimination half life of 3–4 h, but may contribute to nausea and vomiting because it has a relatively long elimination half-life compared for example to alfentanil [190]. However, its analgesic effects carry on into the immediate postoperative period.

Alfentanil has a rapid onset time of 90 s, and is slightly less lipid soluble than fentanyl. This means its volume of distribution is smaller in the steady state, and its

Table 2.8 Some commonly used opioids. After [191]

Drug	Relative potency	Distribution half-life (min)	Elimination half-life (h)	Clearance (ml kg^{-1} min^{-1})	Vol^{SS} (l kg^{-1})
Morphine	1	1–3 rapid 9–20 slow	2–4	10–23	3·4–4·7
Pethidine	0·1	4–30	2·4–7·0	12–22	3·5–5·3
Fentanyl	100	1–2 rapid 10–15 slow	3–4	10–20	3·5–4·4
Alfentanil	15	1–3	1–2	3–8	0·4–1·0
Sufentanil	700	1–3 rapid 10–15 slow	2–4	11–21	1·7–4·0

Vol^{SS}, volume of distribution, steady state.

elimination half-life which is related to clearance and volume of distribution is significantly shorter than the other opioids (1–2 h).

Recovery times and indices have been shown to be significantly shorter with alfentanil than fentanyl [191, 192]. There also seems to be a quicker return to normal activities in the longer term recovery period with alfentanil [193]. The incidence of nausea and vomiting is probably the same when compared to fentanyl [191] although some workers have reported a higher incidence [193].

Recently, Bagshaw *et al.* [194] assessed the addition of alfentanil or placebo in a single dose to propofol–enflurane anaesthesia during day-case dental surgery. They found no significant difference in recovery by critical flicker fusion, or p-deletion tests. They also found no difference in the incidence of nausea and vomiting between the two groups. Despite preoperative intramuscular diclofenac both groups complained of pain after surgery in similar numbers, suggesting that there is very little residual analgesic effect of alfentanil postoperatively.

Because of its short duration of effect alfentanil has suitable characteristics for administration as an infusion. A recommended infusion rate in humans is 1 $\mu g\ kg^{-1}\ min^{-1}$ [195].

Sufentanil is widely used in the USA. It has a slightly shorter elimination half-life than fentanyl (2–4 h vs. 3–4 h). This is again due to its smaller volume of distribution. Phitayakom *et al.* [196] found it to compare favourably with fentanyl in terms of postoperative analgesia and the incidence of nausea and vomiting, when used by an infusion technique. White *et al.* [197], found the optimum dose for sufentanil as a bolus before induction of anaesthesia to be 10–15 $\mu g\ kg^{-1}$. A higher dose caused an increased frequency of nausea and vomiting.

Nalbuphine and *butorphanol* are partial agonists which have been used in a day-case setting. Their effectiveness is similar to morphine for analgesia, and an advantage is that they have a 'ceiling effect' with respect to their respiratory depressant action and a low potential for social abuse. However, both these agents cause a high incidence of dysphoria and postoperative sedation [198, 199] while Pandit *et al.* [199] found butorphanol was associated with the same incidence of nausea and vomiting as fentanyl.

Non-steroidal anti-inflammatory drugs (NSAIDs)

NSAIDs act by inhibiting the cyclo-oxygenase pathway and prostaglandin synthetase. This leads to a decrease in the release of the mediators of pain and inflammation in the tissues. NSAIDs have a latent period during which their effects are minimal, and so have a slow onset of action requiring up to 40 min for the onset of effective analgesia. They have a number of side effects which are well known, e.g. bronchoconstriction in asthmatics; stomach ulceration and haemorrhage; renal failure in those with compromised renal function; and an anticoagulant effect by influencing platelet function.

Given these limitations NSAIDs may still be among the most useful drugs for assisting the management of pain in day-case patients. There are now a wide range of NSAIDs on the market (e.g. diclofenac, ibuprofen, indomethacin and ketorolac).

Ketorolac is a new NSAID with a potent analgesic action—30 mg i.m. is equivalent to 10 mg of morphine i.m. It is also licensed for intravenous use. As outlined above, it has a relatively slow onset and takes 30–40 min to reach peak effect. It does not cause cardiorespiratory depression, though it may induce slight somnolence and a very small incidence of nausea and vomiting [200]. Ketorolac may be a useful agent if it can provide analgesia equivalent to that of morphine, without the opioid side effects of respiratory depression, nausea and vomiting. Alternatively because of its long duration of action with a half-life over 7 h, it could be used to provide an opioid-sparing effect when used in conjunction with conventional μ-opioids.

Recently, however, there has been concern over reported deaths in patients receiving ketorolac (Toradol). Up until December 1992 approximately 16 million patients world-wide, particularly in the USA, received ketorolac and some 923 spontaneous reports of adverse reactions have been reported which are a feature of other NSAIDs. One of the major advantages of ketorolac is its small volume (1 ml alcohol) for parenteral administration.

For these reasons the starting dose for parenteral administration has been reduced to 10 mg i.m. or i.v. from 30 mg [201]. Furthermore, ketorolac should not be given with other NSAIDs or anticoagulant drugs [201]. Arguably these remarks apply to the whole range of NSAIDs. There should be strict adherence to the contraindications to the use of NSAIDs which include:

1 a history of peptic ulceration;
2 bleeding diathesis;
3 confirmed or suspected cerebrovascular bleeding;

4 operations associated with high risk of haemorrhage;
5 a history of asthma;
6 moderate to severe renal impairment;
7 hypovolaemia;
8 dehydration;
9 hypersensitivity to other NSAIDs and aspirin.

Recently a large multicentre double-blind controlled trial by Wong *et al.* [202] in ambulatory surgical patients compared ketorolac tromethamine 30 mg i.v. with fentanyl 50 μg i.v. followed by 60 mg codeine plus 600 mg acetaminophen orally. They found that although ketorolac had a slow onset of action, it had otherwise equivalent analgesic effects. There were no significant differences in the incidence of nausea and vomiting in the early postoperative phase between the groups studied. This may be due to the fact that intraoperative opioids had been given to all patients which may mask the differences between ketorolac and opioids in the postoperative period and in this study fentanyl was given intraoperatively to the ketorolac group. However, ketorolac was associated with a lower incidence of somnolence and nausea in the later postoperative period [202].

Although results with ketorolac are encouraging, a controlled trial avoiding the use of opioids completely is desirable to make a real comparison between the side effects of NSAIDs and other drugs.

Muscle relaxants

Suxamethonium

In the past suxamethonium with its rapid onset of action and short duration of effect was popular for short procedures in ambulatory patients. However, it is associated with well-known side effects, the most important of which in the outpatient or day-case setting is severe myalgia.

There is still debate over whether suxamethonium does cause a true increase in muscle pain after day-case anaesthesia. For example Zahl and Apfelbaum [203] showed that the use of vecuronium, a non-depolarizing agent, compared with suxamethonium did not lower the incidence or severity of muscle pain after laparoscopy. However, other investigators have reported muscle pain associated with suxamethonium lasting up to 4 days after this operation [204].

Atracurium and vecuronium

Newer non-depolarizing agents such as atracurium and vecuronium provide muscle relaxation which may be reversed easily after 20–30 min [205]. There is some recent evidence to suggest that the use of neostigmine for reversal of neuromuscular blockade may increase the incidence of nausea and vomiting after outpatient surgery [206].

Mivacurium

The new muscle relaxant mivacurium may offer significant advantages over both suxamethonium and the currently available short-acting competitive depolarizing relaxants. It has a short elimination half-life of 17 min, due to its degradation by plasma cholinesterase. Although its onset of action is the same as that of atracurium, (about 90–120 s) the time to spontaneous recovery of neuromuscular function in an average adult is much shorter at about 10–20 min [207].

The recommended dosage for mivacurium is 0·07–0·15 mg kg^{-1} in adults. The lowest and highest doses in this range produce clinically effective muscle relaxation for 10–15 min and 15–20 min respectively [207].

It is rapidly metabolized by plasma cholinesterase, and it is important to remember that patients with atypical cholinesterase enzymes will have a prolonged neuromuscular block, similar to that seen with suxamethonium.

Mivacurium releases histamine in similar quantities to atracurium. This may cause hypotension and tachycardia, but is only important when twice the ED_{95} of the drug is administered [208].

Rocuronium

Rocuronium is a rapid-onset analogue of vecuronium, which offers a similar onset time to suxamethonium for good intubating conditions. However, its effects last as long as vecuronium and it may be less useful than mivacurium in the outpatient setting, the rapid offset of action of which, even without reversal with an anticholinesterase, is sudden and is probably more important for brief surgical procedures.

Anti-emetics

As has been suggested throughout this chapter, postoperative nausea and vomiting is a very important cause of morbidity, sometimes resulting in overnight hospital stay [209]. Hitherto the two anti-emetics which have been used most regularly are metoclopramide and droperidol.

Metoclopramide is a chlorinated procainamide derivative, which has a central anti-emetic effect and increases gastrointestinal motility while increasing upper oesophageal sphincter tone. Unfortunately, it is associated with dystonic reactions, usually manifested as oculogyric crises. There is as yet no consensus of opinion regarding its effectiveness as an anti-emetic in outpatient anaesthesia [210].

Droperidol is a butyrophenone derivative which has been studied in outpatient anaesthesia. Like metoclopramide it acts via central dopaminergic D_2-receptor blockade, and as such is associated with sedation and dystonic reactions. Recovery time are significantly delayed when droperidol has been used. Psychomotor skills are also impaired [211, 212]. Prophylactic droperidol may not significantly alter the incidence of nausea and vomiting in day-case anaesthesia when compared to metoclopramide [211] and it may also be associated with delayed dysphoric side effects occurring after discharge [213].

Ondansetron, a 5-hydroxytryptamine-3 receptor antagonist has recently been introduced. Two studies have shown that intravenous ondansetron in doses of 1, 4 and 8 mg were all effective in reducing postoperative emesis when compared to a placebo. There were no significant side effects. In these large studies, ondansetron was highly effective in preventing postoperative nausea and vomiting [214, 215].

A number of 'me too' $5HT_3$ blocking drugs are currently undergoing clinical trials and these drugs combined with the development of minimally invasive therapy and day-case surgery will provide a new impetus for the study of postoperative nausea in the years ahead.

Premedicant drugs

Premedicant drugs may be divided into two main groups. Sedative drugs, which are not used routinely in day-case anaesthesia, except in some paediatric practice. Midazolam is probably the most useful drug in this respect because of its solubility in water and hence its effectiveness by any route of administration. In adults the recommended dose is 0·1 mg kg^{-1} i.m. [160] and its use in paediatric practice is reviewed in Chapter 3.

The second group of drugs are used to reduce gastric acid secretion, and therefore decrease the risk of aspiration pneumonitis in patients at risk, for example hiatus hernia, symptoms of oesophageal rupture or suspected pyloric obstruction, and pregnancy.

H_2-receptor antagonists such as ranitidine, in combination with gastrokinetic agents such as metoclopramide, have been used to give reduced gastric acidity and residual volume which lessens the risk of gastric aspiration [216]. Omeprazole causes selective non-competitive inhibition of the Na^+/K^+ adenosine triphosphate (ATPase) proton pump in the stomach in humans. It has also been shown to increase gastric pH in day-case patients, and again this could be important in the prevention of aspiration pneumonitis [217].

Low molecular weight heparin

In patients at high risk for thrombotic episodes, prophylaxis with heparin (5000 i.u.) administered subcutaneously immediately after the induction of anaesthesia should be considered mandatory. Deep venous thrombosis (DVT) can occur in the legs during virtually any procedure with the potential for a fatal pulmonary embolism during the recovery period in apparently otherwise healthy patients. DVT is an important preventable cause of postoperative mortality and its incidence in the various minimally invasive procedures is unknown.

Conclusions

Day-case anaesthesia for ambulatory surgery is a growth industry throughout the world, particularly the UK and USA. For example, of the 22 million surgical procedures performed in the USA each year approximately 60% take place in outpatient settings. This is being driven by economics, made possible by new technologies, minimally invasive therapy and more appropriate anaesthesia. The search for better anaesthetic drugs and techniques which are effective yet have rapid offset characteristics and few postoperative sequelae continues. The years ahead will see the results, not only of large numbers of clinical trials, but also the development of audit procedures and the acquisition of data on the true effectiveness of new drugs and the incidence of their side effects.

Acknowledgements

Parts of this chapter have been rewritten, with permission, from Whitwam JG. Drugs for sedation. In McCloy R, ed. *Quality Control in Endoscopy. Report of an International Forum*. Berlin: Springer-Verlag, 1991: 3–21. © Springer-Verlag.

References

1 Calvey NT, Williams NE. *Principles and Practice of Pharmacology for Anaesthetists*, 2nd edn. Oxford: Blackwell Scientific Publications, 1991.
2 Whitwam JG. Intravenous induction agents. *Clin Anaesth* 1984; 2: 515–37.
3 Van der Walt JH, Mackay P. Patient safety in the recovery room. *Anaesth Intens Care* 1988; 16: 77–80.
4 Zelcer J, Wells D. Anaesthetic related recovery room complications. *Anaesth Intens Care* 1987; 15: 168–74.
5 Kortilla K. Post anaesthetic cognitive and psychomotor impairment. *Int Anaesth Clin* 1986; 24: 59–74.
6 Royal College of Surgeons of England. *Report of Working Party. Guidelines for Sedation by Non-Anaesthetists*. London: Royal College of Surgeons of England, 1993.
7 Mohler H, Okada T. Benzodiazepine receptor: demonstration in the central nervous system. *Science* 1977; 198: 849–51.
8 Braestrup C, Squires RF. Specific benzodiazepine receptors in rat brain characterised by high-affinity ^{3}H-diazepam binding. *Proc Natl Acad of Sci USA* 1977, 74: 3805–9.
9 Richards JG, Möhler H. Benzodiazepine receptors. *Neuropharmacology* 1984; 23: 233–42.
10 Braestrup C, Nielsen M. Neurotransmitters and CNS disease; anxiety. *Lancet* 1982; 2: 1030–4.
11 Chang LR, Barnard EA. The benzodiazepine/GABA receptor complex: molecular size in brain synaptic membranes and in solution. *J Neurochem* 1982; 39: 1507–18.
12 Schoch P, Richards JG, Häring P, Takacs B, Stähli C, Staehelin T, Haefely W, Möhler H. Co-localisation of GABA and benzodiazepine receptors in the brain. *Nature* 1985; 314: 168–70.
13 Möhler H, Schoch P, Richards JG, Häring P, Takacs B, Stähli C. Monoclonal antibodies: probes for structure and location of the GABA receptor/benzodiazepine receptor/chloride channel complex. In: Olsen RW, Venter JC, eds. *Benzodiazepine-GABA Receptors and Chloride Channels: Structural and Functional Properties*. New York: Alan R Liss, Inc.

14 Schofield PR, Darlinson MG, Fujita N *et al.* Sequence and functional expression of the GABA receptor shows a ligand gated receptor super-family. *Nature* 1987; 328: 221–7.
15 Erdös S. Peripheral GABAergic mechanisms. *Trends Pharmacol Sci* 1985; 6: 205–8.
16 Mestre M, Carriot T, Belin C *et al.* Electrophysiological and pharmacological characterization of peripheral benzodiazepine receptors in a guinea pig heart preparation. *Life Sci* 1985; 35: 953–62.
17 Thomson D (ed.). Midazolam and flumazenil—the agonist–antagonist concept for sedation and anaesthesia. Proceedings of an international symposium, April 1989. *Acta Anaesth Scand* 1990; 34 (suppl 92): 1–109.
18 Braestrup C, Nielsen M, Olsen CE. Urinary and brain β-carboline-3-carboxylates as potent inhibitors of brain benzodiazepine receptors. *Proc Natl Acad Sci USA* 1980; 77: 2288–92.
19 Braestrup C, Nielsen M. GABA reduced binding ^{3}H-methyl β-carboline-carboxylate to brain benzodiazepine receptors. *Nature* 1981; 294: 472–5.
20 Braestrup C, Schiechen R, Neef G, Nielsen M, Petersen EN. Interaction of convulsive ligands with benzodiazepine receptors. *Science* 1982; 216: 1241–3.
21 Guidotti A, Forchetti CM, Corda MG, Konkel D, Bennett CD, Costa E. Isolation, characterization and purification to homogeneity of an endogenous polypeptide with agonist action on benzodiazepine receptors. *Proc Natl Acad Sci USA* 1983; 80: 3531–5.
22 Diazepam binding inhibitor (Editorial). *Lancet* 1987; i: 307–8.
23 Ferrero P, Sahti MR, Conti-Tronconi B, Costa E, Guidotti A. Study of an octadecaneuropeptide derived diazepam binding inhibitor (DBI): biological activity and presence in rat brain. *Proc Natl Acad Sci USA* 1985; 83: 827–31.
24 Marquardt H, Todaro GJ, Shoyab M. Complete amino acid sequences of bovine and human endozepines. *J Biol Chem* 1986; 261: 9727–31.
25 Ferrero P, Guidotti A, Conti-Troncon B, Costa E. A brain octadecaneuropeptide generated by tryptic digestion of DBI (diazepam binding inhibitor) functions as a proconflict ligand of benzodiazepine recognition sites. *Neuropharmacology* 1984; 23: 1359–62.
26 Little HJ, Nutt DJ, Taylor SC. Kindling and withdrawal changes at the benzodiazepine receptor. *J Psychopharmacol* 1987; 1: 35–46.
27 Richards JG, Schoch PO, Möhler H, Haefely W. Benzodiazepine receptors resolved. *Experientia* 1986; 42: 121–6.
28 Darragh A, Lambe R, Kenny M, Brick I, O'Boyle C, Taffe W. Ro15-1788 antagonises the central diazepam in man without altering diazepam availability. *Br J Clin Pharmacol* 1982; 14: 677–82.
29 O'Boyle C, Lambe R, Darragh A, Taffe W, Brick I, Kenny M. Ro15-1788 antagonises the effects of diazepam in man without affecting its bioavailability. *Br J Anaesth* 1983; 55: 349–55.
30 Amrein R, Hetzel W. Pharmacology of Dormicum (midazolam) and Anexate (flumazenil). *Acta Anaesth Scand* 1990; (suppl 92) 34: 6–15.
31 Crevoisier C, Ziegler WH, Heigmann P, Dubuis R. Relation entre l'effet clinique et la concentration plasmatique du midazolam chez des sujets volontaires. *Ann Fr Anesth Reanim* 1984; 3: 162–7.
32 Persson MP, Nilsson A, Hartvig P. Relation of sedation and amnesia to plasma concentrations of anaesthesia in surgical patients. *Clin Pharmacol Ther* 1988; 43: 324–31.
33 Lauven PM, Stoeckel H. Hypnotische wirksame Blutspiegel von Midazolam. *Anasth Intensivther Notfallmed* 1987; 22: 90–3.
34 Raeder JC, Nilsen G, Hole A. Pharmacokinetics of midazolam and alfentanil in outpatient general anaesthesia. *Acta Anaesth Scand* 1988; 32: 467–72.
35 Lauven PM, Schwilden H, Stoeckel H. Greenblatt DJ. The effects of a benzodiazepine antagonist Ro15-1788 in the presence of stable concentrations of midazolam. *Anesthesiology* 1985; 63: 61–4.

36 Riou B, Rimailho A, Galliot M, Bourdon R, Huet Y. Protective cardiovascular effects of diazepam in chloroquine poisoning. *Intens Care Med* 1988; 14: 610–16.
37 Yakel DL, Whittaker SE, Elstad MR. Midazolam-induced angiodema and bronchoconstriction. *Critical Care Med* 1992; 20: 307–8.
38 Sanders LD, Davies-Evans J, Rosen M, Robinson JO. Comparison of diazepam with midazolam as i.v. sedation for outpatient gastroscopy. *Br J Anaesth* 1989; 63: 726–31.
39 Whitwam JG, Al-Khudhairi D, McCloy RF. Comparison of midazolam and diazepam in doses of comparable potency during gastroscopy. *Br J Anaesth* 1983; 55: 773–7.
40 Gamble JAS, Kawar P, Dundee JW, Moore J, Briggs LP. Evaluation of midazolam as an intravenous induction agent. *Anaesthesia* 1981; 36: 868–73.
41 Bell GD, Antrobus JHL, Lee J, Coady T, Morden A. Bolus or slow titrated injection of midazolam prior to upper gastrointestinal endoscopy? Relative effect on oxygen saturation and prophylactic value of supplemental oxygen. *Alim Pharmacol Ther* 1990; 4: 393–401.
42 Swain DG, Ellis DJ, Bradby H. Rapid intravenous low-dose diazepam as sedation for upper gastrointestinal endoscopy. *Alim Pharmacol Ther* 1990; 4: 43–8.
43 Dundee JW, Collier PS, Carlisle RJT, Harper KW. Prolonged midazolam elimination half-life. *Br J Clin Pharmacol* 1986; 21: 425–9.
44 Kassai A, Toth G, Eichelbaum M, Klotz U. No evidence of a genetic polymorphism in the oxidative metabolism of midazolam. *Clin Pharmacokinet* 1988; 15: 319–25.
45 Adams P, Gelman S, Reves JG *et al.* Midazolam pharmacokinetics and pharmacodynamics during acute hypovolemia. *Anesthesiology* 1985; 63: 140–6.
46 Shelly MP, Mendel I, Park GR. Failure of critically ill patients to metabolise midazolam. *Anaesthesia* 1987; 42: 619–26.
47 Kalow W. Ethnic differences in drug metabolism. *Clin Pharmacokinet* 1982; 7: 373–400.
48 Cook PJ, Bennett PN, Lennard-Jones JE, Warnes TW. Premedication for endoscopy. *Scand J Gastroenterol* 1978; 13: 33–9.
49 Swenzen GO, Chakrabarti MK, Sapsed-Byrne S, Whitwam JG. Selective depression by alfentanil of Group III and IV somatosympathetic reflexes in the dog. *Br J Anaesth* 1988; 61: 441–5.
50 Whitwam JG. Summary of meeting. In: Kallar SK, Whitwam JG, eds. *Outpatient Anaesthesia. Proceedings of an International Symposium*. Antwerp, Belgium, 9th June 1988, Amsterdam: Medicom.
51 Ben-Shlomo I, Abd-El-Khalim H, Ezry J, Zohar S, Tverskoy M. Midazolam acts synergistically with fentanyl for induction of anaesthesia. *Br J Anaesth* 1990; 64: 45–7.
52 Vinik HR, Bradley EL, Kissin I. Midazolam–alfentanil synergism for anaesthetic induction in patients. *Anesth Analg* 1989; 69: 213–17.
53 Tverskoy M, Fleyshman G, Bradley EL, Kissin I. Midazolam–thiopental anesthetic interaction in patients. *Anesth Analg* 1988; 67: 342–5.
54 Tverskoy M, Ben-Shlomo I, Ezry J, Finger J, Fleyshman G. Midazolam acts synergistically with methohexitone for induction of anaesthesia. *Br J Anaesth* 1989; 63: 109–122.
55 Short TG, Chui PT. Propofol and midazolam act synergistically in combination. *Br J Anaesth* 1991; 67: 539–45.
56 Tverskoy M, Fleyshman G, Ezry J, Bradley EL, Kissin I. Midazolam–morphine sedative interaction in patients. *Anesth Analg* 1989; 68: 282–5.
57 Tucker MR, Ochs MW, White PW. Arterial blood gas levels after midazolam or diazepam administered with or without fentanyl as an intravenous sedative for outpatient surgical procedures. *J Oral Maxillofac Surg* 1986; 44: 688–92.
58 Dolan EA, Murray WJ, Immediata AR, Gleason N. Comparison of nalbuphine and fentanyl in combination with diazepam for outpatient oral surgery. *J Oral Maxillofac Surg* 1988; 46: 471–3.

59 Sury MRJ, Cole PV. Nalbuphine combined with midazolam for outpatient sedation. An assessment in fibreoptic bronchoscopy patients. *Anaesthesia* 1988; 43: 285–8.
60 Romagnoli A, Keats AS. Ceiling effect for respiratory depression by nalbuphine. *Clin Pharmacol Ther* 1980; 27: 478–85.
61 Vinik HR, Kissin I. Propofol–midazolam–alfentanil combinations: is hypnotic synergism present? *Anesth Analg* 1993; 76: S450.
62 Elwood RJ, Hildebrand PJ, Dundee JW, Collier PS. Ranitidine influences the uptake of oral midazolam. *Br J Clin Pharmacol* 1983; 15: 743–5.
63 Fee JPH, Collier PS, Howard PJ, Dundee JW. Cimetidine and ranitidine increase midazolam bioavailability. *Clin Pharmacol Ther* 1987; 41: 80–4.
64 Knüchel M, Ochs HR, Verbrug-Ochs B, Labedzki L, Greenblatt DJ. Interaktion von Ranitidin und Cimetidin mit Midazolam bei intravenöser und oraler Gabe. *Med Welt* 1987; 38: 244–8.
65 Buckley MMT, Brogden RM. Ketorolac. A review of the pharmacodynamic and pharmacokinetic properties and therapeutic potential. *Drugs* 1990; 39: 86–109.
66 Amrein R, Leishman B, Bentzinger C, Roncari G. Flumazenil in benzodiazepine antagonism. Actions and clinical use in intoxication and anaesthesiology. *Med Toxicol* 1987; 2: 411–29.
67 Klotz U, Kanto J. Pharmacokinetics and clinical use of flumazenil. *Clin Pharmacokinet* 1988; 14: 1–12.
68 Whitwam JG. Flumazenil: a benzodiazepine antagonist. *Br Med J* 1988; 297: 999–1000.
69 Fisher GC, Hutton P. Cardiovascular responses to flumazenil-induced arousal after arterial surgery. *Anaesthesia* 1989; 44: 104–6.
70 Wolff J, Carl P, Clausen TG, Mikkelsen BO. Ro15-1788 for postoperative recovery. A randomised clinical trial in patients undergoing minor surgical procedures under midazolam anaesthesia. *Anaesthesia* 1986; 41: 1001–6.
71 Alon E, Baitella L, Hossli G. Double-blind study of the reversal of midazolam-supplemented general anaesthesia with Ro15-1788. *Br J Anaesth* 1987; 59: 455–8.
72 Ricou R, Forster A, Bruckner A, Chastonay P, Gemperle M. Clinical evaluation of a specific benzodiazepine antagonist (Ro15-1788). Studies in elderly patients after regional anaesthesia under benzodiazepine sedation. *Br J Anaesth* 1986; 58: 1005–11.
73 Sage DJ, Chase A, Boas RA. Reversal of midazolam sedation with Anexate. *Br J Anaesth* 1987; 59: 459–64.
74 Jensen S, Knudsen L, Kirkegaard I. Flumazenil used in the antagonizing of diazepam and midazolam sedation in outpatients undergoing gastroscopy. *Eur J Anaesth* 1988; Suppl 2: 161–6.
75 Rodrigo C, Rosenquist JB. The effect of Ro15-1788 (Anexate) on conscious sedation produced with midazolam. *Anaesth Intens Care* 1987; 15: 185–92.
76 Holloway AM, Logan DA. The use of flumazenil to reverse diazepam sedation after endoscopy. *Eur J Anaesthesiol* 1988; Suppl 2: 191–8.
77 Kirkegaard I, Knudsen I, Jensen S, Kruse A. Benzodiazepine antagonist Ro15-1788. Antagonism of diazepam sedation in outpatients undergoing gastroscopy. *Anaesthesia* 1986; 41: 1184–8.
78 Andrews PJD, Wright DJ, Lamont MC. Flumazenil in the outpatient. A study following midazolam as sedation for upper gastrointestinal endoscopy of sedation and amnesia to plasma concentrations of midazolam in surgical patients. *Clin Pharmacol Ther* 1988; 43: 324–31.
79 Nutt D, Glue P, Lawson C, Wilson S. Flumazenil provocation of panic attacks. *Arch Gen Psychiatry* 1990; 47: 917–25.
80 Louis M, Forster A, Suter PM. Gemperle M. Clinical and haemodynamic effects of a specific benzodiazepine antagonist (Ro15-1788) after open heart surgery. *Anesthesiology* 1984; 513A.
81 Midazolam—is antagonism justified? (Editorial) *Lancet* 1988; i: 140–2.
82 Ashton H. Benzodiazepine withdrawal: an unfinished story. *Br Med J* 1984; 288: 1135–40.

83 Cumin R, Bonetti EP, Scherschlicht R, Haefely WE. Use of the specific benzodiazepine antagonist Ro15-1788 in studies of physiological dependence on benzodiazepine. *Experientia* 1982; 38: 833–4.
84 Savic I, Widen L, Stone-Elander S. Feasibility of reversing benzodiazepine tolerance with flumazenil. *Lancet* 1991; 337: 133–7.
85 Bell GD, Reeve PA, Moshiri M *et al.* Intravenous midazolam: a study of the degree of oxygen desaturation occurring during upper-gastrointestinal endoscopy. *Br J Clin Pharmacol* 1987; 23: 703–8.
86 Mora CT, Torjman M, White PF. Effects of diazepam and flumazenil on sedation and hypoxic ventilatory response. *Anesth Analg* 1989; 68: 473–8.
87 Power SJ, Chakrabarti MK, Whitwam JG. Response to carbon dioxide after oral midazolam and pentobarbitone. *Anaesthesia* 1984; 39: 1183–7.
88 Deham A, Ward DS. Effect of i.v. midazolam on the ventilatory response to substained hypoxia in man. *Br J Anaesth* 1991; 66: 454–7.
89 Forster A, Fardaz JP, Suter PM, Gemperle M. Respiratory depression by midazolam and diazepam. *Anesthesiology* 1980; 53: 494–7.
90 Power SJ, Morgan M, Chakrabarti MK. Carbon dioxide response curves following midazolam and diazepam. *Br J Anaesth* 1983; 55: 837–41.
91 Dundee JW, Wyant GM. *Intravenous Anaesthesia*. Edinburgh: Churchill Livingstone, 1974.
92 Al-Khudhairi D, Askitopoulou H, Whitwam JG. Acute tolerance to the central respiratory effects of midazolam in the dog. *Br J Anaesth* 1982; 54: 953–8.
93 Blouin RT, Conard PF, Perreault S, Gross JB. The effect of flumazenil on midazolam-induced depression of the ventilatory response to hypoxia during isohypercarbia. *Anaesthesiology* 1993; 78: 635–41.
94 Weinbrum A, Geller E. The respiratory effects of reversing midazolam sedation with flumazenil in the presence or absence of narcotics. *Acta Anaesth Scand* 1990; 34 (suppl 92): 65–9.
95 Glen JR. Animal studies of the anaesthetic activity of ICI 35,868. *Br J Anaesth* 1980; 52: 731–42.
96 Glen JB, Hunter SC. Pharmacology of an emulsion of ICI 35,868. *Br J Anaesth* 1984; 56: 617–26.
97 Grattidge P. Patient controlled sedation using propofol in day surgery. *Anaesthesia* 1992; 47: 683–5.
98 Patrick MR, Blain IJ, Feneck RO *et al.* A comparison of the haemodynamic effect of propofol (Diprivan) and thiopentone in patients with coronary artery disease. *Postgrad Med J* 1985; 61 (suppl 3): 23–7.
99 Grounds RM, Twigley AJ, Casli F, Whitwam JG, Morgan M. The haemodynamic effects of intravenous induction. Comparison of the effects of thiopentone and propofol. *Br J Anaesth* 1985; 40: 735–40.
100 Taylor MB, Grounds RM, Mulrooney PP, Morgan M. Ventilatory effects of propofol during induction of anaesthesia. Comparison with thiopentone. *Br J Anaesth* 1986; 41: 816–20.
101 Grounds RM, Maxwell DL, Taylor MB *et al.* Acute ventilatory changes during intravenous induction of anaesthesia with thiopentone and propofol in humans using inductance plethysmograph. *Br J Anaesth* 1987; 59: 1098–102.
102 McKenzie N, Grant IS. Comparison of the new emulsion formulation of propofol with methohexitone and thiopentone for induction of anaesthesia in day cases. *Br J Anaesth* 1985; 57: 725–31.
103 Wells JKG. Comparison of ICI 34868, etomidate and methohexitone for day-case anaesthesia. *Br J Anaesth* 1985; 57: 732–5.
104 Shearer ES. Convulsions and propofol. *Br J Anaesth* 1990; 45: 255–6.

105 Glen JB. Animal studies of anaesthetic activity of ICI 35,868. *Br J Anaesth* 1980; 52: 731–42.
106 Cockshott ID. Propofol (Diprivan). Pharmacokinetics and metabolism—an overview. *Postgrad Med J* 1985; 61 (suppl 3): 45–50.
107 Simons PJ, Cockshott ID, Douglas EJ *et al.* Blood concentration, metabolism and elimination after a sub-anaesthetic intravenous dose of I4C-propofol (Diprivan) to male volunteers. *Postgrad Med J* 1985; 61 (suppl 3): 64–7.
108 Kay NH, Sear JW, Uppington J, Cockshott ID, Douglas EJ. Disposition of propofol in patients undergoing surgery. A comparison in men and women. *Br J Anaesth* 1986; 58: 1073–9.
109 Gray PA, Park G, Cockshott ID *et al.* Propofol metabolism in man during the anhepatic and reperfusion phases of liver transplantation. *Xenobiotica* 1992; 22: 105–14.
110 Dogra S, Isaac PA, Cockshott ID, Foy JM. Pulmonary extraction of propofol in post cardiopulmonary bypass patients. *J Drug Devel* 1989; 2: 133–7.
111 Cassidy MK, Housten JB. *In vivo* assessment of extrahepatic metabolism in first pass effects using the model compound phenol. *J Pharm Pharmacol* 1980; 32: 57–9.
112 Cassidy MK, Houston JB, *In vivo* capacity of hepatic and extrahepatic enzymes to conjugate phenol. *Drug Metab Disp* 1984; 12: 619–24.
113 Mather LE, Selby DG, Runciman WB, McLean CF. Propofol assay and regional mass balance on sheep. *Xenobiotica* 1989; 19: 1337–47.
114 O'Toole DP, Michigan KR, Howe JP *et al.* A comparison of propofol and methohexitone as induction agents for day case isoflurane anaesthesia. *Anaesthesia* 1987; 42: 373–6.
115 Heath PJ, Kennedy DJ, Ogg TW, Gilks WR. Which IV induction agent for day surgery? A comparison of propofol, thiopentone, methohexitone and etomidate. *Anaesthesia* 1988; 43: 365–8.
116 Edelist G. A comparison of propofol and thiopentone as induction agents in outpatient surgery. *Can J Anaesth* 1987; 34: 110–16.
117 Johnston R, Noseworthy T, Anderson B *et al.* Propofol versus thiopentone for outpatient anaesthesia. *Anaesthesiology* 1987; 67: 431–3.
118 Kay B, Hargreaves J, Sivalingam J, Healey TEJ. Intravenous anaesthesia for cystoscopy: a comparison of propofol and methohexitone with alfentanil. *Eur J Anaesth* 1986; 3: 111–20.
119 Winwood MA, Jago RH. Anxiety levels following anaesthesia for day case surgery. *Anaesthesia* 1993; 48: 581–4.
120 Valanne J, Kortilla K. Comparison of methohexitone and propofol for induction of enflurane anaesthesia in outpatients. *Postgrad Med J* 1985; 61: 138.
121 Chittleborough MC, Osborne GA, Rudkin GK *et al.* Double blind comparison of patient recovery after induction with propofol or thiopentone for day case relaxant general anaesthesia. *Anaesth Intens Care* 1992; 20: 169–73.
122 Gupta A, Larsen LE, Sjoberg F. Thiopentone or propofol for induction of isoflurane-based anaesthesia for ambulatory surgery? *Acta Anaesth Scand* 1992; 36: 670–4.
123 Doze VA, Westphal LA, White PF. Comparison of propofol with methohexital for outpatient anaesthesia. *Anesth Analg* 1986; 65: 1189.
124 Millan JM, Jewkes CF. Recovery and morbidity after daycase anaesthesia. A comparison of propofol with thiopentone—enflurane with and without alfentanil. *Anesthesiology* 1988; 43: 738.
125 Doze VA, Shafer A, White PF. Propofol versus thiopental-isoflurane for general anaesthesia. *Anesthesiology* 1988; 69: 63–71.
126 Nightingale JJ, Lewis IM. Recovery from day-case anaesthesia: comparison of total IV anaesthesia using propofol with an inhalational technique. *Br J Anaesth* 1992; 68: 356–9.
127 Nightingale JJ, Lewis IM. Recovery from anaesthesia: A comparison of total intravenous

anaesthesia with an inhalation technique. *Br J Anaesth* 1990; 65: 287–8.
128 Valanne J. Recovery and discharge of patients after long propofol infusion vs. isoflurane anaesthesia for ambulatory surgery. *Acta Anaesth Scand* 1992; 36: 530–3.
129 Zuurmond WWA, van Leeuwen L, Helmers JH. Recovery from propofol infusion as the main agent for outpatient arthroscopy. A comparison with isoflurane. *Anaesthesia* 1987; 42: 356–9.
130 Milligan KR, O'Toole DP, Have JP *et al.* Recovery from outpatient anaesthesia. A comparison of incremental propofol and propofol-isoflurane. *Br J Anaesth* 1987; 59: 1111–14.
131 Marshall CA, Jones RM, Bajorek PA, Cashman JN. Recovery characteristics using isoflurane or propofol for maintenance of anaesthesia; a double blind controlled trial. *Anaesthesia* 1992; 47: 461–6.
132 Borgeat A, Wilder-Smith ON. Subhypnotic doses of propofol possess direct anti-emetic properties. *Anesth Analg* 1992; 74: 539–41.
133 Stark RD, Binks SM, Dutka VN *et al.* A review of the safety and tolerance of propofol (Diprivan). *Postgrad Med J* 1985; 61 (suppl 3): 152–6.
134 Watcha MF, White PF. Postoperative nausea and vomiting. *Anesthesiology* 1992; 77: 162–84.
135 Jones DF. Recovery from anaesthesia. A comparison of a further four techniques including use of the new induction agent Diprivan. *Br J Anaesth* 1982; 54: 629–33.
136 Cullen PM, Turtle M, Prys-Roberts C, Way WL, Dye J. Effect of propofol anaesthesia on baroreflex activity in humans. *Anesth Analg* 1987; 66: 1115–20.
137 Swenzen GO, Chakrabartri MK, Sapsed-Byrne S, Whitwam JG. Selective depression by alfentanil of group III and IV somatosympathetic reflexes in the dog. *Br J Anaesth* 1988; 61: 441–5.
138 Guise PA. Asystole following propofol and fentanyl in an anxious patient. *Anaesth Intens Care* 1991; 19: 116–18.
139 Janicki PK, James MF, Erskine WA. Propofol inhibits enzymatic degradation of alfentanil and sufentanil by isolated liver microsomes *in vitro*. *Br J Anaesth* 1992; 68: 311–12.
140 Short TG, Chiu PG. Propofol and midazolam act synergistically in combination. *Br J Anaesth* 1991; 67: 539–45.
141 Vinik HR. Propofol alfentanil hypnotic interaction. *Anesth Analg* 1990; 71: 65–9.
142 Kortilla K, Linnoila M, Ertama P, Hakkinen S. Recovery and simulated driving after intravenous anaesthesia with thiopental, methohexital, propanidid or alphadione. *Anesthesiology* 1975; 43: 291–9.
143 Biemer DD. Pharmacokinetics of methohexitone following intravenous infusion in humans. *Br J Anaesth* 1976; 48: 643–8.
144 Whitwam JG, Manners JM. Clinical comparison of thiopentone and methohexitone. *Br Med J* 1962; i: 1663–5.
145 Goroszeniuk T, Whitwam JG, Morgan M. Use of methohexitone, fentanyl and nitrous oxide for short surgical procedures. *Anaesthesia* 1977; 32: 209–11.
146 Cooper GM. Recovery from anaesthesia. *Clin Anaesth* 1984; 2: 145–62.
147 White PF. Continuous infusions of thiopentone, methohexital or etomidate adjuvants to nitrous oxide for outpatient anaesthesia. *Anesth Analg* 1984; 63: 282.
148 Steegers PA, Foster PA. Propofol in total intravenous anaesthesia without nitrous oxide. *Anaesthesia* 1988; 46 (suppl): 94–7.
149 Wagner RL, White PF. Etomidate inhibits adrenocortical function in surgical patients. *Anesthesiology* 1984; 61: 647–51.
150 Wagner RL, White PF, Kan PB. Inhibition of adrenal steroidogenesis by the anesthetic etomidate. *New Engl J Med* 1984; 310: 1415–21.
151 Ledingham I, Watt I. Influence of sedation on mortality of critically ill trauma patients. *Lancet* 1983; i: 1270.
152 De Grood PM, Haibas JB, Van Egmond J, Crul JF. Anaesthesia for laparoscopy. A comparison of

five techniques including propofol, etomidate, thiopentone and isoflurane. *Anaesthesia* 1987; 42: 815–23.
153 Kestin IJ, Doije P. Anaesthesia for evacuation of retained products of conception. *Br J Anaesth* 1987; 59: 364–9.
154 Clyburn P, Kay N, McKenzie PJ. Effects of diazepam and midazolam on recovery from anaesthesia in outpatients. *Br J Anaesth* 1986; 58: 875–7.
155 White PF, Ham J, Way WL, Trevor AJ. Pharmacology of ketamine in isomers in surgical patients. *Anesthesiology* 1980; 52: 231–9.
156 White PF. Use of continuous infusion versus intermittent bolus administration of fentanyl or ketamine during outpatient anaesthesia. *Anesthesiology* 1983; 59: 294–300.
157 Toft P, Raner U. Comparison of midazolam and diazepam to supplement total intravenous anaesthesia with ketamine for endoscopy. *Can J Anaesth* 1987; 34: 446–70.
158 Hannallah RJ, Patel RI. Low dose intramuscular ketamine for anaesthesia preinduction in young children undergoing brief outpatient procedures. *Anesthesiology* 1989; 70: 598–600.
159 Veima R, Ramasubiamanian R, Sachar RM. Anaesthesia for termination of pregnancy midazolam compared with methohexital. *Anesth Analg* 1985; 64: 792–4.
160 McAteer EJ, Dixon J, Whitwam JG. Intramuscular midazolam. A comparison of midazolam with papaveretum and hyoscine for intramuscular premedication. *Anaesthesia* 1984; 39: 1177–82.
161 Dundee WJ, Halliday NJ, Laughram PG, Maiper KW. The influence of age on the onset of anaesthesia with midazolam. *Anaesthesia* 1985; 40: 441–3.
162 Phillip BK, Simpson TM, Hauch MA, Mallampati SR. Flumazenil reversed sedation after midazolam induced general anaesthesia in ambulatory surgery patients. *Anesth Analg* 1990; 71: 371–6.
163 Norton AC, Dundas CR. Induction agents for day-case anaesthesia. A double blind comparison of propofol and midazolam antagonised by flumazenil. *Anaesthesia* 1990; 45: 198–203.
164 Tverskoy M, Fleyshman G, Bradley EL, Kissin I. Midazolam–thiopental anaesthetic interaction in patients. *Anesth Analg* 1988; 67: 342–5.
165 Tverskoy M, Ben-Shlomo I, Ezry J, Finger J, Fleyshman G. Midazolam acts synergistically with methohexitone for induction of anaesthesia. *Br J Anaesth* 1989; 63; 109–12.
166 Vinik HR. Co-induction: a practical application of anaesthetic drug interaction. *Curr Op Anaesth* 1993; 6 (suppl 1): S9–S13.
167 Vinik HR, Bradley EL, Kissin I. Midazolam–alfentanil synergism for anaesthetic induction in patients. *Anesth Analg* 1989; 69: 213–17.
168 Yasuda N, Targ AG, Eger EI. Solubility of I-653 sevoflurane, isoflurane and halothane in human tissue. *Anesth Analg* 1989; 69: 370–3.
169 Wrigley SR, Jones RM. Inhalational agents—an update. *Eur J Anaesth* 1992; 9: 185–201.
170 Ghouri AF, Bodmen M, White PF. Recovery profile after desflurane nitrous oxide versus isoflurane nitrous oxide in outpatients. *Anesthesiology* 1992; 74: 419–24.
171 Van Hemlrijk J, Smith I, White PF. Use of desflurane for outpatient anesthesia; a comparison with propofol and nitrous oxide. *Anesthesiology* 1991; 46: 615–22.
172 Wrigley SR, Fairfield JE, Jones RM, Black AE. Induction and recovery characteristics of desflurane in day case patients: A comparison with propofol. *Anaesthesia* 1991; 46: 615–22.
173 Graham SR, Aitkenhead AR. A comparison between propofol and desflurane anaesthesia for minor gynaecological laparoscopic surgery. *Anaesthesia* 1993; 48: 471–5.
174 Pagel PS, Kampine JP, Schmelling WT, Warltier DC. Comparison of systemic and coronary haemodynamic actions of desflurane, isoflurane halothane and enflurane in the chronically instrumented dog. *Anesthesiology* 1991; 74: 539–51.
175 Jones RM, Cashman JN, Mant TGK. Clinical impressions and cardiorespiratory effects of a new fluorinated inhalational anaesthetic desflurane in volunteers. *Br J Anaesth* 1990; 64: 11–15.

176 Hartman SC, Pagel PS, Kampine JP, Schnelling WT, Warltier DC. Influence of desflurane on regional distribution of coronary blood flow in a chronically instrumented canine model of multivessel coronary artery obstruction. *Anesth Analg* 1991; 72: 279–99.
177 Saito S, Goto F, Takahashi T, Fujita T, Mogi K. Comparative clinical study of induction and emergence time in sevoflurane and enflurane anaesthesia. *Acta Anaesth Scand* 1989; 33: 389–90.
178 Holaday DA, Smith FR. Clinical characteristics and biotransformation of sevoflurane in healthy human volunteers. *Anesthesiology* 1981; 54: 100–6.
179 Calvey TN. Chirality in anaesthesia (Editorial). *Anaesthesia* 1992; 47: 93–4.
180 Carter JA, Dye AM, Cooper GM. Recovery from daycase anaesthesia—the effect of different inhalational anaesthetic agents. *Anesthesia* 1985; 40: 545.
181 Cattenole RW, Verghese C, Blain IJ *et al.* Isoflurane and halothane for outpatient dental anaesthesia in children. *Br J Anaesth* 1986; 58: 385.
182 Kingston HGG. Halothane and isoflurane anaesthesia in paediatric out-patients. *Anesth Analg* 1986; 65: 181.
183 National Halothane Study. Summary of the National Halothane Study. Possible association between halothane anaesthesia and postoperative hepatic necrosis. *JAMA* 1966; 197: 775–88.
184 Committee on Safety of Medicines. *Current Problems*, No. 18. London: HMSO, 1986.
185 Muir JJ, Warner MA, Buck CF *et al.* The role of nitrous oxide in producing postoperative nausea and vomiting. *Anesthesiology* 1986; 65: A461.
186 Alexander GD, Skupski JN, Brown EM. The role of nitrous oxide in post operative nausea and vomiting. *Anesth Analg* 1984; 63: 175.
187 Hug CC Jr. Pharmacokinetics and dynamics of narcotic analgesics. In: Prys-Roberts C, Hug CC Jr, eds. *Pharmacokinetics of Anaesthesia*. Oxford: Blackwell Scientific Publications, 1984: 187–234.
188 Horrigan RW, Moyess IR, Johnson BH, Eger EI, Mangolis A, Goldsmith S. Etomidate vs. thiopental with and without fentanyl. A comparative study in man. *Anesthesiology* 1980; 52: 362–4.
189 Rising S, Dodgson MS, Steen PA. Isoflurane vs. fentanyl for outpatient laparoscopy. *Acta Anaesth Scand* 1985; 29: 251–7.
190 White PF, Coe V, Shafer A, Snug ML. Comparison of fentanyl and alfentanil for outpatient anaesthesia. *Anesthesiology* 1986; 64: 99–109.
191 Haley S, Edelint G, Leiback G. Comparison of alfentanil, fentanyl, and enflurane as supplements to general anaesthesia for outpatient gynaecologic surgery. *Can J Anaesth* 1988; 35: 570–5.
192 Raeden JC, Hole A. Outpatient laparoscopy in general anaesthesia with alfentanil, and atracurium, a comparison with fentanyl and pancuronium. *Acta Anaesth Scand* 1986; 30: 30–4.
193 Hull CJ, Jakobson LA. Clinical trial of alfentanil as an adjuvant for short anaesthetic procedures. *Br J Anaesth* 1983; 55: 1735–85.
194 Bagshaw ONT, Singh P, Aitkenhead AR. Alfentanil in day case anaesthesia. *Anaesthesia* 1993; 48: 476–81.
195 Dollery CTD. Alfentanil infusion. In: Dollery CTD, ed. *Therapeutic Drugs*. Edinburgh: Churchill Livingstone, 1991: A43–6.
196 Phitayakom P, Melnick BM, Vicinie AF. Comparison of continuous sufentanil and fentanyl infusions for outpatient anaesthesia. *Can J Anaesth* 1987; 34: 242–5.
197 White PF, Snug ML, Doze VA. Use of sufentanil in outpatient anaesthesia—determining an optimal pre-induction dose. *Anesthesiology* 1985; 63: A202.
198 Garfield JM, Garfield FB, Phillip BK, Earls F, Roaf E. A comparison of clinical and psychological effects of fentanyl and nalbuphine in ambulatory gynaecologic patients. *Anesth Analg* 1987; 66: 1301–12.

199 Pandit SK, Kothary SP, Pandit NA, Mathai MK. Comparison of fentanyl and butorphanol for outpatient anaesthesia. *Can J Anaesth* 1987; 34: 130–3.
200 Buckley MM, Brogden RN. Profile of ketorolac. *Drugs* 1990; 39: 86–109.
201 Committee on Safety of Medicines (UK). Current Problems in Pharmacovigilance. *Ketorolac: new restrictions on dose and duration of treatment.* 19 June 1993: 5–6.
202 Wong MY, Carpenter RL, Kobaez JD *et al.* A randomised double blind evaluation of ketorolac tromethamine for postoperative analgesia in ambulatory surgery patients. *Anesthesiology* 1993; 78: 6–14.
203 Zahl K, Apfelbaum JL. Muscle pain occurs after outpatient laparoscopy despite the substitution of vecuronium for succinylcholine. *Anesthesiology* 1989; 70: 408.
204 Urbach GM, Edelist G. Anaesthetic complications in surgical outpatients. *Can J Anaesth* 1977; 24: 401.
205 Pearce AC, Williams JP, Jones RM. Atracurium for short surgical procedures in day patients. *Br J Anaesth* 1984; 56: 973.
206 King MJ, Milazkiewicz R, Carli F, Deacock AR. Influence of neostigmine on postoperative vomiting. *Br J Anaesth* 1988; 62: 4031.
207 Wrigley SR, Jones RM, Harrop-Griffiths AW, Platt MU. Mivacurium chloride: a study to evaluate its use during propofol nitrous oxide anaesthesia. *Anesthesiology* 1992; 47: 646–53.
208 Hunter JM. Histamine release and neuromuscular blocking drugs. *Anaesthesia* 1993; 48: 561–3.
209 Gold B, Kitz D, Lecky JM, Nehans JM. Unanticipated admission to the hospital following ambulatory surgery. *JAMA* 1989; 262: 3008–10.
210 Kortilla K, Kauste A, Aurinen J. Comparison of domperidone, droperidol, and metaclopramide in the prevention and treatment of nausea and vomiting after balanced general anaesthesia. *Anesth Analg* 1979; 58: 396–400.
211 Cohen SE, Woods WA, Wynen J. Antiemetic efficacy of droperidol and metoclopramide. *Anesthesiology* 1984; 60: 67–9.
212 Valune J, Kortilla K. Effect of small dose droperidol on nausea, vomiting and recovery after outpatient enflurane anaesthesia. *Acta Anaesth Scand* 1985; 29: 359–62.
213 Melnick B, Sawyer R, Karambelkan D *et al.* Delayed side-effects of droperidol after ambulatory general anaesthesia. *Anesth Analg* 1989; 69: 748–51.
214 McKenzie R, Kovac A, O'Connor T *et al.* Comparison of ondansetron vs. placebo to prevent postoperative nausea and vomiting in women undergoing ambulatory gynaecologic surgery. *Anesthesiology* 1993; 78: 21–8.
215 Scuderi P, Wechler B, Yung-fong Sung *et al.* Treatment of postoperative nausea and vomiting after outpatient surgery with the 5-HT_3 ondansetron. *Anesthesiology* 1993; 78: 15–20.
216 Manchikanti L, Colliver JA, Marrero TC, Roush JR. Ranitidine and metoclopramide for prophylaxis of aspiration pneumonia in elective surgery. *Anesth Analg* 1984; 63: 903–10.
217 Haskins DA, Jahr JS, Texidor M, Ramadhyani U. Single dose oral omeprazole for reduction of gastric residual acidity in adults for outpatient surgery. *Acta Anaesth Scand* 1992; 36: 513–15.

Chapter 3
Pharmacological Principles in Paediatric Patients

N. S. Morton and D. Lord

Pharmacokinetics in neonates, infants and children

The absorption, distribution, metabolism and excretion of drugs is significantly different in infants because of variations in metabolic capacity (due to the immaturity of organs and of enzyme systems), and differences in relative body composition.

Absorption

In the neonate there is a relative achlorhydria, gut peristalsis is irregular and the gastric emptying time may be prolonged. The biliary system is immature. There is a very high glucuronidase activity in the neonatal intestine for example, which causes morphine glucuronide to be broken down to morphine. This contributes to problems in using morphine in the newborn.

There is less surface area available for absorption from the rectum than from the upper gastrointestinal tract. However, blood draining via the middle and inferior rectal veins bypasses the liver and a first pass metabolic pathway. Absence of this first pass metabolism means that peak plasma concentrations of drugs administered by the rectal route are rapidly attained. Drugs such as methohexitone, diazepam, midazolam, diclofenac and paracetamol can be given much more effectively by this route in children than in older subjects.

Absorption via the oral, nasal and pulmonary mucosae may all be usefully employed in children [1]. First pass metabolism is avoided and absorption from these highly vascular tissues occurs rapidly. Nasally administered drugs such as midazolam may enter the brain via olfactory neurons. The oral, transmucosal and sublingual routes are feasible for administration of midazolam and fentanyl in children. The pulmonary mucosal route during endotracheal administration is useful for the administration of emergency drugs during paediatric resuscitation, e.g. atropine, adrenaline, lignocaine.

The intraosseous route, where absorption occurs via the vascular bone marrow cavity, has evolved as an efficient method of drug and fluid administration during administration. Percutaneous absorption is enhanced in small infants because of their relatively higher skin water content and thinner stratum corneum. A eutectic mixture of local anaesthetic (EMLA) cream applied to the neonatal skin undergoes significant systemic absorption.

Distribution

The total body water content is proportionately greater in neonates than in older children: 85% of body weight in the premature neonate; 78% in the term neonate; 60% at age 1 year; and approximately 50% from adolescence onwards. Extracellular water contents at these ages are 50, 45, 27 and 20% of body weight respectively.

The neonate has relatively little fat, 12% of body weight compared to the 1-year-old infant (30%) and the older female (20–30%). From adolescence onwards, the male has 10–15% less fat in proportion to the female.

Drugs with limited tissue uptake are distributed throughout the extracellular water. Thus, in neonates and infants, a larger relative dose of such drugs is required to achieve a given concentration at the target tissue.

Plasma proteins

Free, unbound drug is the pharmacologically active component of the drug and when this is increased more active compound reaches the target organs. However, more also reaches other organs and may produce adverse effects. More drug is distributed to extravascular tissues and so the volume of distribution is increased and more drug is immediately available to be metabolized and excreted by the liver and kidneys.

Albumin and α_1-acid glycoprotein are the main drug binding proteins. Their quantity and binding capacity are low in the neonate. For drugs with a high affinity for proteins the low protein binding in the neonate will allow a much higher proportion of the drug to be unbound and hence free. For example, if a drug is normally 98% bound and 2% unbound in older children, a reduction in binding to 96% results in a doubling of the free fraction to 4%. In contrast, for a drug which is normally 22% bound and 78% unbound, a reduction in binding to 20% allows an insignificant increase in free drug.

Metabolism

The main sites of metabolism of drugs are the hepatic microsomal enzyme system, plasma esterases, kidneys and the lungs.

Hepatic metabolism either causes degradation of drugs (by oxidation, reduction or hydrolysis) or results in the synthesis of water-soluble compounds, which are more easily excreted. In neonates, the concentration and activity of enzyme systems is less than in adults, because of the immaturity of the liver at this stage of development. The synthetic reactions, such as conjugation, are more affected by this immaturity. Glucuronide conjugation, for example, does not reach adult values until the age of 3 months. The neonate's plasma and blood enzyme activity is also low and only reaches adult levels at 1 year of age. The rise in plasma enzyme activity tracks the increase in plasma protein levels. The overall effect of these differences is that in the neonate, the elimination half-life of drugs is significantly prolonged.

In contrast, in the infant, the capacity to metabolize drugs, particularly by degradation reactions, is markedly increased. From 3 months of age onwards the relative metabolic rate increases to a maximum between 2 and 3 years of age and then gradually decreases to adult levels in early adolescence. In part this may be due to the relatively large size of the liver in the infant, 4% of body weight compared with 2% in the adult and relative drugs clearance is two- to sixfold greater in infants and young children. Hence local anaesthetics, sedatives and muscle relaxants, for example, all have reduced half-lives in this age group.

Excretion

The main route of drug excretion is via the kidneys. The number of nephrons is the same in neonates as in adults but are neither anatomically or functionally mature until the age of 5–6 months. Therefore, the renal excretion of many drugs and their metabolites is reduced in small infants. Thus, although the initial loading dose needed to produce the same blood or tissue levels is relatively larger to allow for the larger volume of distribution, the interval between incremental doses needs to be longer to prevent accumulation. The relative capacity of the kidneys to excrete drugs increases steadily to a maximum level by 2–3 years old and thereafter steadily declines.

Pharmacology of individual anaesthetic agents in children

Volatile agents

At the time of writing the three principal agents generally available for use in children are halothane, isoflurane and enflurane. The uptake and distribution of volatile anaesthetic agents is relatively faster in children. This is because there is a rapid rise in alveolar concentration due to a higher ratio between alveolar ventilation and functional residual capacity and a higher cardiac index. In addition, a relatively greater proportion of cardiac output is distributed to the brain.

No available drug fulfils all the criteria for an ideal inhalational agent [2]. Halothane remains the most commonly used agent for the inhalational induction of anaesthesia in children. Of the currently available volatile agents it produces the most rapid and smooth induction of anaesthesia [3] due to less irritation of the airway and production of secretions [4–9]. Enflurane and isoflurane with their lower blood:gas solubility coefficients should make both induction and recovery faster, but they are ethers and their unacceptable incidence of breath holding and laryngospasm prolong induction and can be associated with significant desaturation [4, 6, 10]. The incidence of these airway problems has been reported to be reduced by the coadministration of carbon dioxide [11], commencing with a higher concentration of isoflurane [10].

Of all the volatile agents enflurane causes the greatest depression of the respiratory responses to hypoxia and hypercarbia [12]. Neuromuscular blockade is potentiated by enflurane and isoflurane to a greater extent than halothane. All three agents cause cardiovascular depression. Halothane has a relatively greater effect on the myocardium compared to the peripheral vascular system whereas the effect of isoflurane is mainly by peripheral vasodilatation and the cardiac output is maintained in part by an increase in heart rate. Enflurane occupies a mid-position.

All three agents undergo biotransformation. Enflurane releases fluoride which is potentially nephrotoxic, but this occurs to a much lesser extent with isoflurane.

Halothane undergoes metabolism in children but the incidence of halothane-associated hepatitis in children is very low [13] in spite of a great deal of repeated exposure world-wide. It seems likely that in the absence of a safer and more acceptable agent, with fewer side effects, halothane will remain the agent of choice for the inhalational induction of anaesthesia in children: otherwise perhaps sevoflurane will be preferred, being pleasanter than desflurane with a rapid recovery.

Halothane sensitizes the myocardium to the effects of adrenaline to a relatively greater extent than enflurane and isoflurane. However, it is suggested that in the absence of congenital heart disease adrenaline in a dose of 10 $\mu g\ kg^{-1}$ may be used to produce vasoconstriction in the presence of halothane [14].

In a comparison of the recovery characteristics of halothane, isoflurane and enflurane, enflurane allowed significantly faster recovery [3] but the time to discharge of the patient was similar for all three agents.

The use of the new agent sevoflurane (Chapter 2) for paediatric ambulatory surgery has been reported in comparison with halothane [15] and desflurane is also undergoing trials in infants and children [16].

Intravenous agents

Thiopentone is used extensively in paediatric anaesthetic practice [17, 18]. It has been compared with propofol for induction of anaesthesia in children aged between 2 and 11 years using nitrous oxide, halothane and isoflurane for maintenance with regional nerve block for analgesia [19]. In children under 5 only time to open the eyes was shorter in the propofol group; whereas in the 5–11 year age group the differences between the drugs were more obvious, as in adults, with earlier discharge in the propofol group. Laryngeal masks are routinely used in day-case anaesthesia in children [19–21].

Methohexitone is metabolized faster than thiopentone and, for example, is still used routinely in outpatient dental anaesthesia by many anaesthetists. A dose of 1–2 $mg\ kg^{-1}$ is rapidly distributed but its total clearance is much slower than propofol [22]. A drawback to its use has been a high incidence of pain on injection which can be abolished by prior mixing with lignocaine. The incidence of spontaneous movements is no higher than with propofol.

Induction of anaesthesia with rectally administered methohexitone is finding increasing favour in North America and Europe [23–36]. Methohexitone 20–30 mg kg^{-1} in a 10% solution induces sleep in 6·7–7·8 min in 87–93% of patients depending on the dosage, with a slightly faster onset time at the higher dose [34]. The cardiovascular system is stable [32, 34] and oxygen saturation is maintained [36, 37].

Intramuscular injection of methohexitone 6 mg kg^{-1} as a 5% solution induces heavy sedation within 4 min and lasts 40–50 min [38] but the injection is painful and probably not indicated where ready venous access is available.

Propofol

Propofol was first used in children in 1985 [39]. Its use, pharmacokinetics and pharmacodynamics in children have been recently reviewed [22, 40].

The pharmacokinetics of propofol fit a three compartment model [22] and since the central compartment volume is larger in children than adults, with a faster clearance rate, larger doses of propofol are required. In children as in adults it is rapidly metabolized to the inactive glucuronide and the corresponding quinol glucuronide and is excreted in the urine [41–43].

Higher doses of propofol are required, compared with adults, for the induction of anaesthesia in children in the range 2·5–3·5 mg kg^{-1} increasing to 4 mg kg^{-1} in unpremedicated patients [44] and the infusion rate for continuous anaesthesia is also greater than in adults [44–46] with a 50% greater initial bolus dose and a 25% higher infusion rate.

A major disadvantage of propofol is pain on injection which is greater when injected in the small veins on the dorsum of the hand [47]. This can be abolished by adding lignocaine 1 mg per 3 mg propofol [48] with a minimum concentration of lignocaine of 0·2 mg kg^{-1} body weight added immediately prior to injection [49].

Propofol produces a dose-related respiratory depression similar to thiopentone. It facilitates the introduction of an oropharyngeal airway or a laryngeal mask soon after injection. This is a major advantage when using propofol as the sole agent for non-painful diagnostic procedures [50]. Propofol causes an initial transient increase in pulse rate and a 5–25% decrease in blood pressure, which is similar to thiopentone.

Spontaneous movements occur in both adults and children and concern has been expressed about the possible association of propofol with seizure activity. Borgeat *et al.* [51] correlated electroencephalographic (EEG) activity with videotape evidence of spontaneous movements; dystonic movements were associated with δ-waves suggesting a subcortical origin. When propofol was used as the sole agent in over 100 anaesthetics in children for magnetic resonance imaging (age range from 6 weeks to 4 years) there was no increase in seizure activity even in children with severe epilepsy.

As in adults, propofol allows more rapid recovery in older children when compared with thiopentone [52–54]. However, in children under 5 years the differences are not so obvious [19]. The incidence of postoperative nausea and vomiting is less than for propofol–halothane than thiopentone–halothane or halothane alone [53–55].

Neuromuscular blocking agents (Table 3.1)

Suxamethonium

The dose of suxamethonium correlates with extracellular fluid volume which is more accurately related to surface area rather than weight [56]. Infants are more resistant to depolarizing muscle relaxants than older children. The effective dose for 95% twitch depression (ED_{95}) is 0·729 mg kg^{-1} in infants, 0·423 mg kg^{-1} in children and 0·290 mg kg^{-1} in adults [57]. Infants have a lower level of pseudocholinesterase activity but the duration of action of suxamethonium is not significantly prolonged. A dose of 1·5–2 mg kg^{-1} is often required for intubation in infants whereas 1 mg kg^{-1} produces satisfactory conditions in children and adults. Phase 2 block can be demonstrated with administered doses in excess of 4 mg kg^{-1} [58].

Suxamethonium 3–4 mg kg^{-1} i.m. produces complete neuromuscular blockade in 3–4 min with a duration of action of 20 min [59].

Some paediatric centres believe that suxamethonium should be preceded by atropine 0·02 mg kg^{-1} but other centres do not routinely follow this practice. The use of suxamethonium in unpremedicated children has been associated with a higher incidence of bad dreams which can be prevented by pretreatment with non-depolarizing blocking agents [60]. However, this would be regarded by some paediatric anaesthesiologists as unsafe practice. Muscle pains do occur in children after suxamethonium and there are few indications for its use in modern paediatric day-case anaesthesia.

Atracurium

When administered on a dose per weight basis, young children appear to require a larger dose than adolescents and adults. When dosage is on the basis of surface area, children and adults appear to be similar. However, children are relatively more sensitive to the effects of the drug but with a shortened duration of effect. The relative volume of distribution and clearance decrease in older children and adults [61]. The same effective intubating dose of 0·3–0·5 mg kg^{-1} can be given to all patients and this single dose becomes reversible after 15–30 min.

Vecuronium

This drug relies on redistribution and liver metabolism for termination of effect and excretion. Unlike atracurium there is a greater variation of dose requirement and effect in relation to age. Infants are far more sensitive with a smaller dose requirement and a longer duration of effect [62, 63]. Older children require larger doses than adults which is related to a proportionally larger distribution volume. Plasma clearance is similar in all ages. A dose range to facilitate intubation is 0·08–0·12 mg kg^{-1} depending on age.

Table 3.1 Mean ED_{95} in mg kg^{-1} for muscle relaxants in different age groups

Drug	Infant	Child	Adult
Suxamethonium	0·729	0·423	0·290
Mivacurium	—	0·09–0·11	0·07–0·08
Atracurium	0·156	0·26	0·195
Vecuronium	0·045	0·06	0·042

Mivacurium

Mivacurium is a new short-acting non-depolarizing relaxant, related to atracurium and is metabolized mainly by plasma pseudocholinesterase. In equipotent doses, its speed of onset is similar to atracurium and vecuronium. Its duration of action is twice that of suxamethonium but approximately one-half to one-third of that of atracurium and vecuronium [64]. It is readily antagonized by anticholinesterase drugs but its short duration of action [65] should make this unnecessary in the majority of cases. At a dose of 0·1–0·2 mg kg^{-1} there is cardiovascular stability with minimal histamine released. The mean infusion dosage requirement for extended blockade in children has been assessed as 0·315 mg m^{-2} min^{-1} when maintaining anaesthesia with halothane and 0·375 mg m^{-2} min^{-1} for maintenance with added narcotic [66]. In children heterozygous for the pseudocholinesterase gene, a 50% prolongation of activity has been demonstrated. Mivacurium should be avoided in patients with a known pseudocholinesterase deficiency.

Benzodiazepines

The two current benzodiazepines used in paediatric day care are diazepam and midazolam. Midazolam is more rapid in both onset and elimination. It can be administered intravenously, intramuscularly, orally, rectally or intranasally. When administered nasally a peak plasma concentration of 57% of that which occurs with the same dose administered intravenously is achieved after approximately 10 min [67]. Premedication with midazolam, e.g. by the nasal route, can sometimes be advantageous in children, not only by allaying anxiety, but also by producing amnesia for induction purposes.

Local anaesthetic drugs

Lignocaine and bupivacaine are the most common local anaesthetic agents used in paediatric practice. Their clearance is similar to adults [68–70]. Maximum recommended doses for lignocaine alone are 4 mg kg^{-1} and 7 mg kg^{-1} with adrenaline. The recommended total dose of bupivacaine is 2 mg kg^{-1} (3 mg kg^{-1} in the anaes-

Table 3.2 Maximum recommended dosage of commonly used local anaesthetics (mg kg^{-1})

Bupivacaine	2·0 (3·0 in the anaesthetized child)
Lignocaine	7·0
Prilocaine	5·0
Amethocaine	1·5

thetized child). The maximum dose of adrenaline used for vasoconstriction is 0·01 mg kg^{-1}. The maximum recommended doses of several drugs are shown in Table 3.2. Remember, however, that toxicity can occur from rapid injection of a smaller dose into high vascular tissues (see Chapter 21).

Methaemoglobinaemia

Methaemoglobinaemia is a potential problem when using prilocaine. This amide local anaesthetic is metabolized in the liver to *o*-toluidine, an oxidizing agent which induces the formation of methaemoglobin. Foetal haemoglobin is particularly sensitive to oxidation to methaemoglobin. Methaemoglobin in the blood causes an increased affinity of normal haemoglobin for oxygen and a reduced oxygen carrying capacity. Thus the P_{50} and oxygen delivery to the tissues are reduced. Methaemoglobinaemia may persist for longer in the neonate because the enzyme methaemoglobin reductase is less active.

In the context of paediatric day-case anaesthesia, methaemoglobinaemia could arise due to prilocaine given for intravenous regional analgesia (IVRA; Bier's block). Prilocaine is a component of EMLA which is commonly used in the UK and Europe to facilitate painless venepuncture. (If a large amount of EMLA is applied for a prolonged period to eczematous skin or to the skin of a neonate, there is a risk of methaemoglobinaemia.) Silver nitrite dressings used in burns can produce methaemoglobinaemia.

Clinical detection of methaemoglobinaemia may be difficult. A level of 2 g dl^{-1} will produce cyanosis (cf. 5 g dl^{-1} deoxyhaemoglobin). Treatment of methaemoglobinaemia includes stopping the administration of prilocaine, giving 100% oxygen and the administration of intravenous methylene blue (2 mg kg^{-1}) for severe cases.

Anaphylactic reactions

These are reviewed in Chapter 4.

References

1 Malvinorsky JM, Lejus C, Servin F *et al.* Plasma concentrations of midazolam after i.v., nasal, or rectal administration in children. *Br J Anaesth* 1993; 70: 617–20.
2 Heijke S, Smith G. Quest for the ideal inhalation anaesthetic agent. *Br J Anaesth* 1990; 64: 3–6.

3 Simmons M, Miller CD, Cummings GC, Todd JG. Outpatient paediatric dental anaesthesia. A comparison of halothane, enflurane and isoflurane. *Anaesthesia* 1989; 44: 735–8.

4 Sampaio MM, Crean PM, Keilty SR, Black GW. Changes in oxygen saturation during inhalation induction of anaesthesia in children. *Br J Anaesth* 1989; 62: 199–201.

5 Pandit UA, Steude GM, Leach AB. Induction and recovery characteristics of isoflurane and halothane anaesthesia for short outpatient operations in children. *Anaesthesia* 1985; 40: 1226–30.

6 Phillips AJ, Brimacombe JR, Simpson DL. Anaesthetic induction with isoflurane or halothane. Oxygen saturation during induction with isoflurane or halothane in unpremedicated children. *Anaesthesia* 1988; 43: 927–9.

7 Kingston HG. Halothane and isoflurane anesthesia in pediatric outpatients. *Anesth Analg* 1986; 65: 181–4.

8 Fisher DM, Robinson S, Brett CM, Perin G, Gregory GA. Comparison of enflurane, halothane, and isoflurane for diagnostic and therapeutic procedures in children with malignancies. *Anesthesiology* 1985; 63: 647–50.

9 McAteer PM, Carter JA, Cooper GM, Prys-Roberts C. Comparison of isoflurane and halothane in outpatient paediatric dental anaesthesia. *Br J Anaesth* 1986; 58: 390–3.

10 Warde D, Nagi H, Raftery S. Respiratory complications and hypoxic episodes during inhalation induction with isoflurane in children. *Br J Anaesth* 1991; 66: 327–30.

11 Coleman SA, McCrory JW, Vallis CF, Boys RJ. Inhalation induction of anaesthesia with isoflurane: effect of added carbon dioxide. *Br J Anaesth* 1991; 67: 257–61.

12 Wren WS, Allen P, Synnott A, O'Keeffe D, O'Griofa P. Effects of halothane, isoflurane and enflurane on ventilation in children. *Br J Anaesth* 1987; 59: 399–409.

13 Wark H, O'Halloran M, Overton J. Prospective study of liver function in children following multiple halothane anaesthetics at short intervals. *Br J Anaesth* 1986; 58: 1224–8.

14 Karl HW, Swedlow DB, Lee KW *et al.* Epinephrine–halothane interactions in children. *Anesthesiology* 1983; 58: 142–5.

15 Naito Y, Tamai S, Shingu K, Fujimori R, Mori K. Comparison between sevoflurane and halothane for paediatric ambulatory anaesthesia. *Br J Anaesth* 1991; 67: 387–9.

16 Zwass MS, Fisher DM, Welborn LG *et al.* Induction and maintenance characteristics of anesthesia with desflurane and nitrous oxide in infants and children. *Anesthesiology* 1992; 76: 373–8.

17 Sorbo S, Hudson RJ, Loomis JC. The pharmacokinetics of thiopental in pediatric surgical patients. *Anesthesiology* 1984; 61: 666–70.

18 Jonmarker C, Westrin P, Larsson S, Werner O. Thiopental requirements for induction of anesthesia in children. *Anesthesiology* 1987; 67: 104–7.

19 Runcie CJ, Mackenzie D, Arthur DS, Morton NS. Comparison of recovery from anaesthesia induced in children with either propofol or thiopentone. *Br J Anaesth* 1993; 70: 192–5.

20 McGinn G, Haynes SR, Morton NS. An evaluation of the laryngeal mask airway during routine paediatric anaesthesia. *Paediatr Anaesth* 1993; 3: 23–8.

21 Wilson IG. Editorial: The laryngeal mask in paediatric practice. *Br J Anaesth* 1993; 70: 124–5.

22 Propofol. In: Dollery CT, ed. *Therapeutic Drugs*, 2nd edn. Edinburgh: Churchill Livingstone, 1993; in press.

23 Björkman S, Gabrielsson J, Quaynor H, Corbey M. Pharmacokinetics of i.v. and rectal methohexitone in children. *Br J Anaesth* 1987; 59: 1541–7.

24 Goresky GV, Steward DJ. Rectal methohexitone for induction of anaesthesia in children. *Canad Anaesth Soc J* 1979; 26: 213–15.

25 Quaynor H, Corbey M, Björkman S. Rectal induction of anaesthesia in children with methohexitone. Patient acceptability and clinical pharmacokinetics. *Br J Anaesth* 1985; 57: 573–7.

26 Liu LM, Gaudreault P, Friedman PA, Goudsouzian NG, Liu PL. Methohexital plasma concentrations in children following rectal administration. *Anesthesiology* 1985; 62: 567–70.
27 Laishley RS, O'Callaghan AC, Lerman J. Effects of dose and concentration of rectal methohexitone for induction of anaesthesia in children. *Canad Anaesth Soc J* 1986; 33: 427–32.
28 Larsson LE, Nilsson K, Andreasson S, Ekstrom-Jodal B. Effects of rectal thiopentone and methohexitone on carbon dioxide tension in infant anaesthesia with spontaneous ventilation. *Acta Anaesth Scand* 1987; 31: 227–30.
29 Griswold JD, Liu LMP. Rectal methohexital in children undergoing computerised cranial tomography and magnetic resonance imaging scans. *Anesthesiology* 1987; 67: A494.
30 Forbes RB, Vandewalker GE. Comparison of two and ten per cent rectal methohexitone for induction of anaesthesia in children. *Can J Anaesth* 1988; 35: 345–9.
31 Kestin IG, McIlvaine WB, Lockhart CH, Kestin KJ, Jones MA. Rectal methohexital for induction of anesthesia in children with and without rectal aspiration after sleep: a pharmacokinetic and pharmacodynamic study. *Anesth Analg* 1988; 67: 1102–4.
32 Forbes RB, Murray DJ, Dillman JB, Dull DL. Pharmacokinetics of two per cent rectal methohexitone in children. *Can J Anaesth* 1989; 36: 160–4.
33 Forbes RB, Murray DJ, Dull DL, Mahoney LT. Haemodynamic effects of rectal methohexitone for induction of anaesthesia in children. *Can J Anaesth* 1989; 36: 526–9.
34 Khalil SN, Florence FB, Van den Nieuwenhuyzen MC, Wu AH, Stanley TH. Rectal methohexital: concentration and length of the rectal catheters. *Anesth Analg* 1990; 70: 645–9.
35 Audenaert SM, Lock RL, Johnson GL, Pedigo NW Jr. Cardiovascular effects of rectal methohexital in children. *J Clin Anesth* 1992; 4: 116–19.
36 Daniels AL, Cote CJ, Polaner DM. Continuous oxygen saturation monitoring following rectal methohexitone induction in paediatric patients. *Can J Anaesth* 1992; 39: 27–30.
37 Liu LMP, Goudsouzian NG, Liu PL. Rectal methohexital premedication in children: a dose-comparison study. *Anesthesiology* 1980; 53: 343–5.
38 Varner PD, Ebert JP, McKay RD, Nail CS. Methohexital sedation of children undergoing CT scan. *Anesth Analg* 1985; 64: 643.
39 Purcell-Jones G, James IG. The characteristics of propofol (Diprivan) for induction of general anaesthesia for paediatric surgery. *Postgrad Med J* 1985; 61 (suppl 3): 115.
40 Morton NS, Johnston G, White M, Marsh BJ. Propofol in paediatric anaesthesia. *Paediatr Anaesth* 1992; 2: 89–97.
41 Saint-Maurice C, Cockshott ID, Douglas EJ, Richard MO, Harvey JL. Pharmokinetics of propofol in young children after a single dose. *Br J Anaesth* 1989; 63: 667–70.
42 Valtonen M, Iisalo E, Kanto J, Rosenberg P. Propofol as an induction agent in children: pain on injection and pharmacokinetics. *Acta Anaesth Scand* 1989; 33: 152–5.
43 Jones RD, Chan K, Andrew LJ. Pharmacokinetics of propofol in children. *Br J Anaesth* 1990; 65: 661–7.
44 Marsh B, White M, Morton N, Kenny GN. Pharmacokinetic model driven infusion of propofol in children. *Br J Anaesth* 1991; 67: 41–8.
45 Browne BL, Wolf AR, Prys-Roberts C. Dose requirements for propofol in children during total i.v. anaesthesia (Abstract). *Br J Anaesth* 1990; 64: 396.
46 Marsh BJ, Morton NS, White M, Kenny GN. A computer controlled infusion of propofol for induction and maintenance of anaesthesia in children. *Can J Anaesth* 1990; 37: S97.
47 Scott RPF, Saunders DA, Norman J. Propofol: clinical strategies for preventing the pain of injection. *Anaesthesia* 1988; 43: 492–4.
48 Morton NS. Abolition of injection pain due to propofol in children (Letter). *Anaesthesia* 1990; 45: 70.

49 Cameron E, Johnston G, Crofts S, Morton NS. The minimum effective dose of lignocaine to prevent injection pain due to propofol in children. *Anaesthesia* 1992; 47: 604–6.
50 Vangerven M, Van Hemelrijk J, Wouters P, Vandermeersch E, Van Aken H. Light anaesthesia with propofol for paediatric magnetic resonance imaging. *Anaesthesia* 1992; 47: 706–7.
51 Borgeat A, Dessibourg C, Popovic V, Meier D, Blanchard M, Schwander D. Propofol and spontaneous movements: an EEG study. *Anesthesiology* 1991; 74: 24–7.
52 Puttick N, Rosen M. Propofol induction and maintenance with nitrous oxide in paediatric outpatient dental anaesthesia. A comparison with thiopentone–nitrous oxide–halothane. *Anaesthesia* 1988; 43: 646–9.
53 Borgeat A, Popovic V, Meier D, Schwander D. Comparison of propofol and thiopental/halothane for short-duration ENT surgical procedures in children. *Anesth Analg* 1990; 71: 511–15.
54 Watcha MF, Simeon RM, White PF, Stevens JL. Effect of propofol on the incidence of postoperative vomiting after strabismus surgery in pediatric outpatients. *Anesthesiology* 1991; 75: 204–9.
55 Hannallah R, Britton J, Schafer P, Norden J. Effect of propofol anaesthesia on the incidence of vomiting after strabismus surgery in children. *Anesth Analg* 1992; 74: S131.
56 Cook DR. Muscle relaxants in infants and children. *Anesth Analg* 1981; 60: 335–43.
57 Meakin G, McKiernan EP, Morris P *et al.* Dose response curves for suxamethonium in neonates, infants and children. *Br J Anaesth* 1989; 62: 655–8.
58 DeCook TH, Goudsouzian NG. Tachyphylaxis and phase II block development during infusion of succinylcholine in children. *Anesth Analg* 1980; 59: 639–43.
59 Liu LMP, DeCook TH, Goudsouzian NG *et al.* Dose response to intramuscular succinylcholine in children. *Anesthesiology* 1981; 55: 599–602.
60 O'Sullivan EP, Childs D, Bush GH. Peri-operative dreaming in paediatric patients who receive suxamethonium. *Anaesthesia* 1988; 43: 104–6.
61 Fisher DM, Canfell PC. Spellman MJ, Miller RD. Pharmacokinetics and pharmacodynamics of atracurium in infants and children. *Anesthesiology* 1990; 73: 33–7.
62 Meretoja OA. Is vecuronium a long-acting neuromuscular blocking agent in neonates and infants? *Br J Anaesth* 1989; 62: 184–7.
63 Fisher DM, Castagnoli K, Miller RD. Vecuronium kinetics and dynamics in anesthetized infants and children. *Clin Pharmacol Ther* 1985; 37: 402–6.
64 Basta SJ. Clinical pharmacology of mivacurium chloride: a review. *J Clin Anesth* 1992; 4: 153–63.
65 Goudsouzian NG, Alifimoff JK, Eberly C *et al.* Neuromuscular and cardiovascular effects of mivacurium in children. *Anesthesiology* 1989; 70: 237–42.
66 Brandom BW, Sarner JB, Woelfel SK *et al.* Mivacurium infusion requirements in pediatric surgical patients during nitrous oxide–halothane and during nitrous oxide–narcotic anesthesia. *Anesth Analg* 1990; 71: 16–22.
67 Walbergh EJ, Wills RJ, Eckhert J. Plasma concentrations of midazolam in children following intranasal administration. *Anesthesiology* 1991; 74: 233–5.
68 Ecoffey C, Desparmet J, Berdeaux A, Maury M, Giudicelli JF, Saint-Maurice C. Pharmacokinetics of lignocaine in children following caudal anaesthesia. *Br J Anaesth* 1984; 56: 1399–402.
69 Ecoffey C, Desparmet J, Maury M, Berdeaux A, Giudicelli JF, Saint-Maurice C. Bupivacaine in children: pharmacokinetics following caudal anesthesia. *Anesthesiology* 1985; 63: 447–8.
70 Murat I, Montay G, Delleur MM, Esteve C, Saint-Maurice C. Bupivacaine pharmacokinetics during epidural anaesthesia in children. *Eur J Anaesth* 1988; 5: 113–20.

Chapter 4
Anaphylactic and Anaphylactoid Reactions

J. Pepys and M. M. Fisher

There has been a marked increase in reports of adverse reactions to anaesthetic and associated agents due to greater awareness and understanding. Among the most hazardous reactions, apparently unpredictable, are type I, immediate anaphylactic-type reactions, caused mainly, but not exclusively, but the quaternary or tertiary ammonium ion myorelaxants. These are now of general widespread use and most data has been collected on them and other anaesthetic agents because of original detailed clinical and immunological findings [1, 2]. Major contributions have been made by workers; in France [3–5] and in the UK [6–8]. Their reports, and those of others, provide a practical guide to identifying causes of anaphylactic reactions and are possibly of predictive value.

Terminology and mechanisms

The terms anaphylactic and anaphylactoid have often been used interchangeably, reflecting lack of information on or understanding of the mechanisms involved, since there are similar features.

Anaphylaxis is an immunological reaction mediated mainly by the production of specific heat-labile, long-term sensitizing Immunoglobulin E (IgE) antibody which sensitizes mast and basophil cells. Reactions are elicited by the bridging of IgE molecules on the surface of the cell membranes by divalent allergenic epitopes of appropriate size, admirably provided by the quaternary ammonium myorelaxants. The cells rapidly become degranulated, liberating preformed mediators of tissue reactions, such as histamine and chemotactic factors for eosinophil and neutrophil cells. Newly synthesized mediators are also liberated from cell membrane arachidonic acid, such as prostaglandins, leucotrienes and platelet-activating factor, which are up to a thousand times more potent than histamine in eliciting long-lasting broncho-constriction. Mast cell enzymes, particularly tryptase, a marker of mast cell reactions, whatever the cause, are also liberated. An essential feature of such allergic sensitization is that only very small amounts of allergen can suffice to provoke reactions.

A role in anaphylaxis has yet to be determined for heat-stable short-term sensitizing IgG antibodies (IgG-STS), which can also mediate immediate allergic reactions, though at a much less sensitive level than IgE antibody [9]. At present it can be shown by passive transfer tests in humans and primates and awaits the development of more readily applicable tests.

Anaphylactoid reactions are non-immunological and may be so termed by exclusion because immunological mechanisms are not demonstrable. They are elicited by agents which are capable of liberating histamine without the participation of antibodies, but which can often also act as allergens as is the case with the quaternary ammonium myorelaxants. In skin tests these two effects may be distinguished by elicitation of reactions to very low concentrations unlikely to be attributable to histamine liberation *per se*. An attempt has been made to arrive at a safety index based on the concentration causing histamine release in the skin and the neuromuscular effect of the myorelaxants with 300 for pancuronium and vecuronium; 88 for alcuronium and for the most potent histamine liberators of 42 for D-tubocurarine and atracurium [10]. In spite of the low index for atracurium there are few reports of anaphylactic or anaphylactoid reactions to it. An analysis of reactions attributed to myorelaxants suggested that 71% were anaphylactic, 15% anaphylactoid and 10% undiagnosed [11].

Mast and basophil cell reactions can also be elicited by the anaphylatoxins, C3a and C5a, derived from complement activated through the classical pathway by immune complexes of antigen and antibody formed in moderate excess of antigen. Complement products, activated through the alternative pathway without the participation of antibodies, can also be histamine liberating.

Incidence of anaphylactic/anaphylactoid reactions

Uncertainty as to the incidence of such reactions is reflected in the report on 'anaphylactoid reactions to neuromuscular blocking agents', which raised the question of 'a commonly undiagnosed condition' [12]. In comparing reports on immediate adverse reactions associated with anaesthesia, allowances have to be made for differences in clinical criteria ranging from mild erythema to severe life-threatening reactions; in diagnostic procedures and criteria; in the drugs in use; and in anaesthetic methods.

An increase in incidence from 1 in 28000 in 1970 to 1 in 5000 in Australia has been reported [13]. A national study of 200000 anaesthesias in France reported severe reactions in 1 in 4500 cases [14], whereas a study in Germany and The Netherlands cites a reaction rate of 1 in 600 [15]. The importance of the myorelaxants is shown by their identification in over one-half of the cases in France and of these 71% had anaphylactic reactions and 6% were fatal. In a UK survey in 1982, deaths attributed totally to anaesthesia were 1 in 10000 [16] and a separate extrapolation from material submitted to a research laboratory suggested an overall morbidity rate of 1 in 3500 per annum [17].

Clinical features of reactions

Immediate anaphylactic reactions develop within seconds to 1–2 min; with flush, cough, impalpable pulse and ventilatory difficulty. The earliest signs are changes in pulse oximeter due to loss of pulse or desaturation and transient difficulty in inflation. Reactions occurring later, within 4–5 min, are mainly due to bronchospasm and those after 2 h or more show acute hypotension and facial and laryngeal oedema [17]. In an analysis of 200 French cases [18] circulatory collapse was present in 92%; tachycardia in 94%, skin reactions in 79%; bradycardia in 6%; arrhythmia in 4%; cardiac arrest in 14%; and bronchospasm in 39%.

The significance of minor reactions is not known and it is suggested (though without supporting data) that they may be harbingers of future disorders [17].

The severity of reactions has been graded into four groups, ranging from skin reactions to cardiac and/or respiratory arrest, to be discussed later in relation to anaphylaxis to dextran [19].

Predisposing factors

Anaphylaxis to the myorelaxants occurs predominantly in females, the majority of whom have not received them previously. The source of their IgE sensitization is not known. Related ammonium ion compounds are common in the body and in the environment. In 10 suxamethonium sensitive subjects, seven gave positive skin test reactions to cetrimonium [20]. Benzalkonium is also suspect, but only eight of 51 patients referred because of adverse reactions, of whom 46 had immediate anaphylactic reactions and five mainly late skin reactions, gave weak prick test reactions to a high concentration of 100 mg ml^{-1} [21].

There is uncertainty about whether common allergic disorders or atopy are predisposing, due in part to differences in the criteria used for them. Of 29 patients with anaphylaxis attributable to myorelaxants four were atopic only, 11 had both atopy and asthma, two had only asthma; more than would be expected but not remarkably so [21]. Atopics show an increased tendency to histamine release from their basophils and abnormal release in atopics on challenge with thiopentone, Diprivan and chlormethiazole has been reported [22].

Among other possible predisposing causes are the use of β-adrenergic receptor blocking drugs which potentiate anaphylactic reactions causing refractoriness to adrenaline and the mode of administration of the anaesthetic agents. The intravenous administration of a myorelaxant as a bolus causes more marked increases in histamine release, in the heart rate and in the fall in blood pressure, as compared with administration as an infusion [23].

The French workers also lay stress on latent chronic tetany (spasmophilia) as a predisposing factor and found it in 60% of affected patients, mainly female, as against 15% of the control population [24]. They attribute it to lower cellular magnesium levels and report that the irritable state can be confirmed by electromyography after ischaemia and hyperventilation.

Diagnostic procedures

The Association of Anaesthetists [25] advises that 'any patient who has a suspected anaphylactic reaction associated with anaesthesia should be investigated fully'. This entails a detailed record of all the agents used and of the time and nature of adverse reactions. Investigation should have a dual role, to identify the cause or causes on the one hand to provide a guide to possible acceptable alternatives on the other.

Measurement of tryptase in serum within the first few hours provides evidence of a mast cell reaction whether immunological or not. For practical purposes for identification of the cause of type I immediate reactions the skin test comes first, followed by confirmation from serological tests for specific IgE antibody.

Other tests, such as basophil and mast cell reactions, measurement of histamine and other mediators, and tests for complement activation contribute to understanding of mechanisms involved, but are more of research interest.

Skin test methods

It is recommended that skin tests should be made several weeks after a reaction but positive results can be elicited soon after if urgent testing is needed. It is advisable that antihistamine drugs should be avoided before testing, but here too it is not uncommon in spite of their use at the time to elicit positive reactions. These tests are the most useful source of information and should be readily available. The initial tests used in this context were intradermal [26, 27] and are now being superseded by the prick test [5, 28–30].

Skin prick test

This test fulfils the ideal requirements for this purpose. It is safe, simple, inexpensive and of minimal, if any, discomfort. It is rapid in execution and response and minimizes the effects of non-specific irritants. It has high degrees of specificity, giving very few reactions in controls to the anaesthetic agents and a high degree of sensitivity in affected subjects. It should in any case precede intradermal tests, if these are intended, in order to prevent possible systemic reactions. These are very unlikely in relation to prick tests.

The prick test is made by pricking at an angle through a drop of undiluted test material (Table 4.1) [5, 21, 28], readily available as used clinically into the superficial layers of the epidermis with a gentle lifting motion [31]. A separate small hypodermic needle for each test is suitable. The volar surface of the forearm can accommodate 20 or more well-spaced tests.

Table 4.1 Skin prick tests and test concentrations [21]

Alcuronium (Alloferin) 5 mg ml^{-1}	Gelatin (Haemaccel) 35 mg ml^{-1}
Alfentanil (Rapifen) 500 μg ml^{-1}	Hetastarch (Hespan) 60 mg ml^{-1}
Atracurium (Tracrium) 10 ml ml^{-1}	Latex (rubber glove plus saline)
Cefuroxime (Zinnacef) 50 mg ml^{-1}	Pancuronium (Pavulon) 2 mg ml^{-1}
Dextran (Gentran 70) 50 mg ml^{-1}	Propofol (Diprivan) 10 mg ml^{-1}
Droperidol (Droleptan) 5 mg ml^{-1}	Suxamethonium (Anectine) 50 mg ml^{-1}
Fentanyl citrate (Sublimaze) 50 μg ml^{-1}	Thiopentone sodium (Intraval sodium) 50 mg ml^{-1}
Gallamine (Flaxedil) 40 mg ml^{-1}	Tubocurarine (Jexin) 10 ml ml^{-1}
Gelatine (Gelofusine) 40 mg ml^{-1}	Vecuronium (Norcuron) 2 mg ml^{-1}

Control tests should be completely negative, except for dermographism. As a result, even very small wealing reactions, 1–2 mm diameter, together with an erythematous flare and often with itching, can be regarded as positive. It is common and misleading for reactions to be regarded as positive only if 3–5 mm diameter or more in size. This criterion refers to assessment of possible clinical relevance with regard to common allergens encountered in the ordinary way, rather than as in indication of sensitization *per se*. It is not advisable to use this criterion for potent allergens likely to be given intravenously. Even very weak reactions to the myorelaxants in particular, capable of repetition in cases of doubt, should be regarded as suspect [32]. There are problems however with reactions to atracurium which is more histamine liberating, giving small 1–2 mm reactions in 18% of subjects [30] and reactions to D-tubocurarine. The following definite or probable causes were identified by positive prick test reactions in 36 of 46 cases of anaphylaxis: atracurium (eight); gallamine (one); pancuronium (one); suxamethonium (18); vecuronium (one); tubocurarine (one); alfentanil (one); gelofusine (two); latex (two); and cefuroxime (one).

Intradermal tests

This test consists of the intradermal injection of 0·01–0·02 ml of the appropriate dilution of allergen, usually 1 in 1000 to 1 in 10000 of the prick test concentration. This volume of fluid may elicit a swelling at control tests, so that it is necessary to have a convention regarding positivity, namely that the reaction should be 2–3 mm diameter larger than the control. Such a convention is not needed for the prick test as the control should be completely negative, making the prick test more sensitive and precise in this respect. Intradermal tests for myorelaxants are regarded as positive if the weal is 9 mm diameter, the flare 20 mm and the duration of the reaction is more than 30 min [32].

Problems arise with the skin tests in distinguishing between non-immunological, histamine-liberating effects and immunological reactions for which serological findings would be supportive. The use of increasing dilutions for skin tests may be helpful, since allergic reactions can be elicited by concentrations far lower than those capable of histamine liberation. For example in a patient with a clinical history of anaphylaxis attributable to atracurium the prick test with a dilution of 1 in 10000 elicited reproducibly a 1–2 mm wealing reaction, unlikely to be due to a non-immunological liberation of histamine [21].

Concordance of 95–97% of prick and intradermal test reactions, particularly for the myorelaxants [5, 28, 33], supports the use of the prick test by itself. The tests are good for allergy to the gelatins, but less so for the barbiturates, propofol, morphine and morphine-like analgesics and benzodiazepines [32]. The reactions are reproducible notably for the myorelaxants over periods of years [27, 34–37]. Precharged needles have also been used for prick tests [5]. Mixtures of five myorelaxants (suxamethonium, gallamine, alcuronium, pancuronium and vecuronium) gave positive reactions in 10 of 11 subjects sensitive to one or other and negative results in 23 others who had not reacted [37]. In practice the simplicity of the prick tests to each myorelaxant makes individual positives and negatives more informative.

Cross-sensitivity between the myorelaxants is commonly reported; 64% for suxamethonium, 46·3% for gallamine, 22·4% for alcuronium and 14% for pancuronium. The range of anaesthetic and associated agents is provided in Table 4.1, and the skin prick tests identified definite or probable causes in 34 of 46, i.e. seven of 10 cases.

Serological tests for specific IgE antibody

The presence of specific IgE antibodies to a myorelaxant, suxamethonium, was first shown by passive transfer, Prausnitz–Kuestner, tests in humans [38]. This was confirmed later by reports of the serological radio-allergosorbent test (RAST) type which demonstrated specific IgE antibodies against myorelaxants [2] and thiopentone [39] followed by many other such reports [40]. This made it possible by the use of inhibition tests to characterize precisely the chemical nature of the allergenic ammonium ion epitopes [41] and to assess the presence of cross-reactions. The IgE tests correlate moderately well with skin test reactions, though the production of false positives in tests against sera with high levels of IgE and the possible production of false negatives because of blocking by IgG antibodies makes the serological tests less useful for diagnostic and screening purposes than skin tests.

At an inquest on a fatal case of anaphylaxis attributed to suxamethonium, it was suggested that patients undergoing elective surgery should be screened by RAST, notably female patients, or those who had had suxamethonium previously or had other evidence of allergy [42]. Mass screening is controversial because the positive predictive value of a test depends on the prevalence of the abnormality under consideration and this is low for the anaesthetic agents. Other arguments against it are the problems of false positives and the need for considerable resources and cost [43].

In a pilot study for a prospective trial, positive IgE tests were obtained to suxamethonium in 3·4%; to alcuronium in 9·7%; and to thiopentone in 3·9%. There was thus some evidence in support of latent sensitization capable of manifesting itself as any anaphylactic reaction on first exposure. A prospective trial has been made of 373 patients given thiopentone plus suxamethonium and alcuronium in 316 and thiopentone and alcuronium in 57 cases. Blood taken beforehand was tested after the anaesthetic and 22 had a positive RAST to suxamethonium (two), alcuronium (14) and thiopentone (two); with two positive to thiopentone and alcuronium and one to all three agents. There was one anaphylactic reaction in a RAST-negative subject, and another patient had a high RAST for suxamethonium but had no reaction to its use [44]. The conclusion from this was that the RAST is too inaccurate as a screening test.

Predictive tests

The importance of identifying causal agents to avoid a second reaction has been emphasized [45]. Both the skin test and the RAST are of value for providing evidence of specific IgE sensitization. Their results correlate moderately well, but the advantages of the prick test over the intradermal test and the problems of the RAST have been discussed. An important point to be emphasized is that the wealing reaction to the skin test is a biological reaction; so much so that it could be described as 'anaphylaxis in miniature' and it provides evidence to be respected of possible reactions to allergens introduced intravenously. In discussion of the predictive value of skin tests, the problems of penicillin allergy are cited. Some patients with negative results may react adversely to administration of penicillin and others with positive results may tolerate its use. The difference from the myorelaxants is that penicillin allergens are heterogeneous, whereas the epitopes of the myorelaxants are well-defined ammonium ions which give them greater sensitivity and specificity.

The question of whether skin tests should be used for preanaesthetic screening is controversial because of the low rates of sensitization and doubts about the validity of the results. One approach [46] has been to advise tests if two of the following criteria are present: (a) a past history of drug allergy; (b) past exposure to the particular agent or frequent contact with related quaternary ammonium compounds as in hairdressers and medical personnel; or (c) in atopic subjects. The female clients of the hairdressers are also exposed and this may be relevant to sensitization. Three examples of this important aspect in patients who had anaphylactic reactions to myorelaxants consisted of a nurse anaesthetic assistant sensitive to suxamethonium and a hairdresser handling ammonium thioglycolate, both of whom had contact urticaria analogous to skin test reactions, and the third was a client who was sensitized by applications for a 'permanent' and who developed contact dermatitis. These histories were obtained after the anaphylactic events, which stresses the importance of the history in itself, and showed that skin test screening could have predicted their adverse reaction and led to avoidance of potential causes.

The emphasis above has been on the myorelaxants. Other anaesthetic causes of anaphylaxis are also important.

Thiopentone anaphylaxis

The incidence of anaphylaxis to thiopentone is low and has been estimated at 1 in 30000 [8] and in 90% of cases there was a history of previous exposure, sensitivity to other drugs or a history of asthma, hay fever or eczema [47]. Retrospective and prospective studies cite figures of 1 in 22773 to 1 in 29000 [48, 49]. These figures are regarded as uncertain and probable underestimates because of the very large numbers of thiopentone inductions annually, suggesting that anaphylactic reactions may have gone unrecognized or misdiagnosed [50].

A comparison of 203 patients with anaphylaxis to myorelaxants and 31 to thiopentone showed that only one of the latter had not been exposed to thiopentone previously, with an average exposure of 6·8 times and a range of 2–15 times. By contrast, in those with anaphylaxis to myorelaxants, the majority had not been exposed to them previously. Reactions in the past occurred in 22% of the thiopentone reactors and in 5% of the myorelaxant group [51]. In 83 patients studied prospectively, there were no significant differences between intradermal and prick tests to thiopentone and only one of 31 anaphylactic patients who gave a negative skin test reaction, gave a systemic reaction to the testing [51]. Intravenous challenge tests provoked severe and even hazardous reactions [52–54].

The skin test reactions suggested IgE sensitization which has been confirmed by serological tests showing specific antibodies to thiopentone. Previous findings of cross-reactivity with the sera of myorelaxant-affected subjects was clarified by inhibition tests with thiopentone which were effective for thiopentone anaphylaxis but not for myorelaxant anaphylaxis [55].

Propofol anaphylaxis

Adverse reactions to propofol were common when cremophor, polyoxyethylated castor oil, was used as the vehicle—it was abandoned earlier because of its role in reactions to althesin. In its present form using a soya and egg lipid vehicle, to which negative tests were given, 14 patients are reported [56] who had anaphylactic reactions to first administration of Diprivan. Positive intradermal tests, but less frequent prick tests, were given to Diprivan in eight cases, as compared with negative intradermal test reactions in 100 controls. Positive IgE antibody and leucocyte histamine release tests were also given in some of the cases. Whereas there is a great preponderance of females in myorelaxant anaphylaxis, of the above 14 cases six were male. Previous drug reactions, reported in five cases are suggested as a criterion against the use of Diprivan, as well as its use together with a histamine-liberating agent such as atracurium. A reproducible strong, prick test reaction to propofol has been seen in one of 51 subjects, with no history of its having been given at any time [21].

Etomidate adverse reactions

Adverse reactions to etomidate have been mucocutaneous in 90% of cases with less frequent cardiovascular or respiratory symptoms [57]. Two severe reactions have been reported [58] and one anaphylactic reaction [59]. It is, however, a poor histamine liberator and has been considered as suitable for patients at risk [60].

Ketamine adverse reactions

Adverse reactions to ketamine appear to be uncommon and in eight reactions over a period of 20 years five were assumed to be anaphylactic [57]. It causes limited histamine liberation and is considered suitable for patients at risk and recommended for treatment of refractory bronchospasm [61].

Droperidol adverse reactions

Droperidol is an inhibitory of histamine *N*-methyltransferase [62] and is not recommended if there is a risk of histamine release or a history of a previous adverse reaction.

Narcotic analgesic adverse reactions

There appears to be a limited role for morphine and morphinemimetic drugs as causes of anaphylactic or anaphylactoid reactions. An anaphylactoid reaction to fentanyl confirmed by a skin test reaction has been reported [63]. In six of a group of 51 subjects, there were four doubtful and two definitely positive prick test reactions to fentanyl, none of them having received fentanyl at any time and two were positive to alfentanil [21].

Many of these are potent histamine liberators. Morphine and meperidine are the most potent and naloxone, alfentanil and nalbuphine the least. Anaphylactoid reactions to them are rarely described [64, 65]. In a patient having an anaphylactic reaction to papaveretum, confirmed by intradermal test reactions to it, but not to morphine, both morphine and codeine combined with IgE antibodies in the serum [66]. IgE antibodies to meperidine have also been reported in a patient who reacted to it [65]. In another patient with a history suggesting an anaphylactic reaction to an intramuscular injection of morphine and with a history of urticaria due to codeine, unequivocal reactions were elicited by a 1 in 10000 concentration, unlikely to be histamine liberating [21]. It has been suggested that more of the severe 'anaphylactoid' reactions will be found to be IgE mediated [66]. Attention is drawn to a patient in whom a diagnosis of allergy, shown as angioedema and bronchospasm, was made on clinical grounds and attributed to midazolam [85].

Table 4.2 Severity of reactions to different agents [19]

	All grades (%)	Grades 3 & 4 (%)
Dextran		
60–75 kD	0·069	0·017
40 kD	0·007	0·002
Gelatin		
urea-linked	0·146	0·048
modified-fluid	0·066	0·016
Hydroxylethyl starch	0·085	0·006

Anaphylaxis to agents associated with anaesthesia

In a prospective study of the administration of 200906 U of plasma substitutes reactions were recorded to plasma proteins in 0·003%; to gelatins in 0·038%; to dextran 60–75 kD in 0·008%; and to hydroxyethyl starch in 0·006% [19]. The severity of reactions was graded as follows:

1 skin reactions, mild fever;

2 measurable non life-threatening reactions—cardiovascular with tachycardia and hypotension;

3 shock—life-threatening with smooth muscle spasm;

4 cardiac or respiratory arrest.

The severity of reactions to the different agents is outlined in Table 4.2. The recorded death rates from plasma substitutes ranged from 6 to 9% [15]. Whilst reactions to the gelatins are more frequent, the majority of deaths are due to the dextrans.

Dextran reactions

Prevention of reactions to dextran by the use of low molecular weight monovalent dextran 1 kD in order to inhibit reactions to the high molecular weight dextrans 60–75 1 kD has been successful. Intravenous administration of 10 ml 2 min beforehand reduced the reaction rate by 50%; 20 ml reduced it by 90–97%. Grades 3 and 4 reaction rates fell to 1·4 in 10000 as against the expected 25 in 10000. The death rate fell from 1 in 34000 to 1 in 670000 [67–70].

Antibodies not of the IgE class to dextran as shown by passive haemagglutination tests have been found in 60% of Swedish and German subjects with high titres in 14–25% [71], probably present in response to dextrans met in everyday life. Adverse reactions are correlated with the titres which fall after a reaction together with complement activation by the classical pathway, namely representing a form of aggregate anaphylaxis.

Gelatin reactions

The demonstration of the antigenicity of the gelatins for humans [72, 73] supports the possibility of their causing anaphylaxis. Such reactions have been reported together with positive intradermal and prick tests which are not elicited in the normal population [74]. Both the urea-linked gelatin (Haemaccel) and the modified fluid, succinylated gelatin, have been responsible and in two anaphylactic patients both forms elicited strong wealing reactions on prick testing with the materials as used clinically [21].

Latex allergy

Allergic and anaphylactic type reactions to latex (*Hevea brasiliensis*) allergens in rubber gloves and other articles are being increasingly reported. Many hospital personnel have been found to have immediate-type allergy to rubber gloves. Anaphylactic reactions in children with spina bifida who require multiple exposures to rubber have been reported [75–78]. Positive prick tests correlating with positive RAST for specific IgE antibodies are reported [77]. For practical purposes prick tests with saline after being pressed into a piece of rubber glove can elicit vigorous reactions, providing evidence of the ease with which the allergens can become available on exposure to the body. In two urological patients who had had frequent catheterization, strongly positive prick test reactions were obtained in this way [21] and may have been relevant to the reaction during anaesthesia. Cross-reactions are reported between latex, chestnut and banana in subjects having allergic reactions, including anaphylaxis to the latter [79, 80].

Adverse reactions to non-anaesthetic drugs

Depending upon the apparent clinical relevance of a reaction to almost any drug that may have been given, investigation is indicated. For example, a prick test reaction was elicited only to cefuroxime in a patient with a suspect clinical history [21]. Antibiotics, mainly penicillin, are often suspect and others such as protamine have been proven [81–84]. Antibodies to protamine capable of mediating anaphylaxis have been described, not only in the IgE class, but also in the IgG-STS and complement-fixing IgG antibodies and positive prick and intradermal tests have been elicited. A further example is the report of anaphylactic reactions to aprotinin supported by positive skin and IgE tests [86].

Local anaesthetics

Histories of adverse reactions to local anaesthetics are not uncommon. Evidence for an allergic mechanism is, however, rare. Suspicion of allergic sensitivity has arisen mainly from contact sensitization to the ester-linked group such as procaine but not to the amide group, such as lignocaine which has been used in preference. Analysis of patients with a history of adverse reactions concluded that (a) there was a low incidence of reactions compatible with a systemic IgE mechanism; (b) there was a lack of specific and clinically useful information from skin tests with dilutions; and (c) that there was apparent safety in challenging with an alternative preparation [87]. Another study with similar results concluded that the 'vast majority of patients labelled as allergic to local anaesthetics' are in fact not [88]. Most reports settle for provocative challenges with a series of injections of increasing dosage to show acceptability.

Management

Immediate

The majority of cases respond promptly to aggressive early treatment although rarely patients may die in spite of excellent care. The basis of treatment is general supportive measures such as oxygen, external cardiac compression and intermittent positive pressure ventilation with the specific measures of intravenous fluids, and vasoactive and antibronchospastic drugs. The key to treatment is early recognition of the problem and early intervention. Anaphylaxis should be considered as a cause of hypotension and tachycardia particularly after induction, and inspection for a confirmatory rash occur. In a study of simulated anaesthetic accidents Schmid and O'Donnell [89] found 60% of doctors missed the diagnosis of anaphylaxis. Interestingly 100% of 'overseas doctors' made the diagnosis and only 24% of USA trained doctors which may reflect the apparently less common occurrence of such reactions in the USA.

Cardiovascular collapse

The use of adrenaline is most commonly associated with improvement [90] and the drug has the advantage of being useful in bronchospasm as well as cardiovascular collapse [91]. At least 10% of patients will require a second injection [88]. However, it has a number of side effects such as myocardial ischaemia and, possibly in large doses, myocardial necrosis [92]. It has been associated with ventricular arrhythmias, which in our series have been associated largely with intravenous 'push' doses [93].

In patients who are not monitored, direct-acting vasoconstrictors or intramuscular adrenaline may be safer [93]. Noradrenaline will improve blood pressure in a number of patients who do not respond to adrenaline [91]. Recent unpublished data from The Netherlands could suggest that dopamine may be as effective as adrenaline with fewer side effects.

Intravenous fluids are usually necessary and may be sufficient alone in many patients if given in sufficient quantity [94]. The available data supports the use of colloid solutions [91, 94, 95] although less severe cases may respond to crystalloid; 2–3 l or more of colloid may be necessary [91].

In spite of elegant demonstrations of the effects of anaphylactic mediators on myocardial mechanical and electrical function, heart failure is rare in acute anaphylaxis, although patients with cardiovascular disease are more likely to show impaired cardiac function or arrhythmias [91]. Rarely, patients with normal cardiac function prior to a reaction may develop severe global myocardial dysfunction requiring balloon counterpulsation [96] but whether this is due to the pathological process or exogenous catecholamines is uncertain. In patients who do not respond to conventional measures or require continuing sympathomimetics, antishock trousers, naloxone or thyrotropin-releasing hormone, have been advocated. Recent case reports have confirmed the clinical observations that H_2 blockers may lead to improvements when cardiovascular instability persists [97]. In β-blocked patients, in whom anaphylaxis may be refractory to conventional management, glucagon was effective in one case [98].

Bronchospasm

This is the most difficult aspect of acute anaphylaxis to treat. Adrenaline is the sympathomimetic most commonly associated with improvement [91]. To this we routinely add aminophylline and salbutamol by inhalation and intravenous infusion. Steroids are routinely given because whilst they have little immediate effect anaphylactic bronchospasm may be protracted. External chest compression may assist artificial ventilation in severe obstruction [99]. Other therapeutic manoeuvres are the use of volatile anaesthetics, ketamine, endotracheal procaine and magnesium sulphate, which will occasionally produce a dramatic response. When all treatments have been attempted and the patient cannot be mechanically ventilated, the occurrence of barotramua or cardiac arrest should lead to consideration of cardiopulmonary bypass. Extensive care should be exercised with simple anaesthetic ventilators to avoid 'stacking' of breaths with the subsequent risks of barotrauma and cardiovascular collapse [100].

Angioedema

Intubation, adrenaline and H_1 blockade will usually stop oedema progressing or reoccurring [90]. These patients require observation for up to 10 h as oedema may recur.

Pulmonary oedema

The pulmonary oedema of anaphylaxis is usually a membrane oedema responding to positive end expiratory pressure and volume.

Anaphylaxis may be biphasic and recur later [101]. A period of observation is necessary particularly when angiooedema has occurred. Failure to respond rapidly, or the persistence of bronchospasm should lead to transfer to an intensive care unit or major hospital.

References

1 Fisher MM. Intradermal testing in the diagnosis of allergic reactions to intravenous drugs. *Anaesth Intens Care* 1976; 4: 97–104.

2 Baldo BA, Fisher MM. Substituted ammonium ions as allergenic determinants in drug allergy. *Nature* 1983; 306: 262–4.

3 Laxenaire MC, Moneret-Vautrin DA. *Le Risque Allergique en Anesthésie-Réanimation*. Paris: Masson, 1991.

4 Vervloet D, Nizankovska E, Arnaud A, Senft M, Charpin J. Adverse reactions to suxamethonium and other muscle relaxants under general anaesthesia. *J Allergy Clin Immunol* 1983; 71: 552–63.

5 Leynadier F, Sansarricq M, Didier JM, Dry J. Prick tests in the diagnosis of anaphylaxis to general anaesthetics. *Br J Anaesth* 1987; 59: 683–9.

6 Assem E-SK, ed. *Allergic Reactions to Anaesthetics. Clinical and Basic Aspects*. Basel: Karger, 1992.

7 Watkins J. Second report from an anaesthetic reactions advisory service. *Anaesthesia* 1989; 44: 157–9.

8 Clarke RSJ. Epidemiology of adverse reactions to anaesthesia in the United Kingdom. *Klin Wchnschr* 1982; 60: 1003–5.

9 Pepys J, Parish WE, Stenius-Aarniala B, Wide L. Clinical correlations between long-term (IgE) and short term (IgG-STS) anaphylactic antibodies in atopic and 'non-atopic' subjects with respiratory allergic disease. *Clin Allergy* 1979; 9: 645–58.

10 Galletly DC. Comparative cutaneous histamine release by neuromuscular blocking agents. *Anaesth Intens Care* 1986; 14: 365–9.

11 Moneret-Vautrin DA, Laxenaire MC, Hummer-Sigiel M, Mouton C, Guéant JL. Myorelaxants. In: Laxenaire MC, Moneret-Vautrin DA, eds. *Le Risque Allergique en Anesthésie-Réanimation*. Paris: Masson, 1991: 52–8.

12 Youngman PR, Taylor KM, Wilson JD. Anaphylactoid reactions to neuromuscular blocking agents: a commonly undiagnosed condition? *Lancet* 1983; ii: 597–9.

13 Fisher MM. The epidemiology of anaesthetic anaphylactoid reactions in Australasia. *Klin Wchnschr* 1982; 60: 1017–20.

14 Hatton F, Tiret L, Maujol L *et al*. Enquête épidémiologique sur les anesthésies. Premières résultats. *Ann Fr Anesth Réanim* 1983; 2: 333–85.

15 Langrehr D, Newton D, Agoston S. Epidemiology of adverse reactions in anaesthesia in Germany and The Netherlands. *Klin Wchnschr* 1982; 60: 1010–16.

16 Lunn JN, Mushin WW. *Mortality Associated with Anaesthesia*. London: Nuffield Provincial Hospitals Trust, 1982.

17 Watkins J. Markers and mechanisms of anaphylactoid reactions. In: Assem ESK, ed. *Allergic Reactions to Anaesthetics. Clinical and Basic Aspects*. Basel: Karger, 1992: 108–29.

18 Laxenaire MC, Moneret-Vautrin DA, Vervloet D, Alazia M, Francois G. Accidents anaphylactoides graves per anaesthésiques. *Ann Fr Anesth Réanim* 1985; 4: 30–46.

19 Ring J, Messmer K. Incidence and severity of anaphylactoid reactions to colloid volume substitutes. *Lancet* 1977; i: 466–9.

20 Charpin J, Vervloet D, Nizankovska E. Adverse reactions due to muscle relaxants. In: *Proceedings*

of XI International Congress of Allergology and Clinical Immunology, 1982. London: Macmillan, 1983: 67–73.

21 Pepys J, Pepys EO, Baldo BA, Whitwam JG. Anaphylactic–anaphylactoid reactions to anaesthetic and associated agents. Skin prick tests in diagnosis. 1993; in press.

22 Laxenaire MC, Mata E, Guéant JL, Moneret-Vautrin DA, Haberer JP, Basophil histamine release in atopic patients after in vitro provocation with thiopental, Diprivan and chlormethiazole. *Acta Anaesth Scand* 1991; 35: 706–10.

23 Moss J, Philbin DM, Roscan CE, Basta SJ, Gelb C, Savarese JJ. Histamine release by neuromuscular blocking agents in man. *Klin Wchnschr* 1982; 60: 891–5.

24 Moneret-Vautrin DA, Grilliat JP, Laxenaire MC, Sigiel M, Chastel A. Les facteurs de risque d'accidents anaphylactoïdes aux anesthésiques-généraux et substances adjuvantes. *Thérapie* 1980; 35: 335–40.

25 Association of Anaesthetists of Great Britain and Ireland. *Anaphylactic Reactions Associated with Anaesthesia*. London: Association of Anaesthetists of Great Britain and Ireland, September 1990.

26 Fisher MM. Intradermal testing in the diagnosis of allergic reactions to intravenous drugs. *Anaesth Intens Care* 1976; 4: 97–104.

27 Fisher MM. Intradermal testing in the diagnosis of acute anaphylaxis during anaesthesia: results of five years' experience. *Anaesth Intens Care* 1979; 7: 58–61.

28 Moneret-Vautrin DA, Mata E, Widmer S. Intérét des prick-tests pour le dépistage d'une sensibilisation latente aux myorelaxants. *Rev Fr Allergol* 1989; 29: 138–40.

29 Leynadier F. Prick-tests to diagnose anaphylaxis. *Br J Anaesth* 1988; 61: 365–6.

30 Maria Y, Grosdidier R, Haberer JP, Moneret-Vautrin DA. Enquête prospective prèopératoire chez 300 patients per prick-tests aux myorelaxants. *Ann Fr Anesth Reanim* 1989; 8: 301–5.

31 Pepys J. Skin testing. *Br J Hosp Med* 1975; 14: 412–17.

32 Moneret-Vautrin DA, Mouton C, Pupil P, Girard A, Bertrand F. Tests cutanés et tests *in vitro*. In: Moneret-Vautrin DA, Laxenaire MC, eds. *Le Risque Allergique en Anesthésie-Réanimation*. Paris: Masson, 1991: 89–98.

33 Moneret-Vautrin DA, Laxenaire MC. Skin tests in diagnosis of allergy to muscle relaxants and other anaesthetic drugs. In: Assem ESK, ed. *Allergic Reactions to Anaesthetics. Basic and Clinical Aspects*. Basel: Karger, 1992: 145–55.

34 Moneret-Vautrin DA, Laxenaire MC, Guéant JL. Anaphylactic reactions to muscle relaxants. In: Pichler WJ, Stadler BM, Dahinden CA, Pecoud AR, Frei P, eds. *Progress in Allergy and Clinical Immunology*. Toronto: Hofgrefe & Huber, 1989: 450–4.

35 Vervloet D, Benzarti M, Arnaud A, Charpin J. Reproductibilité des tests cutanes aux myorelaxants. *Ann Fr Anesth Réanim* 1985; 4: 184–5.

36 Sage D. Intradermal drug testing following anaphylactoid reactions during anaesthesia. *Anaesth Intens Care* 1981; 9: 381–6.

37 Leynadier F, Sansarricq M, Dry J. Reproductibilité des test cutanes intra-dermiques aprés anaphylaxie aux myorelaxants. *Presse Med* 1987; 16: 523–5.

38 Jerums G, Whittingham S, Wilson P. Anaphylaxis to suxamethonium. *Br J Anaesth* 1967; 39: 73–6.

39 Harle DG, Baldo BA, Wajon P, Fisher MM. Detection of thiopentone reactive IgE antibodies following anaphylactoid reactions during anaesthesia. *Clin Allergy* 1986; 16: 493–8.

40 Guéant JL, Nicholas JP, Moneret-Vautrin DA, Laxenaire MC, Mata E. Tests radio-immunologiques. In: Moneret-Vautrin DA, Laxenaire MC, eds. *Le Risque Allergique en Anesthésie-Réanimation*. Paris: Masson, 1991: 99–105.

41 Harle DG, Baldo BA, Fisher MM. The molecular basis of IgE antibody binding to thiopentone. *Mol Immunol* 1990; 27: 853–8.

42 Sheriff D Kelbie. Sheriffdom of Grampian, Highlands and Islands. Determination given on May 9th 1989. *Lancet* 1989; i: 1400.
43 Noble DW, Yap PL. Screening for antibodies to anaesthetics. No case for doing it yet. *Br Med J* 1989; 299: 2.
44 Reid TMS, Imray JM, Noble DW. Anaesthetic allergy and prospective radioallergosorbent testing. In: Assem ES-K, ed. *Allergic Reactions to Anaesthetics*. Basel: Karger, 1992: 162–73.
45 Fisher MM. The prevention of second anaphylactoid reactions to anaesthetic drugs. *Anaesth Intens Care* 1981; 9: 242–6.
46 Moneret-Vautrin DA, Laxenaire MC, Grilliat JP. Conduite du bilan diagnostiques et prédictif d'un accident anaphylactoïde peranesthésique. In: Moneret-Vautrin DA, Laxenaire MC, eds. *Le Risque Allergique en Anesthésie-Réanimation*. Paris: Masson, 1991: 105–12.
47 Clarke RSJ, Dundee JW, Garrett RT, McArdle GK, Sutton JA. Adverse reactions to intravenous anaesthetics. *Br J Anaesth* 1975; 47: 575–85.
48 Evans JM, Keogh JAM. Adverse reactions to intravenous induction agents. *Br Med J* 1977; 2: 735–6.
49 Beamish D, Brown DT. Adverse responses to i.v. anaesthetics. *Br J Anaesth* 1981; 53: 55–7.
50 Currie TT, Whittingham S, Ebringer A, Peters JS. Severe anaphylactic reaction to thiopentone. *Br Med J* 1966; 1: 1462–3.
51 Baldo BA, Fisher MM, Harle DG. Allergy to thiopentone. *Clin Rev Allergy* 1991; 9: 295–308.
52 Carrie LES, Buchanan RL. Thiopentone anaphylaxis. *Anaesthesia* 1967; 22: 290–5.
53 Barjenbruch KP, Jones JR. Thiopental anaphylaxis: a case report. *Anesth Analg* 1972; 51: 113–16.
54 Fisher MM, Ross JD, Harle DG, Baldo BA. Anaphylaxis to thiopentone: an unusual outbreak in a single hospital. *Anaesth Intens Care* 1989; 17: 361–5.
55 Harle DG, Baldo BA, Wajon P, Fisher MM. Detection of thiopentone reactive IgE antibodies following anaphylactoid reactions during anaesthesia. *Clin Allergy* 1986; 16: 493–8.
56 Laxenaire MC, Mata-Bermejo E, Moneret-Vautrin DA, Guéant JL. Life-threatening anaphylactoid reactions to propofol (Diprivan). *Anaesthesiology* 1992; 77: 275–80.
57 Hummer-Siegiel M, Bois JP, Mata E, Guéant JL. Anesthésiques généraux, benzodiazepines, neuroleptiques, morphiniques. In: Moneret-Vautrin DA, Laxenaire MC, eds. *Le Risque Allergique en Anesthésie-Réanimation*. Paris: Masson, 1991: 46–52.
58 Krumholtz W, Muller H, Gerluch H, Russ W, Hempelmann G. Ein fall von anaphylaktoiden reaktion nach gabe von etomidat. *Anaesthesist* 1984; 33: 161–2.
59 Sold M, Rothhammer A. Lebensbedrochliche anaphylaktoïde reaktion nach etomidat. *Anaesthesist* 1985; 34: 208–10.
60 Watkins J. Etomidate: an 'immunologically safe' anaesthetic agent. *Anaesthesia* 1983; 38 (suppl): 34–8.
61 Fisher MM. Pointers to the treatment of anaphylactoid reactions. In: Watkins T, Levy CJ, eds. *Guide to Immediate Anaesthetic Reactions*. London: Butterworths, 1988: 32–40.
62 Moss J, Verburg KM, Henry DP. Droperidol inhibits histamine *N*-methyl-transferase. *Anesthesiology* 1985; 63: A303.
63 Bennett MJ, Anderson LK, McMillan JC, Ebertz JM, Hanifin JM, Hirshman CA. Anaphylactic reaction during anaesthesia associated with positive intradermal skin test to fentanyl. *Canad Anaesth Soc J* 1986; 33: 75–8.
64 Levy JH, Brister NW, Shearin A *et al.* Wheal and flare responses to opioids in humans. *Anesthesiology* 1989; 70: 756–60.
65 Levy JH, Rockoff MA. Anaphylaxis to meperidine. *Anesth Analg* 1982; 61: 301–3.
66 Harle DG, Baldo BA, Coroneos NJ, Fisher MM. Anaphylaxis following administration of

Papaveretum. Case report: implication of IgE antibodies that react with morphine and codeine, and identification of an allergenic determinant. *Anesthesiology* 1989; 71: 489–94.
67 Ljungstrom KG, Renck H, Strandberg K, Hedin H, Richter W, Widerlov E. Adverse reactions to dextran in Sweden 1970–1979. *Acta Chir Scand* 1983; 149: 253–62.
68 Ljungstrom KG, Renck H, Hedin H, Richter W, Rosberg B. Prevention of dextran-induced anaphylactic reactions by hapten inhibition. *Acta Chir Scand* 1983; 149: 341–8.
69 Ljungstrom KG, Renck H, Hedin H, Richter W, Wiholm BE. Hapten inhibition and dextran anaphylaxis. *Anaesthesia* 1988; 43: 729–32.
70 Messmer K, Ljungstrom KG, Gruber VF, Richter W, Hedin H. Prevention of dextran-induced anaphylactoid reactions by hapten inhibition. *Lancet* 1980; i: 975.
71 Hedin H, Richter W, Messmer K, Rench H, Ljungstrom KG, Laubenthal H. Incidence, pathomechanism and prevention of dextran induced anaphylactoid/anaphylactic reactions in man. *Dev Biol Stand* 1981; 48: 178–89.
72 Maurer P. Antigenicity of oxypolygelatin and gelatin in man. *J Exp Med* 1954; 100: 497.
73 Maurer P, Lebovitz H. Studies of the antigenicity of modified fluid gelatins. *J Immunol* 1956; 76: 335–41.
74 Laxenaire MC, Peignier C, Audibert G, Guéant JL. Substituts colloïdaux du plasma. In: Moneret-Vautrin DA, Laxenaire MC, eds. *Le Risque Allergique en Anesthésie-Réanimation*. Paris: Masson, 1991: 72–81.
75 Turjanmaa K. Incidence of immediate allergy to latex gloves in hospital personnel. *Contact Derm* 1987; 17: 270–5.
76 Leynadier F, Pecquet C, Dry J. Anaphylaxis to latex during surgery. *Anaesthesia* 1989; 44: 547–50.
77 Jaeger D, Kleinhaus D, Czuppon AB, Baur X. Latex-specific proteins causing immediate-type cutaneous, nasal, bronchial and systemic reactions. *J Allergy Clin Immunol* 1992; 89: 759–68.
78 Slater J. Latex allergy—what do we know? *J Allergy Clin Immunol* 1992; 90: 279–80.
79 Rodriguez M, Vega F, Garcia MT *et al.* Hypersensitivity to latex, chestnut and banana. *Ann Allergy* 1993; 70: 31–4.
80 de Corres LF, Moneo I, Munoz D *et al.* Sensitisation from chestnuts and bananas in patients with urticaria and anaphylaxis from contact with latex. *Ann Allergy* 1993; 70: 35–9.
81 Jackson DR. Sustained hypotension secondary to protamine sulphate. *Angiology* 1970; 21: 295–8.
82 Grant JA, Cooper JR, Albyn BS, Buhner D, Farnam J, Yunginger JW. Anaphylactic reactions to protamine in insulin-dependent diabetics after cardiovascular procedures. *J Allergy Clin Dermatol* 1984; 73 (suppl): 180.
83 Lakin JD, Blocker TJ, Strong DM, Yocum MW. Anaphylaxis to protamine sulphate mediated by a complement dependent IgG antibody. *J Allergy Clin* 1978; 61: 102–7.
84 Knape JTA, Schuller JL, de Haan P, de Jong AP, Bovill JG. An anaphylactic reaction to protamine in a patient allergic to fish. *Anesthesiology* 1981; 55: 324–5.
85 Yakel DL, Whittaker SE, Elstad MR. Midazolam-induced angioedema and bronchoconstriction. *Critical Care Med* 1992; 20: 307–8.
86 Wuthrich B, Schmid P, Schmid ER, Tornic M. IgE mediated anaphylactic reaction to aprotinin during anaesthesia. *Lancet* 1992; 340: 173–4.
87 Incaudo G, Shatz M, Patterson R, Rosenberg M, Yamamoto F, Hamburger RN. Administration of local anaesthetics to patients with a history of prior adverse reaction. *J Allergy Clin Immunol* 1978; 61: 339–45.
88 de Shazo R, Nelson HS. An approach to the patient with a history of local anaesthetic hypersensitivity: Experience with 90 patients. *J Allergy Clin Immunol* 1979; 63: 382–94.
89 Schmid HA, O'Donnell D. Anesthesiologists' management of simulated critical incidents.

Anesthesiology 1992; 76: 495–501.
90 Fisher M. Anaphylaxis. *Dis Mon* 1987; 33: 433–79.
91 Fisher MM. Clinical observations on the pathophysiology and treatment of anaphylactic cardiovascular collapse. *Anaesth Intens Care* 1986; 14: 17–21.
92 Soreide E, Buxrud T, Harboe S. Severe anaphylactic reactions outside hospital: etiology, symptoms and treatment. *Acta Anaesth Scand* 1988; 32: 339–42.
93 Fisher MM. Treating anaphylaxis with sympathomimetic drugs. *Br Med J* 1992; 305: 1107–8.
94 Waldhausen E, Kesser G, Marquardt B. Der Anaphlactishe schock (anaphylactic shock). *Anaesthesist* 1987; 36: 150–8.
95 Fisher M. Blood volume replacement in acute anaphylactic cardiovascular collapse related to anaesthesia. *Br J Anaesth* 1977; 49: 1023–6.
96 Raper RF, Fisher MM. Profound reversible myocardial depression after anaphylaxis. *Lancet* 1988; i: 386–8.
97 Yarbrough JA, Moffitt JE, Brown DA, Stafford CT. Cimetidine in the treatment of refractory anaphylaxis. *Ann Allergy* 1989; 63: 235–8.
98 Zaloga GP, DeLacey W, Holmboe E, Chernow B, Glucagon reversal of hypotension in a case of anaphylactoid shock. *Ann Intern Med* 1986; 105: 65–6.
99 Fisher MM, Bowey CJ, Ladd-Hudson K. External chest compression in acute asthma: a preliminary study. *Critical Care Med* 1989; 17: 686–7.
100 Tuxen DV, Lane S. Detrimental effects of positive pressure ventilation during controlled mechanical ventilation of patients with severe airflow obstruction. *Am Rev Respir Dis* 1987; 136: 872–9.
101 Stark BJ, Sullivan TJ. Biphasic and protracted anaphylaxis. *J Allergy Clin Immunol* 1986; 78: 76–83.

Chapter 5
Cardiopulmonary Resuscitation

D. A. Zideman and W. F. Dick

Day-case anaesthesia requires careful patient selection, meticulous surgery and attentive postoperative care. By adhering to these principles, the occurrence of a cardiac arrest in day-case anaesthesia should be minimized, nevertheless the risk will still exist. Quantifying this risk is difficult and it is likely that figures representing the true risk of death related to this form of anaesthesia will not be known for many years to come. Looking at the published data, Keenan and Boyan's study [1] of cardiac arrest during anaesthesia reported an incidence of 1 in 6046 anaesthetics. Tiret *et al.* [2] from France reported a cardiac arrest incidence of 1 in 3358 anaesthetics with a 36% survival rate. In the Confidential Enquiry into Perioperative Deaths (CEPOD) study, 5081 deaths from 485850 operations were analysed [3]. Of the reported deaths, 14·1% were partially related to anaesthesia. In only three cases was anaesthesia the sole cause but the CEPOD study only required the reporting of mortality and not the related morbidity in the study group.

Although the perioperative risk of cardiac arrest is always a matter of concern, it is an event occurring in an otherwise controlled environment. The application of minimal standards of monitoring [4, 5] should ensure the early detection of cardiovascular collapse which will be rapidly treated by experienced medical and nursing staff. In the study by Tiret *et al.* [2] 58% of serious complications were perioperative and 42% postoperative. Of 40 perioperative cardiac arrest patients 18 survived compared with only three of 19 who arrested in the postoperative period. Postanaesthetic respiratory depression and the inhalation of gastric contents were the main causes of postoperative mortality. In the same study only 50% of postoperative complications occurred in the first hour following anaesthesia, while 75% occurred within 5 h. This data must be considered relevant to day-case anaesthesia. Thus the provision of adequate postoperative care for the day-case patient by both the professional hospital staff and the lay relatives or friends out of hospital must be considered of importance. Furthermore, not only must the hospital staff be proficient in resuscitation skills but also the home carers should be aware, as a minimum standard, of how to recognize a potential problem and how to call the emergency services. A day-case can, if required, be allowed to recover and remain under observation all day. Clearly the time of discharge is a matter of clinical judgement (Chapter 22).

Table 5.1 Chain of survival [9]

1	Early access to the emergency services
2	Early basic life support
3	Early defibrillation
4	Early advanced life support

Resuscitation procedures

In 1992, the American Heart Association [6] and the European Resuscitation Council (ERC) [7, 8] published their latest recommendations for cardiopulmonary resuscitation (CPR) and emergency cardiac care. There are only minimal differences between the two series of recommendations which mainly reflect their North American or European origins. Both authorities base their protocols on the concept of the 'chain of survival' (Table 5.1) [9].

No matter where or when the cardiac arrest occurs the strategy of the 'chain of survival' provides the foundation for all resuscitation procedures. The first link of early access requires the recognition of the signs of an imminent cardiac incident together with a rapid assessment of the patient. New to the 1992 protocols is the 'call for help' at this early stage before any further action is taken. The second link early basic life support (BLS) requires the immediate initiation of basic resuscitation. In the hospital situation the medical team should immediately commence BLS and not wait for the arrival of equipment. In the out-of-hospital situation the initiation of BLS will depend on the prior training and experience of the carer. Telephone CPR, i.e. the instruction of a bystander in CPR technique over the telephone, may prove invaluable in this type of situation. The third link of early defibrillation is the key to survival in patients with ventricular fibrillation. The wider availability of automated external defibrillators amongst the emergency medical service responders (paramedical, ambulance personnel) will enhance this link. The fourth link of early advanced cardiac life support is the linchpin of the system. Although early defibrillation will increase survival amongst those in ventricular fibrillation, the enhancement of BLS procedures by the drugs and equipment described in the advanced life support protocols are the only hope of a successful resuscitation for those in asystole, electromechanical dissociation, or when ventricular fibrillation does not respond to the initial defibrillation therapy.

Early access

The early recognition of the symptoms and signs of a cardiac arrest could lead to the prevention of the incident occurring. In the conscious unmonitored patient the occurrence of tightness in the chest, pain, shortness of breath or a rapid change in conscious level should raise the awareness of the observer. In the monitored patient a change of cardiac rhythm, or the ST segment height, a fall in blood pressure or in oxygen saturation, or a change in the expired carbon dioxide level could all indicate impending circulatory collapse. Whatever the environment an assessment of the patient's airway, breathing and circulation will diagnose the problem and should prompt an immediate call for assistance. For the bystander or the out-of-hospital procedure, the situation is more complicated. First, the distinction between sleep and unconsciousness must be made, and a more gentle 'wake up' procedure may be more advisable. Then following the initial shout for help the rescuer should assess the status of the casualty. This is carried out by:

1 Assessing the conscious level by shaking and shouting at the patient;
2 Opening the airway by head tilt and chin lift;
3 Clearing the airway if necessary;
4 Assessing the breathing by looking, listening and feeling for effective breathing;
5 Assessing the circulation by feeling for the carotid pulse. If there is *no* breathing and *no* pulse than the rescuer should immediately leave the patient and quickly activate the emergency medical system, for example dial the emergency telephone number 999 (UK), 911 (USA), 119 (Japan) or the appropriate number to ensure the earliest possibility of external defibrillation without which the patient in ventricular fibrillation cannot survive. The North American Standards require this call to be made before the clinical assessment, the ERC after the assessment. This time difference is irrelevant where more than one rescuer is present as the first rescuer can perform the assessment and commence BLS, the second can go and call for help.

Early BLS

The initiation of early BLS is essential to patient survival. Bystander or professional BLS can 'buy time' but only on a temporary basis as it will rapidly lose its value if the remaining two links in the chain do not follow on rapidly.

Airway

In BLS the airway is opened by head tilt and chin lift or jaw thrust. The importance of maintaining the airway of the postoperative patient cannot be over emphasized. No matter whether the patient has received sedation or general anaesthesia, the airway must always be considered at risk.

Clearing the airway either by suction or by simple finger sweeps also plays an important role. Where surgery has been performed on or in the region of the upper airway, blood and secretions should be carefully removed. It is essential not to discharge from proper medical care any patient until airway bleeding has been controlled and the patient can maintain his or her own airway.

Breathing

In the BLS protocol this refers to expired air respiration by a mouth-to-mouth or mouth-to-mask ventilation technique. Having opened the airway, the rescuer occludes the patient's nose by pinching the nostrils, takes a deep breath and breathes out into the patient, their lips covering the casualty's mouth creating an airtight seal. It is important to observe that the chest of the patient rises with each breath, confirming a satisfactory ventilation technique. Each breath should appear as if the patient were taking a deep breath. Two breaths are given, each inspiration lasting approximately 2 s and delivering 800–1200 ml of gas. Expiration is passive and should be complete 2–4 s following the end of inspiration.

With a mouth-to-mask technique the face-shaped mask is sealed onto the patient's face to form an airtight cover. The rescuer blows through the mask inlet or through the one way valve attached to the mask inlet. The resistance of the valve should be minimal to allow for adequate ventilation. Some masks allow the addition of supplemental oxygen via an oxygen port.

Circulation

Circulation in BLS is maintained by external chest compressions. Chest compressions are performed on the lower third of the sternum two fingers breadth above the xiphisternum using the overlapping heels of both hands. A 4–5 cm vertical compression is sufficient for most adults performed at a rate of 80 min^{-1}. Fifteen compressions are performed followed by two ventilations. External chest compressions can, at best only provide 15–20% of normal cardiac output. Unless a spontaneously beating heart can be restored within a relatively short period of time, recovery is unlikely. Having commenced BLS it should be continued uninterrupted until the arrival of the defibrillation and the advanced life support (ALS) team. No time should be wasted by further checks of the respiration or pulse as it is considered unlikely that BLS alone will be successful in restoring respiration or circulation.

The preceding description is for the full scenario of an adult undergoing resuscitation for a cardiac arrest. Two other situations must also be described.

Respiratory arrest

In this scenario the checks performed under 'early access' indicate:

1 unresponsive;
2 no breathing;
3 pulse present.

In this situation the priority is to restore breathing. Having established the above and opened the airway by head tilt and chin lift, the rescuer performs 10 mouth-to-mouth ventilations and then leaves the casualty to phone for help. On return, the rescuer checks the circulation and continues mouth-to-mouth ventilations at a rate of one breath every 5 s until further help arrives.

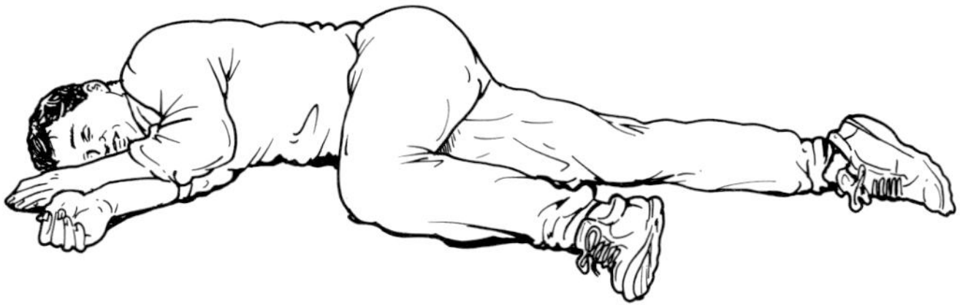

Fig. 5.1 Recovery position.

Unconscious

In the final scenario the checks performed under 'early access' indicate:

1 unresponsive;
2 breathing;
3 pulse present.

In this situation the priority is to protect the airway of the unconscious victim. This is best performed by turning the casualty into the recovery position (see Fig. 5.1) ensuring that having achieved the lateral position the airway remains patent and that breathing and pulse are still present. In this position the casualty can be left while the rescuer goes to phone for help.

Finally, it must be emphasized that what has been described above is the worst scenario of a single unaided rescuer dealing with a single casualty. In most cases, especially within a day-case surgical unit, this should probably not be the situation. Furthermore, the phone will be to hand and an ALS team immediately available. Nevertheless, the early recognition of and the correct primary management of an unconscious patient, a respiratory or a cardiac arrest is the only way of ensuring a successful outcome.

ALS

ALS requires the use of the equipment and drugs for resuscitation. BLS should have been commenced and must continue throughout. Operating theatres, recovery areas, endoscopy and cardiology clinics, and radiology departments should all be self-sufficient in resuscitation equipment, e.g. defibrillator, advanced airway care, 100% oxygen and drugs. Otherwise they must await the arrival of the ALS team and its equipment to commence the definitive management of the resuscitation sequence.

Ventricular fibrillation (VF)

Since most adult cardiac arrests are due to ventricular fibrillation the priority is to defibrillate the patient as soon as possible. The ERC protocol for VF is illustrated in Fig. 5.2.

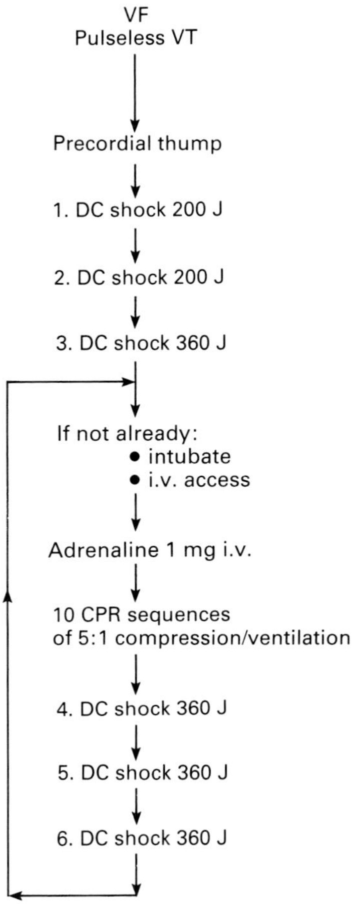

(i) The interval between shocks 3 and 4 should not be > 2 min.
(ii) Adrenaline given during loop approx. every 2–3 min.
(iii) Continue loops for as long as defibrillation is indicated.
(iv) After 3 loops consider: an alkalising agent, or an anti-arrhythmic agent.

Remember – artificial ventilation, once established, should include oxygen therapy

Fig. 5.2 European resuscitation guidelines for VF.

A precordial thump is recommended whilst the initial defibrillation is being established. Caldwell *et al.* [11] converted 23 patients in hospital from ventricular fibrillation using either a cough or a precordial thump. The simplicity of this technique justifies its inclusion in the VF protocol, even though its success rate may be reduced when BLS has been delayed or there is a substantial gap between BLS and the initiation of ALS.

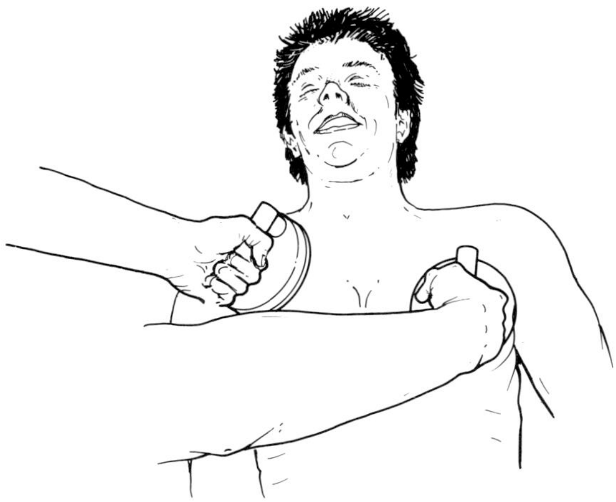

Fig. 5.3 Position of defibrillator paddles.

Defibrillation

The defibrillation paddles are placed on the patient's chest (Fig. 5.3) using a suitable conductive gel to lower electrical impedance. The paddles will monitor the electrocardiogram (ECG) and if a trace of VF (or pulseless ventricular tachycardia) is seen to be present then three defibrillations are performed at 200, 200 and 360 J. The ERC guidelines recommend that defibrillations are performed one after the other only pausing to allow the electrical rhythm to be confirmed and the defibrillator to recharge. No BLS is carried out between these initial defibrillations. Recently, a new type of defibrillator has become available. The automated external defibrillator (AED) is a defibrillator which incorporates a rhythm analysis system. All AEDs are attached to the patient by two large self-adhesive gelled electrodes. The ECG is detected by these electrodes and passed to the defibrillator where it is read and interpreted. The AED [12] follows a preprogrammed algorithm if VF is detected it will charge to 200 J and advise the operator to deliver the defibrillation by pushing the defibrillation button. The 200 J is delivered via the large self-adhesive electrodes and the resulting rhythm reanalysed. The cycle is then repeated for a second 200 J and subsequent 360 J defibrillations. The protocol illustrated in Fig. 5.2 is currently followed in the UK. In the fully automated system the machine will issue an audible or visual warning prior to defibrillation and defibrillate without the need for the operator to initiate the action. Although the potential for out-of-hospital, 'non-expert' defibrillation [13, 14] has already been realized, the use of such machines in hospital is just being developed. Assuming that the argument for early defibrillation is accepted, the AED provides the pathway for any person in the day-care unit, suitably trained, to initiate defibrillation rather than waiting for the ALS team and its equipment to arrive depending on the local arrangements. One further advantage of the AED is that it records and stores its activities for medical audit at a later date. Finally, most AEDs do have the facility to be overridden and placed into the conventional manual mode by means of simple key mechanism. Manually overriding the system usually slows down attempts at defibrillation as it takes longer to assess the ECG rhythm compared with using the AED machine algorithms.

If the initial three attempts at defibrillation are unsuccessful then it is necessary to oxygenate the patient, secure the airway by intubation and to gain venous access by cannulating a large vein. Venous access and tracheal intubation are required to be performed rapidly and accurately. This requires frequent training and practice in these two resuscitation skills. The next step is to administer adrenaline 1 mg i.v. (or 2–3 mg via the tracheal tube if venous access has not yet been established). Adrenaline is an adrenergic receptor agonist. In resuscitation its primary action is via α_1-adrenergic receptors, raising the peripheral vascular resistance and the end diastolic filling pressure, thus improving myocardial perfusion. This α activity also 'stiffens' the major arterial vessels in the chest thus aiding the forward transmission of blood by the raised intrathoracic pressure generated during chest compressions. Adrenaline also has β-adrenergic activity, a positive chronotropic and inotropic effect on the myocardium and a bronchodilator effect on the lungs [15].

Following the establishment of venous access, tracheal intubation and the administration of adrenaline, 10 BLS sequences are performed of five compressions followed by one ventilation. On completion, a further three defibrillations at 360 J are performed. It is suggested that the interval between the third defibrillation (the last of the first cycle of three) and the fourth defibrillation (first of the second cycle of three) should not exceed 2 min. Furthermore, the loop of the DC defibrillation, adrenaline and BLS should be completed every 2–3 min. To achieve this requires training and regular practice in the skills of resuscitation. The loop should be continued for as long as VF is present and defibrillation is indicated. After three loops the use of an alkalizing agent, sodium bicarbonate 50 ml of 8·4% should be considered, together with the administration of a suitable anti-arrhythmic drug, e.g. bretyllium or amiodarone. Resuscitation should continue as long as VF is present but most authorities agree that the chances of a successful event decrease rapidly with the progression of time. Full recovery of cerebral function cannot be anticipated if the restoration of a spontaneously beating heart with an adequate cardiac output is not restored within a few minutes of the start of the arrest.

Asystole

Asystole (Fig. 5.4) is characterized by a flat ECG trace representing ventricular standstill. About 25% of arrests in hospital and 10% of those outside hospital are asystolic. In the perioperative period where hypoventilation, hypoxia and hypercardia are predominant risk factors, asystole or a profound bradycardia should be recognized as the major cause of cardiovascular collapse.

Before asystole is diagnosed it is essential to ensure that the ECG system is correctly connected and that the switches, connections and gain are correctly adjusted. In a

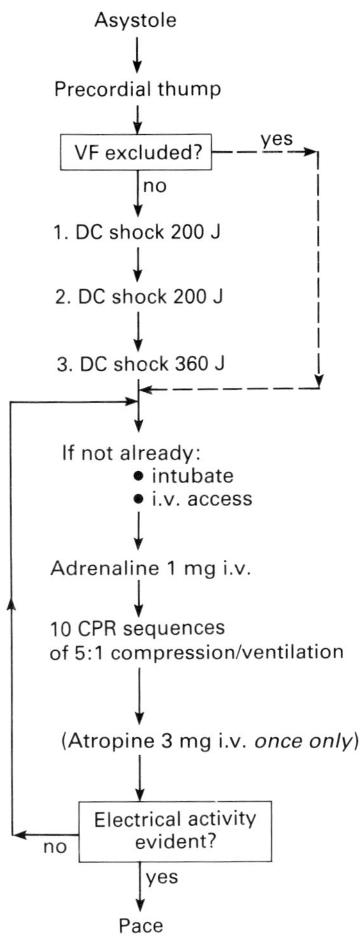

Fig. 5.4 European resuscitation guidelines for asystole.

(i) If no response after 3 cycles consider high dose adrenaline: 5 mg.

pulseless patient, it is very important not to mistake asystole for VF—and thus mistakenly not to provide the definitive treatment for VF, i.e. defibrillation. Thus following a precordial thump if VF cannot be categorically excluded then the sequence should start as described above for VF; three defibrillations at 200, 200 and 360 J. The sequence then continues in the normal recommended way with the establishment of venous access, intubation of the airway and the administration of 1 mg of adrenaline i.v., or 2–3 mg via the tracheal tube. After the 10 CPR sequences of five compressions to one ventilation 3 mg i.v. atropine is given. Atropine is a parasympathetic blocking drug and in the dose recommended will totally block the vagus nerve. In the asystolic situation it is believed that the vagus could be the cause of the severe bradycardia and thus its effects should be eliminated.

Resuscitation from asystole should continue with BLS and repeated doses of 1 mg adrenaline given every 2–3 min. High-dose adrenaline, 5 mg i.v., may be considered during the third or subsequent cycles [16]. Recent studies are showing concern [17, 18] about postresuscitation renal failure when high doses of adrenaline have been administered.

Finally, if there is any evidence of electrical activity myocardial pacing should be attempted. Some modern defibrillators allow transthoracic pacing to be performed. However, the results of pacing have been disappointing. It has been suggested that this may be because it is initiated too late in the resuscitation sequence.

Prolonged resuscitation from asystole will require the correction of acid–base status of the patient. This should be done by titrating the dose of sodium bicarbonate to correct the acidity demonstrated by arterial blood gas results. Sodium bicarbonate can be given as boluses of 50 ml of 8·4% solution (50 mmol) during prolonged resuscitation if arterial blood gas measurements are not directly available.

Electromechanical dissociation (EMD; Fig. 5.5)

EMD is the loss of a palpable pulse despite an ECG demonstrating a recognizable QRS complex. It is probably the most common of all the causes of cardiovascular collapse under anaesthesia or in the immediate postoperative phase. Drug sensitivity, allergy or overdose and hypovolaemia from surgical bleeding must be considered as the primary causes. Tension pneumothorax, cardiac tamponade, pulmonary embolism, hypothermia and electrolyte imbalance must be excluded as additional causes and treated appropriately if detected.

EMD usually has an underlying treatable cause. It is important not only to treat this cause but also to maintain an effective circulation until this specific treatment has been completed. BLS must continue and is supported by early intubation of the airway establishing venous access and the administration of 1 mg i.v. adrenaline. Further doses of adrenaline, high-dose (5 mg) adrenaline [15] and sodium bicarbonate may be needed in prolonged attempts at EMD resuscitation. In addition, where hypocalcaemia, hyperkalaemia or an overdose of a calcium antagonist is suspected, then calcium chloride 10 ml of a 10% solution should be given to support myocardial function.

Postresuscitation care

Following cardiac arrest and resuscitation, the patient must be removed from the day-case unit and carefully observed in an intensive care area. A check of serum electrolytes and arterial blood gases must be made and a 12-lead ECG and chest X-ray performed to assess the overall results of resuscitation and to correct any further underlying anomalies.

Any patient fit enough to undergo day-care surgery must be considered ethically viable for resuscitation. Thus the question of 'Do not resuscitate' does not enter into this discussion. Similarly, it would be hoped that this preoperative 'fitness' together

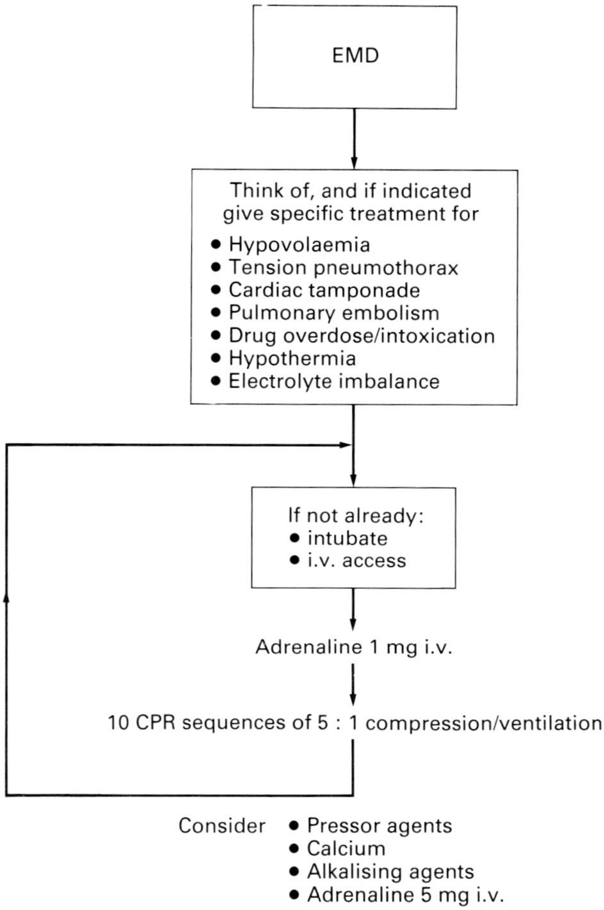

Fig. 5.5 Electromechanical dissociation.

with the immediate availability of resuscitation equipment and expertise would be indicative of an improved survival rate from arrest events in the day-care area. Fortunately, it would appear that these events are rare. Unfortunately, previous evidence has shown that resuscitation whilst under anaesthesia or immediately postanaesthesia, especially when hypoxia or a drug interaction have been the cause of the arrest, carries a poor prognosis [1, 2]. It would be hoped that careful and complete equipment checks and an adequate presurgical history and examination will limit these events to an absolute minimum.

However, there is a need to educate the many non-anaesthetically trained practitioners of sedation (e.g. gastroenterologists, cardiologists, interventional radiologists and surgeons) in the extent and dangerous synergism which may occur when combining an opioid with a benzodiazepine, leading to unintended induction of anaesthesia, loss of the airway and respiratory depression (Chapters 2 and 16).

Paediatric resuscitation

Paediatric day surgery has become more popular over the last 2 years. It is an effective way of dealing with minor or intermediate surgical procedures, hernia, orchidopexy, circumcision, ear, nose and throat and dental procedures, and then allowing the return of the child to the familiar home environment.

However, the decision to perform such surgery as a day case requires careful patient selection and an uncompromising position on not only child suitability but also the suitability of the parent to assume responsibility for the postoperative care.

It would be hoped that those performing day-care anaesthesia would be well versed in paediatric resuscitation techniques. The need for prompt recognition and management of resuscitation is the same as for adults and all the protocols are similar; nevertheless, the differences are important to an eventual successful outcome.

Children do not usually have pure 'cardiac' events. Most require resuscitation following an airway/breathing event. It is important to correct hypoxia or hypoventilation early in children before it can progress to a full circulatory collapse. The paediatric protocols [6, 19] reflect this (Fig. 5.6). In the infant (defined as a child under the age of 1 year) having assessed responsiveness, opened the airway and checked for breathing, the rescuer gives five breaths of mouth-to-mouth and nose ventilation if there is no breathing, before feeling for a pulse. Checking for an infant's pulse is performed by feeling for the brachial pulse. If this is absent or if there is a bradycardia of less than 60 beats min^{-1}, external chest compressions are performed at a rate of 100 min^{-1}, five compressions, to each breath, to a depth of 2 cm using two fingers pressing on the lower half of the sternum. The infant, otherwise healthy apart from its surgical condition, will have a healthy myocardium which will continue to beat, despite circulatory collapse. The patient will gradually become hypoxic causing a bradycardia. Slow heart rates in infants do not adequately support the circulation and this is the reason for initiating chest compression when the pulse rate falls to below 60 beats min^{-1}. After 1 min of BLS the infant is taken to the telephone, while maintaining BLS, and help summoned. In infants the early commencement of BLS before calling for help may well halt the progression of the collapse to a more sinister conclusion.

In children (over the age of 1 year), the same protocol is followed but because of the larger size, ventilation is performed by a mouth-to-mouth technique and the pulse check is performed at the carotid artery. Chest compressions are carried out using the heel of one hand compressing to 3 cm depth but in a ratio of five compressions to one breath. Chest compressions are commenced only if no pulse is felt and not if there is a bradycardia (Fig. 5.6).

Paediatric ALS

It is essential that any day-case unit carrying out paediatric day-care surgery or investigation must be able to perform the practical procedures of paediatric ALS. Not

	Infant (< 1 year old)	Child (> 1 year old)
Check conscious level	Shake, pinch gently shout for help	Shake, pinch gently shout for help
Open airway	Head tilt chin tilt (jaw thrust)	Head tilt chin tilt (jaw thrust)
Check breathing	Look, listen, feel clear airway	Look, listen, feel clear airway
Breathe	5 breaths mouth to mouth and nose	5 breaths mouth to mouth
Check pulse	Feel brachial pulse start compressions if < 60/min	Feel carotid pulse if no pulse start chest compressions
Chest compressions	2 fingers, lower sternum rate 100/min, depth 2 cm 5 compressions : 1 breath	Heel of one hand, lower sternum rate 100/min, depth 3 cm 5 compressions : 1 breath

After 1 min activate emergency medical services

Fig. 5.6 Paediatric resuscitation. Adapted from European resuscitation guidelines.

only must the medical and nursing personnel have the required skills but also the range of equipment needed to implement these skills must be available.

The full range of tracheal tube sizes and a selection of straight and paediatric curved laryngoscope blades are essential equipment. Each tracheal tube is best left uncut until used and is fitted with a 15 mm international standard connector. This 15 mm connector will fit directly into the 22 mm connector of a self-inflating resuscitation bag without the need for an intermediate connection. In experienced hands the size of the self-inflating resuscitation bag is irrelevant as the operator will only squeeze the bag until the chest rises to the equivalent of a deep breath. Ideally, either the child (500 ml) or adult (1200 ml) bag should be available for use. The resuscitation bag should carry an oxygen reservoir and be attached to an oxygen supply of 10–12 l min^{-1} to ensure an F_IO_2 of 1·0. Increasing the inspired oxygen concentration to 100% during the respiratory cycle by using a reservoir bag will improve the chance of survival of infants and children.

Having established an airway and commenced ventilation of the child the next task is to provide venous access for the administration of fluids and drugs. Venous access in

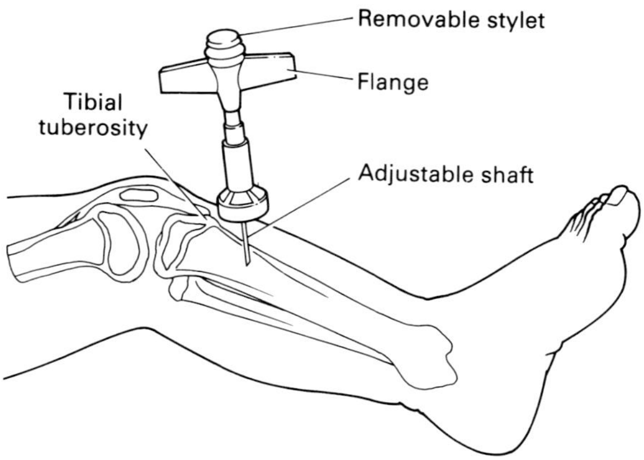

Fig. 5.7 Placement of Illinois sternal or iliac bone marrow–aspiration needle in the proximal tibial location. Reprinted from [20] by permission of the *New England Journal of Medicine*, (322; 1579–81, 1991).

children is probably the most daunting task facing any resuscitator, especially if he or she is not trained in paediatrics. Hence venous access should always be secured at induction of anaesthesia even if a gaseous induction method has been used. This vascular access should remain in place until the child has recovered but it is not unusual for a restless child in recovery to dislodge or even remove the intravenous cannula. A large peripheral vein is usually acceptable, for example, in the antecubital fossa or anterior to the medial malleolus. The establishment of central venous access in children is for experts only. Endotracheal drug administration is a possibility but the volume of fluid for the drugs administered will rapidly exceed that volume which can logistically be put into the lungs. In addition sodium bicarbonate, which plays a major part in paediatric resuscitation, cannot be administered via the tracheal tube.

The intraosseous route is a viable and safe alternative in infants and children for drug administration [20]. The intraosseous needle is placed directly into the tibia, 1 cm below the tibial tuberosity. Fluids and drugs, including caustic drugs such as sodium bicarbonate and calcium chloride, can be injected through the needle into the bone marrow space. Absorption into the circulation is rapid and is complete in about 20–30 s. The intraosseous route should only be regarded as emergency access and a formal venous route established as soon as possible if necessary by cutdown. The complications of intraosseous infusion include drug extravasation, skin infection and osteomyelitis when the needle has been left in place for a prolonged period (Fig. 5.7).

Finally, the correct dose of drug and the appropriate quantity of fluid must be calculated with care and attention to administration. Both drugs and fluid are administered by calculating the dose or volume from the child's weight. Hence all children undergoing anaesthesia need to be weighed preoperatively. If for some reason the child has not been weighed then the dose of drugs can be gauged using the length (height) of the child. The Oakley chart (Fig. 5.8) and the Brasslow tape (Fig. 5.9) are recommended as useful when gauging drug doses based on a child's length.

Endotracheal tube	
Length (cm)	Internal diameter (mm)
18–21	7·5–8·0
18	7·0
17	6·5
16	6·0
15	5·5
14	5·0
13	4·5
12	4·0 3·5
10	3·0–3·5

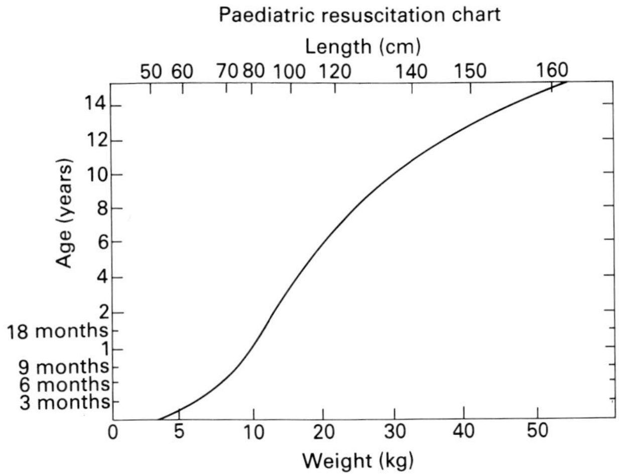

Adrenaline (ml of 1/10 000) intravenous or endotracheal	0·5	1	2	3	4	5
Atropine (mg) intravenous or endotracheal	0·1	0·2	0·4	0·6	0·6	0·6
Bicarbonate (ml of 8·4%) intravenous	5	10	20	30	40	50
Calcium chloride (mmol)* intravenous	1	2	4	6	8	10
Diazepam (mg) Intravenous	1·25	2·5	5	7·5	10	10
Diazepam (mg) Per rectum	2·5	5	10	—	—	—
Glucose (ml of 50%) intravenous	10	20	40	60	80	100
Lignocaine (mg) intravenous or endotracheal	5	10	20	30	40	50
Salbutamol (mg) intravenous	25	50	100	150	200	250
Initial DC defibrillation (J)	10	20	40	60	80	100
Initial fluid infusion in hypovolaemic shock (ml)	50	100	200	300	400	500

* One ml calcium chloride 1 mmol/ml, 1·5 ml calcium chloride 10%, 4·5 ml calcium gluconate 10%

Fig. 5.8 Proposed paediatric resuscitation chart to improve performance. Reproduced from *Br Med J* [21].

Just as in the adult, adequate postresuscitation care is essential and the child must be cared for, in a critical care or intensive care area equipped to treat children. It is worth remembering that all children will be accompanied in a day-case unit by an adult carer. Should a resuscitation event occur then this carer (parent or guardian) must be informed at the earliest available time. Too often the parent or guardian is

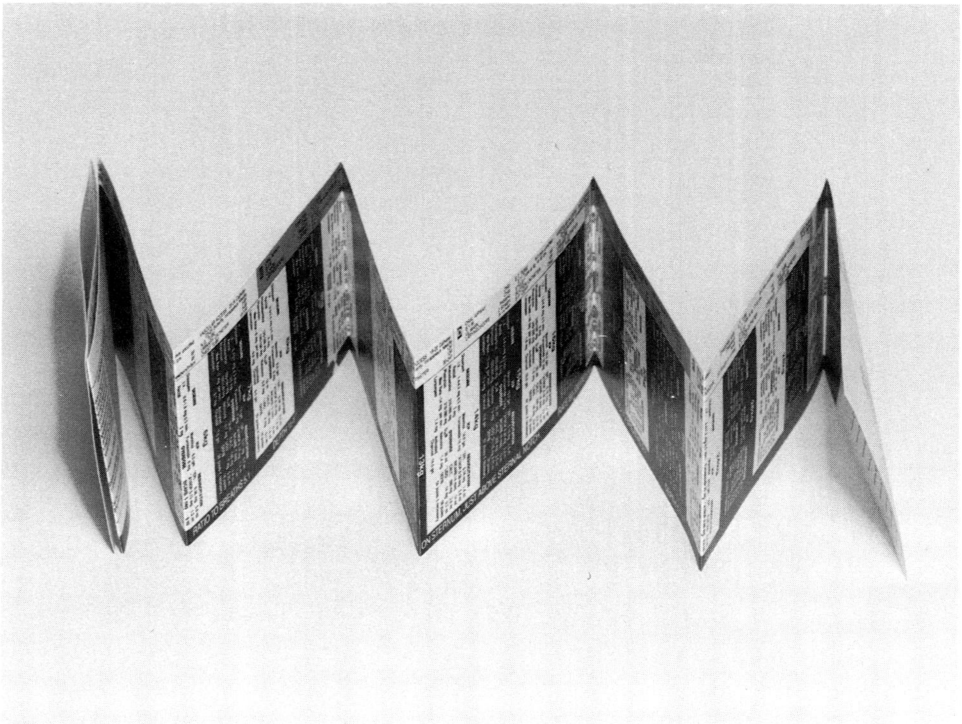

Fig. 5.9 Brasslow Tape indicating drug doses and procedures by weight of child. Tape is extended from feet to vertex to indicate doses of drugs in relation to anticipated weight of the child, together with relevant procedures.

forgotten until the resuscitation event has been terminated, making the incident a distressing occurrence for all concerned.

Before concluding this chapter it is necessary to mention briefly the ethical aspects of resuscitation in a day-care unit. Although the vast majority of the patients attending for day-case procedures will be fit and well with no long-standing medical problems, there may be some who have clinical end stage disease but require a minor surgical procedure. Despite firmly advocating a full resuscitation policy, it is necessary to realize that some of these chronically ill patients may not wish to be resuscitated should they collapse under anaesthesia. In these circumstances, and after direct full discussion and counselling of the parent, or guardian and the patient prior to anaesthesia, a 'Do not resuscitate' order should be carefully recorded in the patient's notes and the patient's wishes respected. Furthermore, it should be deleted on the successful completion of the procedure and should not remain in place for subsequent treatment, but be recorded for each subsequent anaesthetic.

Day-case anaesthesia when carefully and properly practised is a safe procedure. Relatively few resuscitation events occur in the day-case area but the professional staff must be fully equipped and properly trained to recognize and treat such occurrences.

The resuscitation protocols should not be dismissed as of minimal importance just because the surgical and investigative procedures of a day-case area are minor. All patients undergoing anaesthesia are entitled to a gold standard of medical care.

References

1 Keenan RL, Boyan C. Cardiac arrest due to anaesthesia. A study of incidence and cause. *JAMA* 1985; 253: 2373–7.

2 Tiret L, Desmonts JM, Hutton F, Vourch G. Complications associated with anaesthesia—a perioperative study in France. *Canad Anaesth Soc J* 1986; 33: 336–40.

3 Buck N, Devlin HB, Lunn JN. *The Report of a Confidential Enquiry into Perioperative Deaths* (CEPOD). London: Nuffield Provincial Hospital Trust/King's Fund, 1987.

4 Eichorn JH, Cooper JB, Cullen DJ *et al.* Standards for patient monitoring during anaesthesia at Harvard Medical School. *JAMA* 1986; 256: 1017.

5 Sykes MK. Essential monitoring. *Br J Anaesth* 1987; 59: 901–12.

6 American Heart Association. Guidelines for cardiopulmonary resuscitation and emergency cardiac care. *JAMA* 1992; 268: 2171–2302.

7 European Resuscitation Council. Guidelines for basic life support. *Resuscitation* 1992; 24: 103–10.

8 European Resuscitation Council. Guidelines for advanced life support. *Resuscitation* 1992; 24: 111–21.

9 Cummins RO, Ornato JP, Thies, WH, Pepe PE. Improving survival from sudden cardiac arrest: the 'chain of survival' concept. *Circulation* 1991; 83: 1832–47.

10 National Association of EMS Physicians. Emergency medical dispatching. *Prehosp Disaster Med* 1989; 4: 163–5.

11 Caldwell G, Miller G, Quinn E, Vincent R, Chamberlain DA. Simple mechanical methods of cardioversion: defence of the precordial thump and cough version. *Br Med J* 1985; 291: 627–8.

12 Cummins RO, Eisenberg MS, Bergner L. Automatic external difibrillation. Evaluation of its role in the home and in emergency medical services. *Ann Emerg Med* 1984; 13: 798–804.

13 Moore JE, Eisberg MS, Cummins RO *et al.* Layperson use of automatic external defibrillation. *Ann Emerg Med* 1987; 16: 669–75.

14 Weaver WD, Hill D, Farbruch CE *et al.* Use of automatic external defibrillator in the management of out of hospital cardiac arrest. *N Engl J Med* 1988; 319: 661–6.

15 Redding JS, Pearson JW. Evaluation of drugs for cardiac resuscitation. *Anaesthesiology* 1963; 24: 203–8.

16 Koscove EM, Paradis NA. Successful resuscitation from cardiac arrest using high-dose epinephrine therapy. Report of two cases. *JAMA* 1989; 261: 989–91.

17 Callahan M, Barton CW, Kayser S. Potential complications of high dose epinephrine in patients resuscitated from cardiac arrest. *JAMA* 1991; 265: 1117–9.

18 Mattara J, Singhad PC. Acute renal failure following cardiopulmonary resuscitation. *Clin Res* 1992; 40: 251A.

19 European Resuscitation Council. Paediatric resuscitation protocols. *Resuscitation* 1993; in press.

20 Fiser D. Intraosseous infusion. *N Engl J Med* 1990; 322: 1579–81.

21 Oakley PA. Inaccuracy and delay in decision making in paediatric resuscitation and a proposed reference chart to reduce error. *Br Med J* 1988; 297: 817–19.

22 Luter RC, Wears RL, Broselow J *et al.* Length based endotracheal tube and emergency equipment selection in paediatrics. *Ann Emerg Med* 1992; 21: 900–4.

Chapter 6
Methods for Assessment of Recovery

G. G. Lockwood

Early recovery can be assessed by observing landmarks in the return of normal behaviour such as eye opening. Later, specific tests are required to quantify drug effects on brain function. Some of these attempt to emulate real-life tasks, others are more abstract. The most obvious example of the first approach is the driving simulator. Such tests generally require sophisticated equipment and risk influencing the subject by creating interest and therefore increasing arousal and commitment. More commonly psychomotor function is tested by the performance of idealized tasks such as simple reaction time, or of abstract tasks such as critical flicker fusion. This approach can provide evidence of depression of isolated aspects of brain activity, and if they are interpreted using a model of psychomotor function they can provide an overview of the effect of depressant agents on the whole mental state.

Formal tests

Scoring systems

The early stages of recovery can be evaluated by noting the time at which fixed events occur (e.g. open eyes, obey commands, state date of birth) [1]. Alternatively, the state of recovery can be evaluated at fixed times by a scoring system. Steward [2] described a simple system of this type (Table 6.1) which has since been widely used. Recovery to the maximum score, as evaluated by these methods, shows that the patient can be moved from the recovery suite, but does not imply full recovery. However, they may be the only practicable method for assessing recovery in young children.

Subjective assessment of later recovery may be made by the patient, the general nursing staff or a specific investigator. The patient may be asked to score various aspects of their mental state and mood, or mark appropriately labelled visual analogue scales. Some investigators have found these to be as sensitive as commonly used objective tests [3, 4]. They are simple to perform and require no elaborate equipment, but recent work has tended to emphasize the results of objective testing because of the fear that residual anaesthesia may reduce patients' insight into their own mental impairment.

Table 6.1 The Steward simplified postanaesthetic recovery score [2]

Consciousness	
awake	2
responding to stimuli	1
not responding	0
Airway	
coughing on command or crying	2
maintaining a good airway	1
airway requires maintenance	0
Movement	
moving limbs purposefully	2
non-purposeful movements	1
not moving	0

Objective testing

There are a huge number of objective tests of recovery from anaesthesia, and only some of the most common or promising are described here (Table 6.2). Different tests are said to measure different aspects of psychomotor function. It is possible to define a model of psychomotor function with a spectrum of sensory, central processing and motor components, and then devise a minimal set of tests which assesses it completely [5]. In practice such a set will be excessive, perhaps because the drugs used in anaesthesia depress all aspects of mental activity to some extent, or because the tests are not very specific, with considerable overlap.

With any test of mental activity, there are certain precautions which must be taken. Individuals vary considerably in their baseline abilities, and so each must be used as his or her own control. The time of day and position in the menstrual cycle have significant effects on performance and should be controlled. Finally, practice effects must be reduced either by allowing sufficient learning time before collecting results, or by having a control group of subjects not undergoing anaesthesia. The improvement in performance of some psychomotor tests that comes with practice means that a return to initial baseline values actually represents residual impairment, for by that time those in a control group would have improved their own baseline scores [6].

Tests of sensory processes

The inspection time is the least time that a stimulus must be maintained in order to be recognized [7]. The subject is asked to say which of two lines appearing on a computer screen or LED display is the longer. This is not a test of discrimination because the two lines are presented side by side and one line is twice the length of the other. However, the subject may not be able to say which was the longer when the presentation time is very short. The test is repeated over 100 times with the side on which the longer line

Table 6.2 A classification of the psychomotor tests discussed in the text

Sensory	Central	Memory	Motor	Mixed	Physiological
Inspection time	Critical flicker fusion	Digit span	Finger tapping	Simple response time	Maddox Wing
Perceptive accuracy	Stroop phenomenon	Word lists	Pronation/supination	Choice response time	Saccadic eye movements
Block recognition	Coin counting	Picture tests	Body sway	Trieger dot test	
Visualization	Serial sevens		Wire and loop	Pursuit rotor	
P-deletion	Digit–symbol substitution		Blind pointing	Mazes	
Perceptual speed			Pegboard	Driving simulations	
Vigilance			Ball bearing		
			Shape sorter		

appears and the presentation time (10–500 ms) randomized. The inspection time is the presentation time associated with 85% correct answers, and it is increased by cerebral depressants. The test requires special apparatus, but has the advantage that there is little learning effect. It has been used recently to quantify the effects of midazolam [8].

Analogous tests have been used to study recovery from anaesthesia. The perceptive accuracy test (PAT) displays a number at a random position on a computer screen for 500 ms, and the subject responds by typing the number into the computer in his or her own time [9]. This test also includes a motor component of gaze fixation and cannot be thought of as simply a test of perception. The block pattern recognition test is closer to inspection time [3]. A pattern is flashed on a computer screen for a period of 20–100 ms, followed by a finer, random pattern to act as a backward mask. Two seconds later the subject picks the stimulus pattern from a selection of four patterns displayed on the screen.

A visualization test requiring the subject to identify the ends of 10 interwoven lines drawn across a page has been used to detect residual effects of a range of drugs used in anaesthesia [10, 11]. It is an inexpensive test but subjects must be allowed adequate practice if results are to be useful. A more commonly used test is p-deletion. The subject is presented with a page of closely typed letters in 58 rows of 38 random characters. The test lasts 3 min and the score is the number of lines completed. There seems to be no advantage in the more tedious scoring system of counting the number of 'p's overlooked [12]. Although there is a motor component to this test, it is generally agreed that the crucial step in the process of deleting a 'p' is recognizing it. The test can show significant changes following general anaesthesia [13] and sedation [14]. The perceptual speed test is similar, but the subject marks every character which matches the character at the beginning of that row [15]. This small change seems to remove the learning effect inherent in the p-deletion test. The score is the number of correct responses in 1 min.

Vigilance to sensory inputs is best tested by a simple but boring task. In one such test the subject listens to brief 1 kHz tones which come every 2 s in a background of white noise. These tones usually last for 500 ms, but 375 ms tones are substituted at random, and the subject is required to press a button to show he or she has noticed this. The difference in duration is easy to detect under ideal conditions, but the task is so boring and the short tones so rare (every 40 tones or so) that it is difficult to detect every one. The test is very sensitive but takes at least 10 min to perform. It has demonstrated the effects of oral diazepam, measuring for 1 h [16], but has not been used in recovery studies.

Tests of central processes

Central activity can be subdivided into arousal and integration, processing, short-term memory and learning (or longer term memory) [5]. The simplest and most effective test of overall integrative activity of the central nervous system is critical flicker fusion threshold. If a light is made to flicker at increasing frequency, there comes a time when the observer can no longer detect the flickering; to the observer it seems to be on all the time. Similarly, if the frequency of flickering is reduced from this high value, there is a moment when it appears to start flickering again. The mean of several such critical fusing and flickering frequencies is noted. It is a simple test to apply, there is no practice effect, the equipment required is inexpensive and it can easily be controlled by a computer. It is affected by ambient lighting, pupillary size and the angle subtended by the light at the eye (i.e. the size of the light and its distance from the eye). These problems can be minimized by positioning the light at the end of a long, black, non-reflective tube. The subject peers in from the other end through a small hole 2 mm in diameter. This creates an artificial pupil which negates the effect of changes in pupillary size. As an alternative, the conditions of the test may simply be held constant, and the pupil size measured. This will allow valid comparisons between results provided it can be shown that the pupil size does not vary. Critical flicker fusion has been used to detect statistically significant residual effects of benzodiazepines [17], propofol [18], barbiturates, inhalational agents [19] and opiates [20]. However, some workers have found it difficult to implement, and abandoned its use [21]. Recently a new methodology has been described which is said to be easier to implement [22].

Central processing is easily tested by simple arithmetic tasks. Coin counting is a simple example. The subject is given seven coins and is asked to pick up each in turn, stating its value and the cumulative total. The score is the time taken. This test has been used to discriminate between recovery from propofol, thiopentone and etomidate [23]. Another simple assessment is the serial sevens test, in which the subject is required to repeatedly subtract seven from an initial number [14].

A test of perceptual processing is provided by the digit symbol substitution test (DSST), a subset of the Weschler adult intelligence test. It is a sensitive test of the effect of many drugs on perceptual coding skills [3, 24–27]. The subject is presented with a piece of paper on which the numbers 0 to 9 are matched to simple nonsense symbols. The task is to copy the appropriate symbols into boxes labelled randomly by the ordinary digits. The score is the number of symbols correctly transcribed in a given time. If the test is to be repeated then a new set of symbols must be used to prevent learning effects.

The Stroop phenomenon is the impairment of response caused by a conflict in the stimulus, illustrated by the difficulty reading the word 'pink' if it is presented suddenly written in blue ink. Tests of this phenomenon are said to assess the ability to concentrate, and have been used following general anaesthesia [11, 28].

Short-term memory may be assessed by digit span [29]. A three-digit number is read to the subject, one digit per second, and he or she is immediately asked to repeat it. If the response is correct the subject is tested with another three-digit number, then with the first of two four-digit numbers and so on up to nine-digit numbers (i.e. 14 numbers in all) unless he or she fails both numbers of a given length first. The test is then repeated, but this time the subject has to repeat the numbers backwards. The score is the total number of correct recalls. Recall of numerical information may involve different processes to the recall of words or pictures; these can be assessed by the immediate recall of a list of simple, bland words [30] or a series of pictures of everyday objects [14].

Longer term memory is tested by late recall of events that occurred in the recovery period. Subjects may be shown a standard picture at a fixed time during their recovery and asked to say what it was the following day [31]. In one study, free recall of pictures after several minutes distraction was found to be the most sensitive of the tests applied [14]. Alternatively subjects may be asked to learn word associations; words are read to the subjects in pairs during recovery, and later they are asked to recall the other word in each pair in response to being told the first one. The link between the words may be obvious or random, and the test results obviously vary accordingly [17]. Finally, a deliberate painful stimulus has been used during sedation to assess amnesia [32].

Tests of motor processes

Tests of motor function include finger tapping, body sway, co-ordination and manipulation. Finger tapping is affected by motivation, and so the test should be short—certainly less than 1 min. The detection device should be designed so that it does not interfere with the tapping, as a springy switch might. It has been used following midazolam sedation [27] and general anaesthesia [33]. A test along similar lines requiring rapid supination and pronation of the forearm has also been described and shown to be sensitive to propofol and thiopentone [33].

Body sway can be measured objectively with a simple device described by Vickers [34]. A string is attached to the subject's collar, is run directly backwards to one pulley, turns horizontally to another pulley, and then dangles freely with a small weight at the end. The string runs through a loop on its horizontal path, and as the subject sways backwards and forwards, the loop pushes two loosely attached markers apart. It has been shown sensitive to barbiturate induction agents [34] and benzodiazepines [35]. Wright has designed a portable system for measuring sway [36].

Co-ordination has been assessed by asking the subject to pass a loop along a bent wire without touching the two together [10, 11]. Another psychomotor test battery included blind pointing from nose to a target set in a touch-sensitive screen [33]. These tests have shown significant changes following general anaesthesia and sedation.

An early test of the recovery of manipulation skills was the pegboard test [34]. The subject has to transfer a set of pegs from one end of a pegboard to the other as quickly as possible. Another test requires the subject to transfer ball bearings from one container to another using a pair of tweezers [37]. The score is the number transferred. Impairment of manipulation has also been measured by the time taken to post objects into a child's shape sorter following midazolam or propofol [38]. These tests are all subject to significant learning effects, but are very simple to implement and have been used to demonstrate impairment following general anaesthesia and sedation.

Tests of more than one psychomotor process

Although all the preceding tests must involve sensory, central and motor processes to some extent, they are designed so that one element is rate limiting (e.g. symbol coding in the DSST). Many tests of psychomotor function are more general. Sensory and motor processes are both important in the simple reaction time. In this test a button is pressed as quickly as possible in response to some stimulus, which may be audible (a beep) or more commonly visual (a light coming on). The stimuli appear randomly, and their mean frequency influences the response time. Rapid stimulation occurring every 1–4 s taxes concentration, but if this is extended to intervals of 15 s or more then the subject's vigilance becomes important. It is another test which is inexpensive and easy to computerize. It is simple and quick to perform, and has been used extensively in recovery studies [32, 39–42].

The choice reaction time test presents the subject with an array of four to six lights, each with an adjacent button. Two forms of the test are described. In the first, one light goes out as the subject presses its button and another lights up immediately, so that a jumping light is chased around the apparatus [43]. In the other, the subject waits with his or her finger on a central 'home' button with lights arranged in an arc around it. When one of the lights comes on the subject presses the button next to it as quickly as possible. This technique allows the response to be divided into perceptual and central processing time (the time between the light coming on and the home button being released) and motor time (the time between release of the home button and pressing the target button) [44]. The equipment required for these tests is more sophisticated than is required for the simple response time, but it can easily be incorporated into a computer system. There is a small learning effect. Although it tests more brain function than the simple response test, recent assessments of recovery from anaesthesia using both tests have not found a significant result with the choice reaction test in the absence of a significant result in the simple test [35, 39].

The Trieger dot test requires the subject to draw a figure by joining up dots placed at 12 mm intervals. Sensory processes are involved because the subject needs to be able to 'see' the figure in the dots, and motor co-ordination is needed because the test is scored by measuring deviations from the correct figure. This has been used to investigate the effects of inhalational and intravenous anaesthetics [45, 46] and benzodiazepines [28, 47, 48].

Visuomotor co-ordination has been assessed using tracking tasks. The Lafayette pursuit rotor presents a moving target which the subject has to trace with a photoelectric wand. The score is the length of time required to keep the wand on target for a total of 30 s. More recently tests have been devised which require the subject to track a moving target on a computer screen using a mouse. In maze tracking tasks the subject must draw a path through a maze drawn on a sheet of paper without touching the walls. The Bender Gestalt track tracer is an electric version of this test. The score is determined by the time taken to complete the task and by the number of errors. The rotary pursuit, track tracer and pegboard tests have been compared following general anaesthesia in volunteers [49]. The results of the rotary pursuit and pegboard tests were influenced by training, but the track tracer was found to be free of such effects and was recommended as reliable, valid, objective, non-invasive, inexpensive, easily understood by patients and of short duration.

Sophisticated driving simulators have been used to assess recovery from anaesthesia. The equipment required for a realistic simulation is extremely expensive and is not available to many workers, but it has been used to demonstrate impaired driving skills for 8 h after a single dose of thiopentone or methohexitone [50]. Some of the tests described above can be modified to simulate driving practice by, for example, using foot switches in the reaction time tests or controlling tracking tasks with a steering wheel [51]. There is no evidence that such adaptations provide more useful results.

Physiological tests of recovery

Electroencephalography (EEG) has been used to detect residual drug effects following general anaesthesia. It appears to be a very sensitive technique, being able to detect differences in EEG between propanidid and methohexitone anaesthesia for up to 12 h [52]. The measurements require expensive equipment, careful preparation, at least 15 min recording and skilled interpretation: it is impractical as a routine tool. Auditory evoked potentials have also been used [53]. This technique is less demanding than EEG, but is no more sensitive than critical flicker fusion or choice reaction time following midazolam.

In 1970 Hannington-Kiff used the Maddox Wing test to assess recovery from anaesthesia [54]. This is a quick test of ocular divergence. The subject looks into an instrument in which the two eye fields are separated. The right eye sees an arrow and the left sees a scale, and the subject states where the arrow seems to point to on the scale. The test is affected by opiates [25], benzodiazepines [32] and general anaesthetics [44]. It is sensitive and not subject to learning effects.

Saccadic eye movements (the rapid ocular movements which change the point of gaze form one object to another) can be measured by electro-oculography, using external electrodes. The subject moves his or her gaze from one target to another as quickly as possible, and the latency, acceleration, peak velocity and accuracy of the saccade is measured [55]. Although the test requires specialized equipment, it is simple to perform and is not subject to learning effects. It has been used to assess recovery from general anaesthesia [40].

Choice of tests

How does one choose an objective measure of recovery from anaesthesia? The ideal test will be quick and simple to perform with no learning effect, requiring inexpensive equipment which can be used by an unskilled operator. It will be sensitive to all the residual effects of all drugs used in anaesthesia, and the results will be sufficiently reproducible that firm conclusions may be drawn from individual measurements, perhaps with reference to a preanaesthetic baseline.

There is no ideal test at present. The condition that a test measure all the effects of an anaesthetic cannot be satisfied: it would mean that all conscious, unconscious and automatic processes could be assessed, but these are not as yet identified and understood. We must be content with testing the processes of the psychomotor model with the tools available. It is not necessary to perform every test. A recent study concluded that critical flicker fusion and the processing component of the choice reaction time are probably different measures of the same process, that the tapping test is assessing the same functions as the motor component of the choice reaction time, but that the Maddox Wing and p-deletion each measure other processes [44]. Two other works in which several individual tests have been performed allow plausible conclusions to be drawn about other test equivalences [24, 32], though there is an implicit extension here from group results to the individual. With that proviso it would seem that the Maddox Wing, body sway, tests of co-ordination and 'action judgement' (a steering test) all measure processes of unconscious motor control which are affected equally by thiopentone, propofol and benzodiazepines, and that choice reaction time and divided attention tests are also equivalent when used after these drugs.

A complete set of testable psychomotor functions can be postulated (Fig. 6.1). It would comprise perception, co-ordination and central activity (which would always be more sensitive to drug effects than conscious motor processes). It remains to choose tests for each. Tests of co-ordination least affected by practice are the Maddox Wing, body sway and possibly saccadic eye movements, though there is as yet little experience with this test during the period of recovery from general anaesthetics. Pure sensory processes could be assessed by inspection time but this too is new to recovery studies, as is vigilance testing. The best established tests for this function are probably the perceptual speed test and p-deletion, but inspection time or block pattern recognition may supplant them. There are several independently testable central processes, and there are few tests of these which are free of learning effects. Most workers have found that critical flicker fusion gives repeatable results, and digit symbol substitution is another sensitive test, independent of flicker fusion [3]. Visual analogue scales could be included in this category as a measure of subjective experience. The problem of finding a test of memory is even more difficult. There is no established test covering all aspects of memory, and none of those described above has clear advantages over others. Furthermore, the inevitable effects of practice makes the interpretation of any individual's results difficult. Tests of memory, more than any other tests of recovery, only indicate failure to recover.

In summary, if a psychomotor test suite comprising body sway, inspection time, critical flicker fusion, digit symbol substitution and a picture recall test was used for a study of recovery from anaesthesia, it is unlikely that additional tests would reveal an effect not shown by that suite, except possibly in particular aspects of memory.

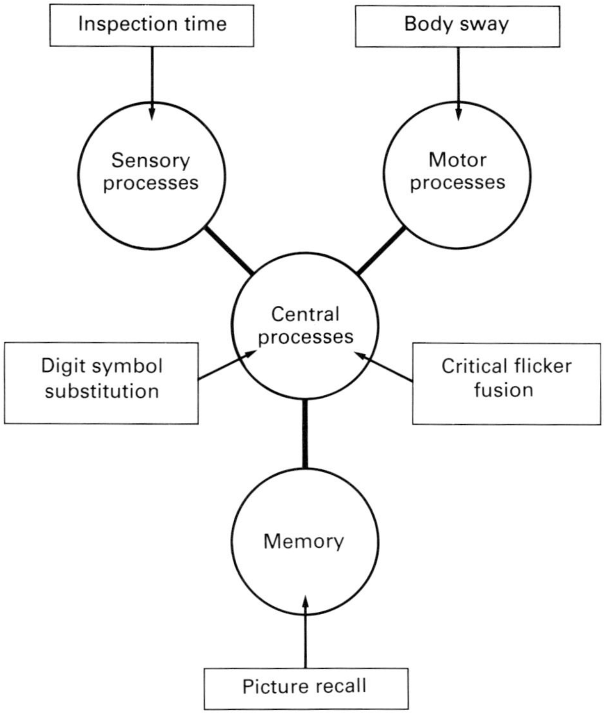

Fig. 6.1 An idealized model of human psychomotor function, with a postulated minimal test set for its objective assessment. Though a great oversimplification, it is unlikely that a clinical study of recovery from general anaesthesia and sedation would detect residual impairment which was not demonstrated by the illustrated test suite.

The role of psychomotor tests

In practice, the decision to discharge patients after day surgery is commonly taken by nursing staff without formal testing. Provided that the patient's initial recovery is grossly satisfactory, he or she will be discharged at the usual time for that list, with a reluctance to allow discharge earlier even if the patient seems to be of perfectly sound mind. The particular arrangements in any hospital are established on the basis of clinical judgement and common sense and are deemed to be reasonable and safe. If it were proposed to introduce an objective test to allow discharge for those patients who seem to be ready earlier than average, how could the test be validated? It could never be certain that the test assessed all aspects of mental function, and if a patient discharged early was to suffer an accident on the way home, they might blame the hospital. The possibility of expensive litigation will be an effective deterrent against the introduction of such a test.

If, on the other hand, a test was introduced to ensure that patients discharged by the usual criteria were indeed ready to leave the hospital, would if find favour then? As it could only prolong patient stay and block beds, it would not be considered useful by those holding department budgets and in any case, if one had to chose between the long-standing arrangements and the result of a new test, most would go along with established wisdom. It seems that there is no role for psychomotor tests in deciding the time of discharge of individual patients.

What, then, is the place of such testing? It is to enable comparison between treatment regimens. If a new anaesthetic technique is associated with a more rapid recovery of psychomotor function than the current standard, it is a fair assumption that the higher intellectual functions will return more rapidly too. If the new technique was adopted by the institution, it would be in a position to reconsider its guidelines for discharging patients.

It is probable that no day patient has fully recovered from anaesthetic at the time of discharge. Street fitness is an ill-defined term meaning that the patient has recovered enough to be discharged unaccompanied from the day unit. (In practice, most units insist on an escort.) It implies that the subject is able to cross roads and use public transport, but he or she is forbidden to drive or use heavy machinery for 24 h, at which time recovery is assumed to be complete. The essential feature of a street-fit patient is the ability to make decisions about everyday events under everyday circumstances. The decision of when to cross a road safely is vital, but how is this ability to be assessed prior to discharge? Decision-making was not one of the testable psychomotor functions discussed above, and the relationship between it and any of those tests is at best obscure. It is hard to see how any objective test could fulfil this role, as its very performance would remove the patient from the everyday circumstances he or she will be operating in later. Even more difficult is the problem of when recovery is sufficient to allow resumption of everyday duties—this will clearly depend upon the patient's occupation. For the time being, these matters remain in the realm of clinical judgement.

References

1 White PF. Studies of desflurane in outpatient anesthesia. *Anesth Analg* 1992; 75 (suppl 4): S47–53.

2 Steward DJ. A simplified scoring system for the postoperative recovery room. *Canad Anaesth Soc J* 1975; 22: 111–13.

3 Armstrong PJ, Morrison LM, Noble D, Sinclair WA, Tiplady B, Wildsmith JA. Effects of i.v. lignocaine on psychological performance and subjective state in healthy volunteers. *Br J Anaesth* 1991; 67: 532–8.

4 Short TG, Galletly DC. Residual psychomotor effects following reversal of midazolam sedation with flumazenil. *Anaesth Intens Care* 1989; 17: 290–7.

5 Hindmarch I. Psychomotor function and psychoactive drugs. *Br J Clin Pharmacol* 1980; 10: 189–209.

6 Marshall CA, Jones RM, Bajorek PK, Cashman JN. Recovery characteristics using isoflurane or propofol for maintenance of anaesthesia: a double-blind controlled trial. *Anaesthesia* 1992; 47: 461–6.

7 Deary IJ. Inspection time. In: Klepper ID, Sanders LD, Rosen M, eds. *Ambulatory Anaesthesia and Sedation. Impairment and Recovery*. Oxford: Blackwell Scientific Publications, 1991: 129–39.

8 Sanders LD, Whitehead C, Gildersleve CD, Rosen M, Robinson JO. Interaction of H_2-receptor antagonists and benzodiazepine sedation. *Anaesthesia* 1993; 48: 286–92.

9 Larsen LE, Gupta A, Ledin T, Doolan M, Linder P, Lennmarken C. Psychomotor recovery following propofol or isoflurane anaesthesia for day-care surgery. *Acta Anaesth Scand* 1992; 36: 276–82.
10 Sanders LD, Davies Evans J, Rosen M, Robinson JO. Comparison of diazepam with midazolam as i.v. sedation for outpatient gastroscopy. *Br J Anaesth* 1989; 63: 726–31.
11 Sanders LD, Isaac PA, Yeomans WA, Clyburn PA, Rosen M, Robinson JO. Propofol-induced anaesthesia. Double-blind comparison of recovery after anaesthesia induced by propofol or thiopentone. *Anaesthesia* 1989; 44: 200–4.
12 Dixon RA, Thornton JA. Tests of recovery from anaesthesia and sedation: Intravenous diazepam in dentistry. *Br J Anaesth* 1973; 45: 207–15.
13 Wrigley SR, Fairfield JE, Jones RM, Black AE. Induction and recovery characteristics of desflurane in day case patients: a comparison with propofol. *Anaesthesia* 1991; 46: 615–22.
14 Kestin IG, Harvey PB, Nixon C. Psychomotor recovery after three methods of sedation during spinal anaesthesia. *Br J Anaesth* 1990; 64: 675–81.
15 Gelfman SS, Gracely RM, Driscoll EJ, Wirdzek PR, Butler DP, Sweet JB. Recovery following intravenous sedation during dental surgery performed under local anesthesia. *Anesth Analg* 1980; 59: 775–81.
16 Hart J, Hill HM, Bye CE, Wilkinson RT, Peck AW. The effects of low doses of amylobarbitone sodium and diazepam human performance. *Br J Clin Pharmacol* 1976; 3: 289–98.
17 Sanders LD, Piggott SE, Isaac PA, Okell RW, Roberts B, Rosen M, Robinson JO. Reversal of benzodiazepine sedation with the antagonist flumazenil. *Br J Anaesth* 1991; 66: 445–53.
18 Hickey S, Asbury AJ, Millar K. Psychomotor recovery after outpatient anaesthesia: individual impairment may be masked by group analysis. *Br J Anaesth* 1991; 66: 345–52.
19 Fletcher JE, Sebel PS, Murphy MR, Smith CA, Mick SA, Flister MP. Psychomotor performance after desflurane anesthesia: a comparison with isoflurane. *Anesth Analg* 1991; 73: 260–5.
20 Wall RJ, Zacharias M. Effects of alfentanil on induction and recovery from propofol anaesthesia in day surgery. *Anaesth Intens Care* 1990; 18: 214–18.
21 Cashman JN, Power SJ. An evaluation of tests of psychomotor function in assessing recovery following a brief anaesthetic. *Acta Anaesth Scand* 1989; 33: 693–7.
22 Salib Y, Plourde G, Alloul K, Provost A, Moore A. Measuring recovery from general anaesthesia. *Can J Anaesth* 1992; 39: 1045–50.
23 Boysen K, Sanchez R, Krintel JJ, Hansen M, Haar PM, Dyrberg V. Induction and recovery characteristics of propofol, thiopental and etomidate. *Acta Anaesth Scand* 1989; 33: 689–92.
24 Korttila K, Nuotto EJ, Lichtor JL, Ostman PL, Apfelbaum J, Rupani G. Clinical recovery and psychomotor function after brief anesthesia with propofol or thiopental. *Anesthesiology* 1992; 76: 676–81.
25 Zacny JP, Lichtor JL, de Wit H. Subjective, behavioral, and physiologic response to intravenous dezocine in healthy volunteers. *Anesth Analg* 1992; 74: 523–30.
26 Ghouri AF, Bodner M, White PF. Recovery profile after desflurane–nitrous oxide versus isoflurane–nitrous oxide in outpatients. *Anesthesiology* 1991; 74: 419–24.
27 Birch BR, Anson K, Gelister J, Parker C, Miller RA. The role of midazolam and flumazenil in urology. *Acta Anaesth Scand* 1990; 92 (suppl): 25–32.
28 Sanders LD, Clyburn PA, Rosen M, Robinson JO. Propofol in short gynaecological procedures. Comparison of recovery over 2 days after anaesthesia with propofol or thiopentone as sole anaesthetic agent. *Anaesthesia* 1991; 46: 451–5.
29 Dyck JB, Chung F. A comparison of propranolol and diazepam for preoperative anxiolysis. *Canad J Anaesth* 1991; 38: 704–9.
30 Korttila K, Ghoneim MM, Jacobs L, Mewaldt SP, Petersen RC. Time course of mental and psychomotor effects of 30 per cent nitrous oxide during inhalation and recovery. *Anesthesiology* 1981; 54: 220–6.

31 Shafer A, White PF, Urquhart ML, Doze VA. Outpatient premedication: use of midazolam and opioid analgesics. *Anesthesiology* 1989; 71: 495–501.
32 Nuotto EJ, Korttila KT, Lichtor JL, Ostman PL, Rupani G. Sedation and recovery of psychomotor function after intravenous administration of various doses of midazolam and diazepam. *Anesth Analg* 1992; 74: 265–71.
33 Ryom C, Flarup M, Suadicani P, Palm T, Mikkelsen S, Gyntelberg F. Recovery following thiopentone or propofol anaesthesia assessed by computerized coordination measurements. *Acta Anaesth Scand* 1992; 36: 540–5.
34 Vickers MD. Measurement of recovery from anaethesia. *Br J Anaesth* 1965; 37: 296–302.
35 Lichtor JL, Zacny J, Apfelbaum JL *et al.* Alcohol after sedation with i.v. midazolam–fentanyl: effects on psychomotor functioning. *Br J Anaesth* 1991; 67: 579–84.
36 Wright BM. A simple mechanical ataxia-meter. *J Physiol* 1971; 281: 27S–8S.
37 Short TG, Galletly DC. Residual psychomotor effects following reversal of midazolam sedation with flumazenil. *Anaesth Intens Care* 1989; 17: 290–7.
38 Vuyk J, Hennis PJ, Burm AG, de Voogt JW, Spierdijk J. Comparison of midazolam and propofol in combination with alfentanil for total intravenous anesthesia. *Anesth Analg* 1990; 71: 645–50.
39 Nightingale JJ, Lewis IH. Recovery from day-case anaesthesia: comparison of total i.v. anaesthesia using propofol with an inhalation technique. *Br J Anaesth* 1992; 68: 356–9.
40 Bellaiche S, Bonnet F, Sperandio M, Lerouge P, Cannet G, Roujas F. Clonidine does not delay recovery from anaesthesia. *Br J Anaesth* 1991; 66: 353–7.
41 Boysen K, Sanchez R, Ravn J, Pedersen E, Krintel JJ, Dyrberg V. Comparison of induction with and first hour of recovery from brief propofol and methohexital anesthesia. *Acta Anaesth Scand* 1990; 34: 212–15.
42 Cashman JN, Power SJ. An evaluation of tests of psychomotor function in assessing recovery following a brief anaesthetic. *Acta Anaesth Scand* 1989; 33: 693–7.
43 Scott WA, Whitwam JG, Wilkinson RT. Choice reaction time. A method of measuring postoperative psychomotor performance decrements. *Anaesthesia* 1983; 38: 1162–8.
44 Zuurmond WW, Balk VA, van Dis H, van Leeuwen L, Paul EA. Multidimensionality of psychological recovery from anaesthesia. Analysing six recovery tests. *Anaesthesia* 1989; 44: 889–92.
45 Randel GI, Levy L, Kothary SP, Pandit SK. Propofol versus thiamylal–enflurane anesthesia for outpatient laparoscopy. *J Clin Anesth* 1992; 4: 185–9.
46 Kashtan H, Edelist G, Mallon J, Kapala D. Comparative evaluation of propofol and thiopentone for total intravenous anaesthesia. *Can J Anaesth* 1990; 37: 170–6.
47 Norton AC, Dundas CR. Induction agents for day-case anaesthesia. A double-blind comparison of propofol and midazolam antagonised by flumazenil. *Anaesthesia* 1990; 45: 198–203.
48 Young ER, Kestenberg SH, Toal CB. The effect of flumazenil on the recovery time of dental patients sedated with diazepam. *Anesth Prog* 1989; 36: 46–51.
49 Denis R, Letourneau JE, Londorf D. Reliability and validity of psychomotor tests as measures of recovery from isoflurane or enflurane anesthesia in a day-care surgery unit. *Anesth Analg* 1984; 63: 653–6.
50 Kortilla K, Linnoila M, Ertama P, Hakkinen S. Recovery and simulated driving after intravenous anesthesia with thiopental, methohexital, propanidid, or alphadione. *Anesthesiology* 1975; 43: 291–9.
51 Korttila K, Linnoila M. Skills related to driving after intravenous diazepam, flunitrazepam or droperidol. *Br J Anaesth* 1974; 46: 961–9.
52 Doenicke A, Kugler J, Schellenberger A, Gurtner TL. The use of electroencephalography to measure recovery time after intravenous anaesthesia. *Br J Anaesth* 1986; 38: 580–90.

53 Milligan KR, Lumsden J, Howard RC, Howe JP, Dundee JW. Use of auditory evoked responses as a measure of recovery from benzodiazepine sedation. *J Roy Soc Med* 1989; 82: 595–7.
54 Hannington-Kiff JG. Measurement of recovery from outpatient general anaesthesia with a simple ocular test. *Br Med J* 1970; 3: 132–5.
55 Griffiths AN, Marshall RW, Richens A. Saccadic eye movement analysis as a measure of drug effects on human psychomotor performance. *Br J Clin Pharmacol* 1984: 18: 73S–82S.

Chapter 7
Safe Endoscopy

E. B. Keeffe

Gastrointestinal (GI) endoscopy remains remarkably safe, in spite of the proliferation of new procedures and the extraordinary increase in the performance of endoscopy over the past 30 years [1]. A number of large retrospective surveys document low complication rates for specific endoscopic procedures (Table 7.1) [2–11]. These reports may suffer from a number of deficiencies such as falsely low reported complication rates (from retrospective methodology, or from failure to record complications occurring after discharge from the endoscopy unit), local institutional experiences not representative of general endoscopic practice, and inclusion of older data from the earlier experience with endoscopy when complications may have been more frequent. On balance, however, the figures in Table 7.1 are reasonably representative and reproducible among different surveys. It is also apparent in this tabulation of complications that each procedure may have its own inherent complication rate, e.g. diagnostic procedures are safer than therapeutic procedures, and upper endoscopy is safer than endoscopic retrograde cholangiopancreatography (ERCP) [12]. In addition, complications may be arbitrarily divided into those that are procedure-related (e.g. bleeding, perforation) or those that are generic to endoscopy (e.g. cardiopulmonary adverse events related to conscious sedation). This chapter will focus on the generic aspects of endoscopic safety and avoid discussion of the technical complications of specific endoscopic procedures.

In spite of the low complication rate associated with the performance of most endoscopic procedures, it is certainly feasible that the practice of endoscopy may be made yet safer by attention to all aspects of the safe performance of endoscopy (Table 7.2) [12]. This chapter will review and update potential factors that have been proposed as determinants of the safety of endoscopy, particularly sedation and monitoring protocols and standardization of endoscopic training and practice [12]. In this analysis, it will become apparent that some of the determinants of the safe performance of endoscopy are relatively fixed, e.g. the specific procedure being performed or the medical condition of the patient, while other determinants are variable, e.g. who performs the procedure or what conscious sedation or monitoring are used. Much of this review of the safety of endoscopy is based on the consensus opinion of endoscopists expressing themselves in textbooks, journals or endoscopy society practice guidelines, rather than scientific data.

Table 7.1 Complications of upper endoscopy and colonoscopy. Modified from [1]. Estimated average figures from large retrospective reviews [2–11]

Procedure	Major complication (%)	Death (%)
Upper endoscopy		
diagnostic	0·2	0·01
oesophageal dilation*	0·5	0·01
variceal sclerotherapy	8·0	1·5
Colonoscopy		
diagnostic	0·4	0·02
polypectomy	2·0	0·05

* Mercury bougies or metal olives; pneumatic dilation excluded.

Table 7.2 Potential determinants of the safe performance of endoscopy. Modified from [12]

What	Procedure is performed
	diagnostic vs. therapeutic
	Conscious sedation or anaesthesia is used
	benzodiazepine alone vs. with narcotic
	bolus vs. titration
	Supplemental oxygen is provided
	Level of monitoring is employed
	personnel (GI nurse) assisting
	electronic equipment (oximetry, ECG) used
	resuscitation equipment available
Who	Undergoes endoscopy
	young vs. elderly
	medically fit vs. unfit
	consultation vs. checklist
	antibiotic prophylaxis used appropriately
	Performs endoscopy
	training and experience
	competence and judgment
Why	Endoscopy is performed
	indicated vs. contraindicated
Where	Endoscopy is performed
	fully staffed hospital endoscopy unit vs. small hospital vs. clinic or office
	elective (endoscopy unit) vs. emergency (ICU or other hospital ward)
How	The patient is recovered
	The outpatient is discharged

ECG, electrocardiogram; GI, gastrointestinal; ICU, intensive care unit.

Procedure-related safety

Each endoscopic procedure has its own safety record, which is documented by published complication rates that usually fall within a narrow range. Specific complication rates vary from one endoscopic procedure to another and predictably depend upon whether the procedure is simple or complex, and whether it is diagnostic or therapeutic (see Table 7.1). It is certainly possible that these usual complication rates might be lowered by attention to the factors outlined in Table 7.2, such as limiting the performance of endoscopy to individuals who have completed full training, having qualified GI nurses to assist during endoscopy and adhering to proper conscious sedation and monitoring recommendations. In addition, further improvements in endoscopic instrumentation and techniques might further lower the complication rates of specific procedures. The recent emergence of quality assurance programmes may provide better future data on complication rates of procedures that are performed using current practices and equipment.

Choice of conscious sedation or anaesthesia

Conscious sedation, the use of intravenous (i.v.) drugs, primarily benzodiazepines in combination with narcotics, to produce a state of depressed consciousness which will facilitate the performance of both diagnostic and therapeutic endoscopic procedures, has become standard practice in most countries. Conscious sedation is defined as a state of depressed consciousness that allows protective reflexes to be maintained, permits the patient to maintain independently a patent airway, and leaves intact appropriate responses to physical or verbal stimulation [13]. Deep sedation is defined by the condition in which the patient is not easily aroused but can independently maintain a patent airway and respond to stimulation.

Even though GI endoscopy, particularly esophagogastroduodenoscopy (EGD), can be performed without conscious sedation, surveys in the USA [14, 15] and the UK [16] indicate that both endoscopists and patients prefer premedications. Some reasons to use sedation include allaying anxiety regarding the procedure, assuring co-operation with manoeuvres performed during endoscopy, and facilitating compliance with repeat procedures when necessary [17]. A membership survey of the American Society for Gastrointestinal Endoscopy (ASGE) of endoscopic sedation and monitoring practices conducted in 1989 confirmed that most American endoscopists routinely use sedation for endoscopic procedures, excluding flexible sigmoidoscopy [14]. Drugs used regularly included meperidine (pethidine, demerol) (87%), midazolam (73%), diazepam (49%) and naloxone (30%). Midazolam was used approximately twice as often as diazepam, a preference confirmed by a later survey from the USA [15]. The majority of endoscopists had intravenous access established prior to endoscopy, and medications were typically administered by the endoscopist (83%) or by a GI nurse (43%). The later survey also found that approximately 65% of endoscopists use a benzodiazepine in combination with an opioid, typically meperidine [15]. In contrast to these American surveys, reports from Iraq and Greece demonstrate that diagnostic EGD can be adequately performed without sedation in 94–98% of patients [18, 19]. Whether or not the performance of upper endoscopy without sedation decreases complications is unknown. In fact, patient co-operation induced by conscious sedation may decrease morbidity, particularly complications related directly to instrumentation. On the other hand, data which demonstrate that more than 50% of deaths from EGD are related to cardiopulmonary complications suggest that endoscopy without sedation may in fact be safer [20].

As noted in national surveys and published literature reviews, medications typically used for GI endoscopy are administered intravenously and include benzodiazepines, either diazepam or midazolam, given alone or with an opioid such as meperidine [14–16, 20, 21]. In routine practice, the combination of a benzodiazepine with meperidine is most often used for colonoscopy, therapeutic EGD and ERCP. Many endoscopists are not aware of the major drug interaction between these agents and the attendant increased incidence of respiratory depression, or of the need to substantially reduce the dosage of both drugs when used together [15, 17, 20, 22–24]. In the survey of complications of endoscopy by Arrowsmith *et al.* (1991) only two factors were associated with an increased risk of cardiorespiratory complications: (a) the combination of a benzodiazepine and opioid for conscious sedation; and (b) the performance of an emergent procedure [15]. In a study published in the anaesthesia literature, none of 12 healthy volunteers developed hypoxaemia ($SaO_2 < 90\%$) or apnoea when midazolam was given alone; six of 12 developed hypoxaemia with fentanyl alone; and 11 of 12 volunteers developed hypoxaemia and six of 12 had apnoea with the administration of both drugs in combination [25]. In the practice of endoscopy, it is generally recommended that the opioid be given first when both agents are being used intravenously, that a reduced dose of opioid (25% of usual) be used, and that 3–5 min be allowed for the opioid to take effect before the reduced dose of benzodiazepine (25% of usual) is administered [23, 24].

The technique of drug administration used for conscious sedation is also likely an important factor related to the safety of endoscopy. For example, bolus administration of midazolam is associated with greater oxygen desaturation than administration by slow titration [26]. The preferred titration rate of each drug used for conscious sedation that will minimize hypoxaemia is not known, and adjustments must be made according to the age and condition of the patient. If a bolus technique is used for conscious sedation, it is recommended that only one-half to two-thirds of the usual dose required when using the titration technique be administered [24]. It also has been recommended that endoscopists revise their previously used sedation end-points of ptosis and hypnosis to anxiolysis and amnesia, i.e. a patient with eyes open rather than closed in sleep [17]. Many endoscopists do not appreciate that an unco-operative and restless patient after sedation is more likely to be oversedated and/or hypoxaemic rather than undersedated.

A final factor regarding conscious sedation that impacts safety is training and experience with the drugs that are commonly used to sedate patients. A needed innovation that would likely increase the safety of endoscopy is the development of a formal curriculum in GI endoscopy training programmes in conscious sedation, including drug pharmacokinetics, drug interactions, end-points, reversal agents, monitoring and response protocols for specific adverse events.

A decrease in oxygen saturation is one of many physiological changes that may occur during GI endoscopy [22]. Several studies have demonstrated that oxygen saturation decreases during EGD and colonoscopy, but it is surprising that no correlation is generally seen between the fall in oxygen saturation and the type or dose of medication used and the age or sex of the patient [22]. On the other hand, a fall in oxygen saturation has been related to the use of larger diameter upper endoscopes, the combination of an opioid and benzodiazepine and the presence of chronic pulmonary disease [22].

The impact of using preoxygenation 1–2 min before an endoscopic procedure with supplemental oxygen during endoscopy, or supplemental oxygen alone, on the safety of endoscopy is unknown. It is clear that significant hypoxaemia during upper and lower endoscopic procedures can be prevented by preoxygenation and/or supplemental nasal oxygen during the procedure [27–29]. Age, anaemia and obesity are independent risk factors for the occurrence of arterial oxygen desaturation during EGD [30]. Since the majority of patients breath through the mouth rather than the nose as soon as the endoscope is passed into the oesophagus [31], oral oxygen delivery systems have been developed and studied [32, 33]. In one study, oxygen administration via a mouth guard alleviated but did not prevent hypoxia [32]. In another study, delivery of oxygen via the oral route was as effective as delivery via nasal cannulae [33]. In addition, the latter study showed that preoxygenation for 1–2 min before endoscopy significantly reduced episodes of desaturation as defined by $SaO_2 < 90\%$.

Some endoscopists recommend that prevention of hypoxaemia by use of supplemental oxygen is preferable to correction of hypoxaemia after it occurs, and preoxygenation or supplemental oxygen should be considered not only in high-risk subjects but also in all patients undergoing endoscopy [34]. The weight of published studies indicates that 2–3 l of supplemental oxygen is safe, with the only exception being patients with severe chronic obstructive pulmonary disease [35]. It remains to be proven whether or not these different strategies will impact the rate of cardiopulmonary complications associated with endoscopy.

The level of monitoring employed

The standard monitoring of patients undergoing GI endoscopy traditionally has included clinical assessment of tolerance to the procedure and the determination of vital signs at variable times before, during and after the procedure [36]. Ideally, monitoring should be carried out by a qualified GI nurse whose primary responsibility is monitoring the patient rather than assisting the endoscopist with the technical aspects of the procedure [36, 37]. Complex or therapeutic endoscopic procedures generally require two GI nurses, one nurse to attend the patient and another nurse to assist the endoscopist [36, 37].

In recent years, there has been an expanded use of electronic monitoring equipment during endoscopy, particularly pulse oximetry and continuous electrocardiography (ECG), even though their usefulness and impact on the safety of endoscopy remains unknown and may be impossible to prove scientifically given the very low baseline rate of cardiopulmonary complications [14, 15, 22]. At the time of the ASGE survey in 1989, 65% of endoscopists used pulse oximetry and 55% used continuous ECG monitoring [14]. A disturbing finding from this study was an apparent double standard, i.e. most electronic monitoring was done in hospitals (99·5%) rather than in private offices (27%). Although the majority of endoscopists use electronic monitoring selectively for high-risk patients, 42% used it universally for all patients. Finally, another disturbing finding from the ASGE survey was that only 76% of endoscopists were certified in basic life support and 30% in advanced life support techniques, a deficiency whose correction might also influence the safety of endoscopy.

Since this survey, a number of factors have influenced the standard of care for monitoring during conscious sedation, including the standards for anaesthesia care promulgated by the Joint Commission on Accreditation of Healthcare Organizations (JCAHO), the standards for basic intraoperative monitoring of the American Society of Anesthesiologists (ASA), as well as state regulations and the standards of insurance carriers in the USA [13, 38]. It is generally now believed that electronic monitoring should be used universally for all patients and for all endoscopic procedures performed using conscious sedation [39].

The ASGE and the British Society of Gastroenterology (BSG) have published guidelines for sedation and monitoring [36, 37]. The key elements of the ASGE guideline are as follows:

1 The use of electronic monitoring equipment may be helpful addition but should not be a substitute for clinical assessment.

2 Standard clinical monitoring should include the determination of heart rate, blood pressure and respiratory rate before sedation, immediately after the endoscopic procedure, and at the time of discharge from endoscopy unit.

3 The appropriate role of pulse oximetry and continuous ECG monitoring during endoscopic procedures is evolving.

4 Pulse oximetry and ECG monitoring may be beneficial for certain high-risk patients and/or procedures.

The BSG recommendations regarding sedation and monitoring during GI endoscopy are stronger and more specific [32]. Recommendations are as follows:

1 Monitoring should be a part of a quality assurance programme.

2 Resuscitation equipment and drugs must be available in endoscopy and recovery areas.

3 All endoscopy staff should be trained in resuscitation methods.
4 A qualified nurse should monitor the patient's condition during procedures.
5 Risk factors should be identified prior to endoscopy by a checklist.
6 Dosage of drugs used for sedation should be kept to a minimum.
7 Antagonists for benzodiazepines and opioids should be available.
8 Intravenous access should be established for 'at risk' patients.
9 Supplemental oxygen is recommended for 'at risk' patients.
10 Monitoring techniques such as pulse oximetry are recommended.
11 Clinical monitoring of the patient must be continued into the recovery area.

In addition to the recommendations of these two societies, the American Academy of Pediatrics has published a guideline for the management and monitoring of the paediatric patient undergoing conscious sedation [40]. The choice of sedative agents and doses employed for paediatric patients is less uniform than for adults, and adherence to this guideline may enhance the safety of endoscopy in the paediatric population.

Taking into account these published guidelines and personal experience, as well as current information regarding technical monitoring [41], appropriate current sedation

Table 7.3 Recommendations for sedation and monitoring during gastrointestinal endoscopy. Modified from [41]

Standard endoscopy unit quality assurance programme in place
Written endoscopy unit protocol regarding sedation and monitoring established
Code cart with equipment and drugs, including opioid and benzodiazepine reversal agents, present in endoscopy unit
Personnel trained in cardiopulmonary resuscitation and advanced cardiac life support
Prior consultation or patient checklist for risk factors performed
One or two nurses in attendance during endoscopy, including one nurse continuously responsible for clinical monitoring
Running intravenous line established
Routine clinical monitoring performed
Electronic monitoring with pulse oximetry used routinely, and blood pressure, heart rate and ECG monitoring used selectively
Drugs used for sedation given in minimal doses and small increments
Opioids (25% of usual dose) given before benzodiazepine (25% of usual dose), waiting 3–5 min between drugs, when both drugs used together
If SaO_2 falls below 90%, regardless of patient's appearance
withhold further drugs
stimulate patient verbally and/or physically
if patient not on oxygen, administer nasal or oral oxygen
If patient is receiving supplemental oxygen, do not equate $SaO_2 > 90\%$ with adequate ventilation—if even transient $SaO_2 < 90\%$ occurs while patient is receiving oxygen supplementation, patient is severely hypoventilating and further sedation should be withheld
Standard postprocedure protocol for monitoring and discharge established—monitor patient with pulse oximetry until $SaO_2 > 90\%$ and stable

ECG, electrocardiogram.

and monitoring practices for endoscopy, in the opinion of the author, are outlined in Table 7.3.

Who undergoes endoscopy?

The safety of an endoscopic procedure is obviously dependent upon the medical condition of the patient undergoing the procedure. A young and medically stable patient is likely to tolerate an endoscopic procedure better than an elderly or unstable patient. Endoscopists typically assess risk based on prior consultation or immediate preprocedure evaluation by checklist. The risk of endoscopy, however, might be better defined by routine use of standard risk classifications, such as ASA physical status or APACHE II score [42, 43].

The importance of familiarity with the patient's medical history prior to a procedure on the overall safety of endoscopy is uncertain. An endoscopic procedure might be performed on a patient seen beforehand for complete consultation or on a patient who is new to the endoscopist and simply completes a brief checklist immediately prior to the procedure. The typical checklist contains facts such as current medications, allergies, bleeding disorders, infectious disease, and heart or lung disease. It is possible that performance of a full consultation rather than completion of a brief checklist would increase the safety of a procedure, particularly for older patients, patients with significant chronic illnesses or patients undergoing more than routine diagnostic EGD.

The education, reassurance and preparation of patients before endoscopy may also be factors that are important for safe endoscopy. Certainly education allays anxiety and may enhance patient co-operation and the likelihood of an uncomplicated procedure. An empty stomach or clean colon facilitates a smoother, and probably safer, endoscopy or colonoscopy. Avoidance of aspirin or non-steroidal anti-inflammatory drugs for several days prior to endoscopy may decrease the incidence of bleeding after manoeuvres such as polypectomy or sphincterotomy. Finally, special considerations, such as protecting the airway during massive upper GI bleeding, may prevent specific procedural complications such as aspiration pneumonia.

Identification of patients who warrant antibiotic prophylaxis is another factor that may contribute to the safety of endoscopy, although the effectiveness of prophylaxis has never been established by controlled trials [44]. Moreover, reports of bacterial endocarditis following GI endoscopy are exceedingly rare. In fact, whether or not endoscopy is a real risk factor for endocarditis is even debated. Although the benefit of using prophylactic antibiotics for the prevention of bacterial endocarditis has not been clearly established, adherence to standard recommendations, such as those of the American Heart Association [44] or a consensus of several societies [45–48], seems appropriate (Table 7.4). Fortunately, current recommendations are more simplified than previous recommendations. There is growing consensus that only patients with high-risk cardiac conditions (prosthetic heart valves or a history of bacterial endocarditis) or lower risk cardiac patients undergoing procedures having a high risk

Table 7.4 Consensus recommendations for antibiotic prophylaxis of bacterial endocarditis prior to endoscopic procedures [45–48]. Modified from [44]

Condition	Endoscopic procedure(s)
Antibiotic prophylaxis recommended	
High-risk cardiac condition prosthetic heart valves previous bacterial endocarditis	All endoscopic procedures*
Low-risk cardiac condition most congenital cardiac malformations rheumatic and other acquired valvular disease hypertrophic cardiomyopathy mitral valve prolapse with valvular regurgitation or echocardiographic findings of thickening or redundancy of the leaflets	Only oesophageal dilatation and variceal schlerotherapy†
Surgically constructed systemic pulmonary shunts	All endoscopic procedures†
Vascular prosthetic graft within 1 year of initial placement	All endoscopic procedures†
Known/suspected obstruction of the biliary tree	ERCP**
Need for feeding tube placement	PEG/PEJ‡
Antibiotic prophylaxis optional	
Leukopenia or immunosuppression (transplant recipients)	All endoscopic procedures§
Cirrhosis with ascites	All endoscopic procedures, especially variceal sclerotherapy and oesophageal dilation ‖
Antibiotic prophylaxis not routinely recommended	
Cardiac conditions other than those listed above	
Orthopaedic prostheses	
Other non-cardiac and non-vascular prostheses	

* Single dose of parenteral ampicillin 2·0 g and gentamicin 1·5 mg kg^{-1} (not to exceed 80 mg), 30 min prior to procedure (vancomycin, 1 g, infused i.v. over 1 h, should be substituted for the ampicillin/penicillin-allergic patient); followed by oral amoxicillin 1·5 g 6 h after initial dose; alternately, the parenteral regimen may be repeated once 8 h after initial dose.

† For these lower risk patients, an alternative oral regimen of amoxicillin 3·0 g 1 h before procedure, followed by 1·5 g 6 h after initial dose is acceptable.

** A parenteral aminoglycoside and cephalosoprin 1–2 h before the procedure and 8–12 h later if obstruction is confirmed; if drainage is inadequate, antibiotics are continued until obstruction is relieved.

‡ A single dose of parenteral cefazolin 1 g 30 min prior to the procedure.

for bacteraemia (sclerotherapy and oesophageal dilation) warrant prophylactic antibiotics.

Who performs endoscopy?

Endoscopic training and experience are major determinants of subsequent competence in practice. Physicians and surgeons who practice GI endoscopy should meet a number of standards related to training, practice, hospital privileges, continuing education and performance review [49]. The specific methods of granting hospital privileges to perform GI endoscopy, including minimum numbers of procedures performed in training and the role of proctoring, has been published by the ASGE [50, 51]. Physicians who perform endoscopy in out-of-hospital locations, e.g. private offices, should meet all of the same requirements for the performance of endoscopy in hospitals.

The Standards of Training Committee of the ASGE has analysed the training process in depth and recently published a revised guideline defining how endoscopic skills are gradually acquired under appropriate supervision, which is initially complete and later periodic [52]. Training in standard GI endoscopic procedures (e.g. EGD, colonoscopy) is distinguished from advanced training (e.g. ERCP), and it may be appropriate that trainees who qualify for advanced endoscopic training extend their period of training for an additional year and that this advanced training be recognized by a formal third-tier certification [52, 53]. The most controversial aspect of the ASGE document on training is the definition of a relatively high threshold number of procedures below which it would be unlikely that trainees could acquire adequate skill and experience to be considered competent. This recommendation has in fact been supported by a prospective, cross-sectional study in a training programme which demonstrated that more than 100 supervised EGDs or colonoscopies were necessary to achieve technical competence [54]. For example, oesophageal intubation did not reach 90% until more than 100 EGDs were performed, and caecal intubation remained at 84% after 100 procedures were done. This study is an important first step in the study of training and competence, even though cognitive endoscopic skills were not addressed.

The safety of endoscopy will be enhanced by the comprehensive training of physicians and surgeons in both the cognitive and technical aspects of endoscopy, which should take place in the setting of a training programme in gastroenterology or

---

§ Prophylaxis appears reasonable, particularly for severely neutropenic or immunosuppressed patients; oral amoxicillin may be adequate.

|| Prophylaxis for all endoscopic procedures, particularly oesophageal dilation and sclerotherapy, with a parenteral cephalosporin or oral amoxicillin; the use of a parenteral cephalosporin is encouraged if there is a history of previous procedure-related or spontaneous bacterial peritonitis.

ERCP, endoscopic retrograde cholangiopancreatography; PEG, percutaneous endoscopic gastroscopy; PEJ, percutaneous endoscopic jejunostomy.

GI surgery. Comprehensive training in endoscopy cannot be acquired outside of an accredited training programme; in particular, endoscopic hospital privileges for endoscopy should not be given to physicians who cite short courses as their sole training experience [55]. It is also important that hospital privileges be granted for each separate procedure for which training and competence is documented rather than globally for all endoscopic procedures.

Quality assurance with periodic assessment of ongoing competence in GI endoscopy is another determinant of the safe endoscopy [56]. Quality assurance should be used for recredentialing for continued performance of specific endoscopic procedures and for the identification and correction of deficiencies in practice. The major elements of a quality assurance programme in GI endoscopy are: (a) the procedure report; (b) the endoscopic unit record; and (c) procedure review. The endoscopy unit record serves as the source of data for procedure review. Clinical indicators such as the appropriateness of indications, absence of contraindications, completion of a procedure or incidence of complications are factors that should be periodically reviewed.

It is unknown what minimum number of procedures should be performed annually to maintain competence in endoscopy. Several societies are beginning to address this issue and develop a consensus regarding maintenance of competence. For example, performance of less than 10 endoscopic sphincterotomies per year is probably not adequate to maintain proficiency. Depending upon the complexity of an individual procedure, endoscopists require variable ongoing procedural experience from very little to considerable to maintain competence.

A final consideration impacting on the safety of endoscopy is physician judgment regarding when to abandon a difficult procedure. The clinical situation, including the alternative diagnostic and therapeutic approaches and risks, must be weighed against continued efforts to complete a technically difficult endoscopy.

Contraindications

Procedural safety is also influenced by adherence to the indications and contraindications for individual procedures [57]. Avoidance procedures that are contraindicated should obviously result in safer endoscopy. Upper GI endoscopy is generally contraindicated when: (a) the risk of the procedure outweighs the potential benefit; (b) the patient is unable to co-operate; and (c) a perforated viscus is known or suspected [57]. Lower endoscopy is contraindicated in fulminant colitis and acute severe diverticulitis [57].

Clinical environment

The safety of endoscopy may be influenced by where the procedure is performed, i.e. a large hospital endoscopy unit versus a small rural hospital versus an outpatient clinic or office. In addition, elective endoscopic procedures are typically safer than those performed as an emergency, usually in a hospital area other than the endoscopy unit. A guideline for the establishment of GI endoscopy areas, including issues such as equipment, space and personnel, has been published [58].

Endoscopy is increasingly being performed in ambulatory endoscopy or surgery centres in the USA. The ASGE guideline on the establishment of GI endoscopy areas emphasizes that the standards for out-of-hospital endoscopic practice should be identical to the guidelines followed in the hospital [58]. The recent ASGE survey of endoscopic sedation and monitoring practices, however, revealed that usage of electronic monitoring devices was much higher for hospital procedures as opposed to office procedures [14]. There are no published data comparing complications, in particular cardiopulmonary complications, in various hospital settings versus out-of-hospital settings, but differences in monitoring practices or the availability of resuscitation equipment and trained personnel may affect the safety record in the various areas where endoscopy is performed.

The important role played by trained GI endoscopy nurses in the safety of endoscopy cannot be overemphasized. Since the endoscopist is usually focused on the technical aspects of the procedure, the primary responsibility for patient monitoring rests with the GI nurse. When complex or therapeutic procedures are performed, one nurse should be assigned primary responsibility for monitoring the patient, while the other nurse can assist the endoscopist. Adequate staffing of trained nurses is particularly important after hours when emergency and therapeutic procedures are often performed.

Another issue related to where endoscopy is performed is the appropriate cleaning, sterilization and disinfection of endoscopic instruments [59]. Regular adherence to strict protocols to clean mechanically and chemically disinfect instruments is important to reduce or eliminate the likelihood of transmission of infection to patients undergoing endoscopic procedures.

Patient recovery and discharge

Recovery and discharge policies after completion of endoscopic procedures should be standard. The risk of conscious sedation extends beyond completion of the endoscopic procedure, and clinical and electronic monitoring should be maintained until the patient is awake and alert.

A patient is generally discharged from the recovery area when monitoring is no longer necessary by the above criteria, and the patient has met the additional requirement of ambulation. Discharge policies for patients undergoing outpatient endoscopy should be standard, and patients should be given written instructions. A patient having conscious sedation should be accompanied home by a responsible adult and instructed not to drive, operate machinery or drink alcohol for 24 h.

References

1 Keeffe EB, Schrock TR. Complications of gastrointestinal endoscopy. In: Sleisenger MH, Fordtran JS, eds. *Gastrointestinal Disease*, 5th edn. Philadelphia: WB Saunders, 1993: 301–8.

2 Shahmir M, Schuman BM. Complications of fiberoptic endoscopy. *Gastroint Endosc* 1980; 26: 86–91.

3 Mandelstam P, Sugawa C, Silvis SE, Nebel OT, Rogers BHG. Complications associated with esophagogastroduodenoscopy and with esophageal dilation. An analysis of the 1974 ASGE survey. *Gastroint Endosc* 1976; 23: 16–19.

4 Andersen KE, Clausen N. Outpatient gastroscopy risks. *Endoscopy* 1978; 10: 180–3.

5 Schiller KFR, Cotton PB, Salmon PR. The hazards of digestive fibre-endoscopy: a survey of British experience (Abstract). *Gut* 1972; 13: 1027.

6 Sanowski RA, Waring JP. Endoscopic techniques and complication in variceal sclerotherapy. *J Clin Gastroenterol* 1987; 9: 504–13.

7 Sivak MV Jr. Esophageal varices. In: Sivak MV Jr, ed. *Gastroenterologic Endoscopy*. Philadelphia: WB Saunders, 1987: 342–72.

8 Rogers BHG, Silvis SE, Nebel OT, Sugawa C, Mandelstam P. Complications of flexible fiberoptic colonoscopy and polypectomy. An analysis of the 1974 ASGE survey. *Gastroint Endosc* 1975; 22: 73–7.

9 Gilbert DA, Hallstrom AP, Shaneyfelt SL, Mahler AK, Silverstein FE. The national ASGE colonoscopy survey—complications of colonoscopy (Abstract). *Gastroint Endosc* 1984; 30: 156.

10 Smith LE. Fiberoptic colonoscopy. Complications of colonoscopy and polypectomy. *Dis Col Rect* 1976; 19: 407–12.

11 Macrae FA, Tan KG, Williams CB. Towards safer colonoscopy: a report on the complications of 5000 diagnostic or therapeutic colonoscopies. *Gut* 1983; 24: 376–83.

12 Keeffe EB. Endoscopic procedural safety. In: McCloy R, ed. *Quality Control in Endoscopy*. Berlin: Springer-Verlag, 1991: 33–45.

13 Joint Commission on Accreditation of Healthcare Organizations. *Accreditation Manual for Hospitals, 1990*. Chicago: Joint Commission on Accreditation of Healthcare Organizations, 1989.

14 Keeffe EB, O'Connor KW. 1989 ASGE survey of endoscopic sedation and monitoring practices. *Gastroint Endosc* 1990; 36: S13–18.

15 Arrowsmith JB, Gerstman BB, Fleischer DE, Benjamin SB. Results from the American Society for Gastrointestinal Endoscopy/US Food and Drug Administration collaborative study on complication rates and drug use during gastrointestinal endoscopy. *Gastroint Endosc* 1991; 37: 421–7.

16 Daneshmend TK, Bell GD, Logan RFA. Sedation for upper gastrointestinal endoscopy: results of a nationwide survey. *Gut* 1991; 32: 12–15.

17 McCloy R. Asleep on the job: sedation and monitoring during endoscopy. *Scand J Gastroenterol* 1992; 27(Suppl): 97–101.

18 Al-Atrakchi HA. Upper gastrointestinal endoscopy without sedation: a prospective study of 2000 examinations. *Gastroint Endosc* 1989; 35: 79–81.

19 Ladas SD, Giorgiotis C, Pipis P *et al.* Sedation for upper gastrointestinal endoscopy: time for reappraisal. *Gastroint Endosc* 1990; 36: 417–18.

20 Bell GD. Review article: premedication and intravenous sedation for upper gastrointestinal endoscopy. *Aliment Pharmacol Ther* 1990; 4: 103–22.

21 Ross WA. Premedication for upper gastrointestinal endoscopy. *Gastroint Endosc* 1989; 35: 120–6.

22 Fleischer D. Monitoring the patient receiving conscious sedation for gastrointestinal endoscopy: issues and guidelines. *Gastroint Endosc* 1989; 35: 262–6.

23 Whitman JG. Drugs for sedation. In: McCloy R, ed. *Quality Control in Endoscopy*. Berlin: Springer-

Verlag, 1991: 3–21.

24 Geller E. Report of workshop on drugs for sedation. In: McCloy R, ed. *Quality Control in Endoscopy*. Berlin: Springer-Verlag, 1991: 22–9.

25 Bailey PL, Pace NL, Ashburn MA, Moll JW, East KA, Stanley TH. Frequent hypoxemia and apnea after sedation with midazolam and fentanyl. *Anesthesiology* 1990; 73: 826–30.

26 Bell GD, Antrobus JHL, Lee J, Coady T, Morden A. Bolus or slow titrated injection of midazolam prior to upper gastrointestinal endoscopy? Relative effect on oxygen saturation and prophylactic value of supplemental oxygen. *Aliment Pharmacol Ther* 1990; 4: 393–401.

27 Bell GD, Brown NS, Morden A, Coady T, Logan RFA. Prevention of hypoxaemia during upper gastrointestial endoscopy by means of oxygen via nasal cannulae. *Lancet* 1987; i: 1022–4.

28 Gross JB, Long WB. Nasal oxygen alleviates hypoxemia in colonoscopy patients sedated with midazolam and meperidine. *Gastroint Endosc* 1990; 36: 26–9.

29 Crantock L, Cowen AE, Ward M, Roberts RK. Supplemental low flow oxygen prevents hypoxia during endoscopic cholangiopancreatography. *Gastroint Endosc* 1992; 38: 418–20.

30 Dhariwal A, Plevris JN, Lo NTC, Finlayson NDC, Heading RC, Hayes PC. Age, anemia, and obesity-associated oxygen desaturation during upper gastrointestinal endoscopy. *Gastroint Endosc* 1992; 38: 684–8.

31 Bell GD, Antrobus JHL, Lee J, Coady TJ, Morden A. Pattern of breathing during upper gastrointestinal endoscopy—implications for administration of supplemental oxygen. *Aliment Pharmacol Ther* 1991; 5: 399–404.

32 Brandl S, Borody TJ, Andrews P, Morgan A, Hyland L, Devine M. Oxygenating mouthguard alleviates hypoxia during gastroscopy. *Gastroint Endosc* 1992; 38: 415–17.

33 Bell GD, Quine A, Antrobus JHL *et al.* Upper gastrointestinal endoscopy: a prospective randomized study comparing continuous supplemental oxygen via the nasal or oral route. *Gastroint Endosc* 1992; 38: 319–25.

34 Bell GD. Who is for supplemental oxygen? (Editorial) *Gastroint Endosc* 1992; 38: 514–16.

35 Davies RJO, Hopkin JM. Nasal oxygen in exacerbations of ventilatory failure: an underappreciated risk. *Br Med J* 1989; 299: 43–4.

36 Standards of Practice Committee. American Society for Gastrointestinal Endoscopy. Monitoring of patients undergoing gastrointestinal endoscopic procedures. Guidelines for clinical application. *Gastroint Endosc* 1991; 37: 120–1.

37 Bell GD, McCloy RF, Charlton JE *et al.* Recommendations for standards of sedation and patient monitoring during gastrointestinal endoscopy. *Gut* 1991; 32: 823–7.

38 American Society of Anesthesiologists. *ASA Standards for Basic Intraoperative Monitoring*. Park Ridge, IL: American Society of Anesthesiologists.

39 Fleischer D. Monitoring during gastrointestinal endoscopy: how much is necessary? *Endoscopy* 1991; 23: 344–5.

40 Committee on Drugs. American Academy of Pediatrics. Guidelines for monitoring and management of pediatric patients during and after sedation for diagnostic and therapeutic procedures. *Pediatrics* 1992; 89: 1110–15.

41 Keeffe EB. Technical monitoring during radiologic interventions—what can be done and what must be done. In: Steinbrick W, Gross-Fengels W, eds. *Interventional Radiology—Adjunctive Medication and Monitoring*. Berlin: Springer-Verlag, 1993: 71–8.

42 Schneider AJL. Assessment of risk factors and surgical outcome. *Surg Clin N Am* 1983; 63: 1113–16.

43 Knaus WA, Draper EA, Wagner DP, Zimmerman JE. APACHE II: a severity of disease classification system. *Critical Care Med* 1985; 13: 818–29.

44 Keeffe EB. Antibiotic prophylaxis: who, when and how. *Gastroint Endosc Clin N Am* 1993; 3: 431–45.

45 Dajani AS, Bisno AL, Chung KJ *et al.* Prevention of bacterial endocarditis. Recommendations by the American Heart Association. *J Am Med Ass* 1990; 264: 2919–22.
46 Endocarditis Working Party of the British Society for Antimicrobial Chemotherapy. Antibiotic prophylaxis of infective endocarditis. *Lancet* 1990; 335: 88–9.
47 Standards of Training and Practice Committee. American Society for Gastrointestinal Endoscopy. Infection control during gastrointestinal endoscopy: Guidelines for clinical application. *Gastroint Endosc* 1988; 34 (suppl): 37S–40S.
48 Standards Task Force. American Society of Colon and Rectal Surgeons. Practice parameters for antibiotic prophylaxis to prevent infective endocarditis or infected prosthesis during colon and rectal endoscopy. *Dis Col Rect* 1992; 35: 277–85.
49 Standards of Training and Practice Committee. American Society for Gastrointestinal Endoscopy. Standards of practice of gastrointestinal endoscopy. Guidelines. *Gastroint Endosc* 1988; 34: 8S.
50 Standards of Training and Practice Committee. American Society for Gastrointestinal Endoscopy. Methods of granting hospital privileges to perform gastrointestinal endoscopy. *Gastroint Endosc* 1988; 34: 28S–9S.
51 Standards of Practice Committee. American Society for Gastrointestinal Endoscopy. Proctoring and hospital endoscopy privileges. *Gastroint Endosc* 1991; 37: 666–7.
52 Standards of Training Committee. American Society for Gastrointestinal Endoscopy. Principles of training in gastrointestinal endoscopy. *Gastroint Endosc* 1992; 38: 743–6.
53 Cohn S, Sachar DB, Ertan A, Lee W, Sorrell MF, Duane W. Training and third-tier certification in gastroenterology. *Gastroenterology* 1988; 94: 1083–6.
54 Cass OW, Freeman ML, Peine CJ, Zera RT, Onstad GR. Objective evaluation of endoscopy skills during training. *Ann Intern Med* 1993; 118: 40–4.
55 Standards of Training and Practice Committee. American Society for Gastrointestinal Endoscopy. Statement on role of short courses in endoscopic training. *Gastroint Endosc* 1988; 34: 14S–15S.
56 American Society for Gastrointestinal Endoscopy. *Quality Assurance of Gastrointestinal Endoscopy.* Manchester, Massachusetts: American Society for Gastrointestinal Endoscopy.
57 Committee on Endoscopic Utilization and Standards of Practice Committee. American Society for Gastrointestinal Endoscopy. *Appropriate Use of Gastrointestinal Endoscopy.* Manchester, Massachusetts: American Society for Gastrointestinal Endoscopy, August, 1992.
58 Standards of Practice Committee. American Society for Gastrointestinal Endoscopy. Guidelines for establishment of gastrointestinal endoscopy areas. *Gastroint Endosc* 1991; 37: 661–2.
59 Standards of Training and Practice Committee. American Society for Gastrointestinal Endoscopy. Infection control during gastrointestinal endoscopy. Guidelines for clinical application. *Gastroint Endosc* 1988; 34: 37S–40S.

Chapter 8
Management of Diabetic Day-Case Patients

K. Shotliff and E. M. Kohner

Diabetes mellitus is a common condition affecting approximately 1% of the population in the UK [1] and up to 6·6% of those aged 20–74 years in the USA [2]. Three-quarters of cases are of the non-insulin-dependent type (NIDDM) which becomes more common with advancing age; affecting up to 9% of those over the age of 65 years in the UK [3] and approximately 18% of those aged 65–74 years in the USA [2]. The type of diabetes, the current treatment, recent glycaemic control, the presence of complications and the surgical procedure to be performed are important in determining the most appropriate form of anaesthesia. The high prevalence of diabetes and the potential problems from both acute metabolic disturbances and chronic complications highlights the importance of a careful preoperative assessment before considering a day-case surgical procedure.

Glycaemic control should be optimized prior to surgery and long-acting insulin (e.g. Ultratard and Humulin Zn) and long-acting oral hypoglycaemic agents (e.g. chlorpropamide and glibenclamide) should be avoided. The use of metformin should also be reviewed as this increases the risk of lactic acidosis. A general medical assessment should be performed for diabetes-related pathology particularly cardiac, peripheral vascular, renal and neurological disease. Autonomic neuropathy is especially important as it is often overlooked and can be a cause of perioperative mortality even in day-case procedures due to perioperative hypotension [4, 5]. Coexisting disease resulting in difficulty lying flat or still will also influence the form of anaesthesia required. The involvement of a diabetologist in such an assessment may be useful as many day-case procedures are not emergencies and outpatient optimization of glycaemic control may take some time [6]. Even for minor procedures patients with brittle insulin-dependent diabetes (IDDM) and those with persistently poor control, i.e. glycosylated haemoglobin $\geqslant 9\%$ or elevated blood glucose levels, may be better managed as inpatients for stabilization on a suitable multiple dose insulin regimen.

For the purpose of day-case surgery diabetic patients fall into three main groups; those taking insulin, those taking oral hypoglycaemic agents, e.g. sulphonylureas, and those treated with diet alone. The different physiological reactions to the stress of surgery between a young insulin-dependent diabetic with no insulin reserves and an NIDDM patient receiving insulin with some reserves should however not be forgotten. This lack of insulin to counteract the catabolic effect of stress hormones explains the need for peroperative administration of both insulin and glucose in IDDM subjects for all but the most minor procedures. Even minor surgery will adversely affect diabetic control. Several factors are important in this; anxiety, starvation, metabolic and hormonal reactions to the procedure, the diabetogenic effect of anaesthetics. For instance, isofluorane depresses insulin secretion [7]. Midazolam does not inhibit insulin secretion in isolated rat pancreatic islet cells [8], but in patients where anaesthesia is induced and maintained with midazolam and halothane the maximum insulin concentration was 12 mmol. This compared with 20 mmol when thiopentone and halothane were used [9]. While a modest loss of diabetic control is undesirable, the major complication of day-case surgery in diabetic patients is hypoglycaemia due to decreased oral intake with starvation and postoperative nausea and vomiting. The risk of this will be minimized by careful patient selection and suitable observation before, during and after such procedures.

Day-case procedures can be subdivided into three main groups, although the majority are presently performed under a general anaesthetic [10].

The first group includes those procedures using a local anaesthetic with no intention of immediately proceeding to a general anaesthetic if complications arise. The presence of an anaesthetist is desirable in some but is not possible for all of these procedures. No alteration in normal diabetic therapy is usually made. However, some experts would argue that for safety and also particularly in a medicolegal sense, since adverse life-threatening reactions can occur acutely and unpredictably in response to the administration of local anaesthetic drugs, that all patients should have the same preparation in terms of stomach content to prevent potential aspiration during the ensuing resuscitation, irrespective of the type of anaesthetic. This is currently an area of critical debate. Clearly such reactions are rare and whatever preparation is undertaken careful monitoring of the blood glucose is required before, during and after such operations. Nausea, vomiting or postoperative pain should be treated appropriately; however, the patient may require admission if such complications do not settle. The use of relatively expensive drugs, such as HT_3 antagonists, e.g. ondansetron, are clearly cost effective if overnight admission of the patient in a hospital or 'hotel' facility can be avoided.

The second group are those procedures using a local anaesthetic where a general anaesthetic may be required if problems arise, for example due to inadequacy of the local block or the patients inability to tolerate the procedure. These patients are starved as for a general anaesthetic but will be able to take both dietary and oral medication soon after the procedure. Such operations are best performed in the morning and the use of glucose-containing intravenous fluids is not recommended. In those patients treated with diet alone blood glucose monitoring is sufficient and the use of small doses of short-acting insulin are recommended if control is poor. Intravenous insulin either with dextrose and potassium in the same solution [11, 12] or by a separate intravenous line [13, 14] are preferred to subcutaneous insulin, although the later route is suitable postoperatively. At the present time a continuous infusion of insulin via a syringe driver is the most popular method of intravenous administration [14].

In NIDDM patients taking oral hypoglycaemic agents these should be omitted on the morning of the procedure. Long-acting agents are best avoided in the days immediately prior to the procedure as significant hypoglycaemia may still occur several days after the withdrawal of such agents in fasting patients, particularly in the elderly [15]. In most cases, careful observation of blood glucose levels is adequate but if these are high, e.g. in poorly controlled patients, insulin will be required to ensure rapid control.

Oral hypoglycaemic agents should be restarted with the first postoperative meal. Adequate treatment of nausea and pain prior to discharge home is important to reduce the risk of readmission due to hypoglycaemia caused by a decreased oral intake, or increased catabolic hormones and vomiting causing hyperglycaemia and the development of ketosis. On discharge all patients should be told to seek medical advice if nausea, vomiting or poor oral intake subsequently occurs.

If intravenous fluids are required, those containing lactate, e.g. Hartmann's solution, should be avoided as it is well known that diabetic patients do not metabolize lactate normally, leading to a rise in the blood glucose level.

In patients treated with insulin the use of long-acting forms will increase the likelihood of hypoglycaemia during fasting and these are therefore best avoided. Insulin requirements will rise with most surgical procedures even minor ones. The lack of insulin reserve in a young IDDM patient is important as the stress of even a minor surgical procedure may cause the release of hormones requiring increased insulin to counteract their catabolic effects. On the day of operation the patient is starved and surgery is best performed in the morning. It is advisable to stop all solids from midnight with oral fluids allowed until 3 h preoperatively [16]. Insulin regimens vary but in general on the morning of the operation short-acting insulin is omitted with a reduced dose of intermediate-acting insulin given subcutaneously providing the blood glucose is $\geqslant 6{\cdot}5\ \text{mmol}\ l^{-1}$, 50% of the usual dose in many protocols [13]. Preoperative assessment of blood glucose will then determine the initial dose of intravenous short-acting insulin needed using either of the regimens above. Perioperative blood glucose estimation will aid subsequent adjustments. Postoperatively, once oral intake is tolerated the remainder of the morning insulin should be given 30 min prior to a normal meal, with additional insulin required if the blood glucose is high at this time.

The final and more common form of day-case surgery requires a general anaesthetic. The patient is starved and the initial management is therefore identical to that already described. The main differences between this form of anaesthesia and those previously described is the high prevalence of postoperative nausea and vomiting seen after a general anaesthetic [17] which accounts for a fairly significant number of unexpected hospital admissions after day-case surgery [18]. Diabetic patients require overnight admission if they continue to be severely nauseated or continue vomiting long into the recovery period. Postoperative drowsiness and a longer duration of decreased oral intake make the use of intravenous fluid and insulin regimens more appropriate, particularly in IDDM subjects. However, anaesthesia with propofol and the use of HT_3 antagonists will decrease the incidence of postoperative sickness in these patients.

In summary, although much attention is paid to perioperative insulin regimens, with good reason, the most important steps in the management of day-case diabetic patients are: (a) careful selection and preparation of the patient; and (b) adequate postoperative observation and treatment of nausea and pain. Once a patient has been selected for a day-case procedure many regimens are available [11–14] and an example is given in Table 8.1. It should be remembered that the reaction of diabetic patients will differ and any regimen should be individually tailored to the needs of each patient. If

Table 8.1 Protocol for diabetic day-case patients

On arrival
Diabetes well controlled—proceed
Diabetes poorly controlled or control unknown—cancel procedure until control optimized or admit to hospital to do so

Diabetes controlled by diet alone
Monitor blood glucose levels hourly
Rarely need insulin

Diabetes controlled by oral hypoglycaemic agent
Operation in the morning if possible
Omit sulphonylurea on morning of procedure
If fasting blood glucose < 7 mmol l^{-1} treat as for diabetes controlled by diet alone (above)
If fasting blood glucose > 7 mmol l^{-1} give intravenous dextrose and insulin as for diabetes controlled by insulin (below)
Treat postoperative nausea/vomiting aggressively and admit if not tolerating oral fluid/food

Diabetes controlled on insulin
Aim for blood glucose of 7–11 mmol l^{-1}
Give half normal dose of intermediate-acting insulin
Give intravenous dextrose and a sliding scale of insulin administered intravenously, e.g. 50 U of soluble insulin in 50 ml of 0·9% saline as a continuous infusion based on blood glucose readings

Blood glucose (mmol l^{-1})	Insulin (U h^{-1})
< 4·5	Nil
4·5–7	1
7–9	2
9–11	3
11–17	4
17–28	6
> 28	6 + review regimen

Postoperatively remainder of normal insulin dose is given once tolerating food
Admit overnight if nausea/vomiting or poor oral intake persist postoperatively

these steps are carried out carefully diabetic patients should tolerate a day-case procedure as well as their non-diabetic counterparts.

References

1 Gatling W, Houston AC, Hill RD. An epidemiological survey: the prevalence of diabetes mellitus in a typical English community. *J Roy Coll Phys Lond* 1985; 4: 248–50.
2 Harris MI, Hadden WC, Knowler WC, Bennett PH. Prevalence of diabetes and impaired glucose tolerance and plasma glucose levels in the US population aged 20–74 years. *Diabetes* 1987; 36: 523–34.
3 Samanta A, Burden AC, Fent B. Comparative prevalence of non-insulin-dependent diabetes in Asian and White Caucasian adults. *Diab Res Clin Pract* 1987; 4: 1–6.
4 Page MMcB, Watkins PJ. Cardiorespiratory arrest with diabetic autonomic neuropathy. *Lancet* 1978; i: 14–16.
5 Burgoss LG, Ebert TJ, Asiddao C *et al.* Increased intraoperative cardiovascular morbidity in diabetics with autonomic neuropathy. *Anaesthesiology* 1989; 70: 591–7.
6 Podolsky S. Management of diabetes in the surgical patient. *Med Clin N Am* 1982; 66: 1361–72.
7 Desborough JP, Jones PM, Persaud SJ, Landon MJ, Howell SL. Isoflurane inhibits insulin secretion from isolated rat pancreatic islets of Langerhans. *Br J Anaesth* 1992; 69: 532P.
8 Desborough JP, Jones PM, Persaud SJ, Howell SL. Effects of midazolam on insulin secretion from isolated rat pancreatic islets of Langerhans. *Br J Anaesth* 1993; 70: 221–2.
9 Desborough JP, Hall GM, Hart GR, Burrin JM. Midazolam modifies pancreatic and anterior pituitary hormone secretion during upper abdominal surgery. *Br J Anaesth* 1991; 67: 390–6.
10 White PF. Outpatient anesthesia: an overview. In: White PF, ed. *Outpatient Anesthesia*. New York: Churchill Livingstone, 1990.
11 Alberti KGMM, Thomas DJP. The management of diabetes during surgery. *Br J Anaesth* 1979; 51: 693–710.
12 Gill GV, Alberti KGMM. The care of the diabetic patient during surgery. In: Alberti KGMM, Defronzo RA, Keen H, Zimmet P, eds. *International Textbook of Diabetes Mellitus*. Chichester: John Wiley, 1992: 1173–83.
13 Meyers EF, Alberts D, Gordon MO. Perioperative control of blood glucose in diabetic patients: a two-step protocol. *Diab Care* 1986; 9: 40–5.
14 Clark JD, Currie J, Hartog M. Management of diabetes in surgery: a survey of current practice by anaesthetists. *Diab Med* 1992; 9: 271–4.
15 Aspuld K, Wiholm BF, Lither F. Glibenclamide associated hypoglycaemia: a report of 57 cases. *Diabetalogia* 1983; 24: 412–17.
16 Strunin L. How long should patients fast before surgery? Time for new guidelines. *Br J Anaesth* 1993; 70: 1–3.
17 White PF, Shafer A. Nausea and vomiting: causes and prophylaxis. *Sem Anesth* 1987; 6: 300–8.
18 Gold BS, Kitz DS, Lecky JH, Neuhaus JM. Unanticipated admission to the hospital following ambulatory surgery. *J Am Med Ass* 1989; 262: 3008–10.

Chapter 9
Pain Treatment in the Day-Care Unit

W. W. A. Zuurmond

The institutionalization of day-care units was beneficial for the effective development of pain treatment. After applied invasive techniques, control of the patient is required for two reasons:

1 To monitor the patient adequately after the blockade.

2 To evaluate the effects of the blockade.

The blockades for benign and malignant pain treatment may be administered for diagnostic, prognostic or therapeutic reasons.

Applying diagnostic blockades, the anaesthetist may be able to differentiate the localization and aetiology of the pain complaints by using placebo or local anaesthetics. Prognostic blockades allows the patient and doctor to predict the effects of a destructive block or denervation by operative intervention. Reversible blocks may be performed with placebo, local anaesthetics with or without corticosteroids, sympathetic blocking drugs or opioids. Irreversible, destructive blocks may be performed using neurolytic agents, thermocoagulation or by making cryolesions.

For pain treatment in the day-care unit the following measures should be advocated:

1 Patients should be informed about the procedure and the effects.

2 The anaesthetist has to take account of the physical and psychological aspects of pain. An interdisciplinary evaluation including psychological assessment of the pain complaints is often required.

3 A nerve stimulator should be used routinely in all blockades for pain relief. Using X-ray facilities, e.g. lateral and posteroanterior plain films, fluoroscopy or a C-arm with image intensifier for radiographic verification of the needle tip and if possible administration of a radio-opaque dye, the incidence of failures and complications decreases. Patients, suffering from chronic benign pain may show unpredictable behaviour during and after invasive procedures. During and after the procedure the anaesthetist has to be certain about the proper positioning of the needle(s) and the predictable effects of the blockade.

4 A destructive block has to be preceded by a prognostic injection with a local anaesthetic to predict the efficacy of the blockade and acceptance by the patient. Evaluating the beneficial and harmful effects of the prognostic block, the decision to perform an irreversible blockade should be made by both the patient and the doctor.

5 Destructive blockades with potential late side effects such as hypotension and

urinary retention, must not be performed in a day-care unit. After destructive procedures such as percutaneous cordotomy, coeliac plexus block and bilateral sympathectomy, the patient has to be observed for more than 12 h.

6 Chronic pain is commonly defined as pain which exists longer than 6 months [1]. However, many acute diseases or injuries heal in a shorter period and if pain is then still present, it must be considered as chronic pain [2].

Therapeutic reversible blocks with local anaesthetics with or without corticosteroids

Infiltration techniques

Trigger point injections

These consist of infiltration of a local anaesthetic directly into the trigger points, every day or every 2–3 days. Recommended drugs and dosage are 1–2 ml lidocaine 1% for each trigger point.

Indications include the myofascial pain syndrome, fibrositis, or non-articular rheumatism, which is associated with marked tenderness of discrete points (trigger points) within affected skeletal muscles; and pain which is referred to areas some distance from the trigger point and the appearance of tight, ropy bands of skeletal muscle [3]. In patients with myofascial pain syndromes, the administration of trigger point injections is a valuable therapy in combination with physical therapy. Contraindications include those cases where there is a known allergy to local anaesthetics.

There are no known complications.

The combination of trigger point injections and physical therapy may be successful, provided that the time between the trigger point injections does not exceed 2 or 3 days.

Painful shoulder injection

The technique according to the general principles of Cyriax [4] is as follows:

1 To restore the function of painless mobility of the joint: intra-articular local anaesthetic combined with corticosteroid.

2 To restore the painless function of the tendon: infiltration of the lesion with local anaesthetic and corticosteroid. In patients suffering from 'a painful arch' infiltration of the supraspinatus tendon is to be recommended. The needle is advanced from the cranioventral side of the endorotated arm.

3 To abolish tenderness of a bursa: puncture of the bursa. In patients suffering from 'a painful arch', the subacromial bursa has to be punctured from a posterolateral angle between the acromion and the humerus. Aspiration of the fluid from the bursa has to be followed by injection of local anaesthetic and corticosteroid.

4 To dissolve calcified material: repeated injections with local anaesthetics dissolve the deposits.

Recommended drugs and dosage are 5–10 ml lidocaine 1% combined with 10–50 mg triamcinolone or 40–80 mg methylprednisolone.

Indications include pain in the shoulder—the painful arch is defined as pain in the shoulder during glenohumeral abduction between 45 and 160°.

Contraindications include (a) a known allergy for local anaesthetics; and (b) patients from whom the administration of corticosteroids is contraindicated.

Complications are rare.

The methods of treatment are simple. The making of a diagnosis is more difficult. After the blockade the patient is managed in the day-care unit, and the functions are evaluated.

Epicondilitis humeri

Epicondilitis of the lateral ('tennis elbow') or the medial ('golfer's elbow') condyle may be treated with injections at the site of maximum pain, using a solution of 2–5 ml lidocaine 1% containing methylprednisolone 40–80 mg. The immediate results should be evaluated after 20 min. The patient must be instructed that pain may return. The effect of the steroids may be expected after 2 or 3 days.

Peripheral nerve and plexus blocks in day-care units

Occipital block

Occipital headache may be relieved by a series of three occipital nerve blocks with local anaesthetic and corticosteroid (5 ml lidocaine 1% with 40–80 mg methylprednisolone). The occipital nerve is found in the suboccipital triangle, 1·5 cm lateral to the external occipital protuberance and 0·5 cm below the superior nuchal line.

Intercostal block

Intercostal neuralgia may follow rib fractures or chest surgery. A diagnosis must be made before commencing treatment: many medical and surgical conditions may present as chest wall pain [5]. Moreover, deafferentation pain may be treated less harmfully with medication or transcutaneous nerve stimulation. The intercostal block may be performed 7 cm from the spine. The needle is introduced and advanced slowly until the point rests on the lower border of the rib. The needle is then advanced caudally until contact with the rib is lost. The needle is then slowly advanced forward 0·3 cm, and 5 ml of lidocaine 1% is injected.

Whilst performing these blocks, pneumothorax may occur, thus creating a major complication. Symptoms of pneumothorax may arise insidiously after the discharge of the patient. Neurolytic blocks may cause pain from neuritis, which can overwhelm the original pain.

Inguinal block

To relieve inguinal pain after trauma or surgery, ilioinguinal or genitofemoral blocks may be performed, provided the original complaint is not an indication for the operation. The iloinguinal nerve can be localized 2·5 cm medially to the anterosuperior iliac spine at the line connecting the anterosuperior iliac spine to the umbilicis. After fanwise injection with local anaesthetic below the fascia lata, an effective block may be expected. The use of a neurotracer is recommended.

Block of lateral femoral cutaneous nerve

In patients suffering from entrapment of the lateral femoral cutaneous nerve, meralgia paraesthetica, 10–25 ml of lidocaine 1% may be injected 2·5 cm medially and 2·5 cm caudally from the anterosuperior spine of the iliac bone, fanwise below the fascia lata. The use of a nerve stimulator is recommended. Corticosteroid may be added to the injection solution.

Recommended drugs and dosage are 5–10 ml lidocaine 1% combined with 10–50 mg triamcinolone or 40–80 mg methylprednisolone.

Contraindications include (a) a known allergy for local anaesthetics; and (b) patients in whom the administration of corticosteroids is contraindicated.

Brachial plexus block, single-dose or continuous

Brachial plexus block may be performed for prognostic, diagnostic and therapeutic reasons in the day-care unit. In patients suffering from intractable pain from reflex sympathetic dystrophy or vasospastic diseases, a continuous brachial plexus block may result in pain relief and improvement of circulation to the arm.

An axillary catheter is placed into the brachial plexus sheath and tunnelled subcutaneously to the anterior side of the shoulder. The catheter is connected to a portable external pump delivering bupivacaine. In co-operation with the general practitioner and the district nurse, the patient can be controlled at home. The recommended dosage of bupivacaine varies between 2 and 4 ml h^{-1} of bupivacaine 0·25%.

The use of neurolytic solutions for denervations of peripheral nerves is not recommended. Peripheral nerve blocks have a low success rate in treating peripheral neuralgias and neuropathies. The neurolytic agents may lead to pain caused by neuritis. The continuous administration of local anaesthetics at home may be a promising non-destructive procedure in the treatment of chronic pain.

Central neural blockade

Single dose epidural anaesthesia with local anaesthetics with or without corticosteroids

The lumbar technique is covered in Chapter 15. Cervical and thoracic epidural anaesthesia is performed with a 23 G 60 mm pole needle connected to a syringe. Constant pressure over the plunger of the syringe is exerted during the forward displacement. The loss of resistance may then be detected. Sluyter and Mehta [6] recommend for the cervical epidural procedure the application of a peripheral nerve stimulator, connected to the pole needle, at a setting of 100 Hz and 1·3 V. If the needle is advanced inadvertently beyond the dura, pain is experienced below the level of needle puncture. Also, deviations of the needle may be detected.

Acute herpes zoster. The administration of a single dose local anaesthetic and corticosteroid in the epidural space corresponding to the affected segmental area may have a positive effect in preventing postherpetic pain. In a prospective study, Berger and Perkins [7] compared the efficacy of epidural methylprednisolone alone or combined with lidocaine for treatment of postherpetic neuralgia. They concluded that both techniques are effective in relieving pain of postherpetic neuralgia. The study of Perkins and Hanlon [8] suggest that local anaesthetic alone was effective and that the inclusion of corticosteroids did not increase benefits.

The recommended dosage is 1–5 ml lidocaine 1% with 40–80 mg methylprednisolone or triamcinolone 20–50 mg. After evaluation and recovery the patient may be discharged from the day-care ward.

Neck pain and low back pain. In neck or low back pain the epidural administration of local anaesthetics combined with corticosteroids is still controversial.

Kepes and Duncalf [9], and the Quebec Task Force on Spinal Disorders [10] conclude in their reviews that the rationale for the use of local spinal analgesics or steroids have not been scientifically proven. Nevertheless, the clinical use of applying epidurals with corticosteroids continues with 1–5 ml lidocaine 1% and 40–80 mg methylprednisolone or 10–50 mg triamcinolone.

Subarachnoid block with local anaesthetics

The indication for performing spinal anaesthesia for pain relief in a day-care unit is restricted to diagnostic and prognostic procedures. The same measures described in Chapter 15 have to be taken. Administration of corticosteroids into the subarachnoid space is contraindicated: meningitis followed by arachnoiditis frequently occurs [9, 11, 12].

Sympathetic blockades

Stellate ganglion blockade

The stellate ganglion is usually formed by the fusion of the inferior cervical and the first thoracic ganglia. The inferior cervical ganglion lies in front of the seventh cervical transverse process and the first thoracic ganglion is situated on the anterior surface of the neck of the first rib. The patient is placed with the head extended by a small pillow behind the neck. The blockade has to be performed using radiographic verification techniques.

The anterior paratracheal approach includes the retraction of the large vessels by the index and middle fingers of the left hand and advancing the needle horizontally from a point 3 cm above the sternoclavicular joint. The needle is placed on the anterior tubercle of C6 or anterior to the transverse process of C7, anterior to the paravertebral fascia. Using radio-opaque dye, the proper position of the advancing needle can be verified.

Recommended drugs and dosage are 5–10 ml lidocaine 1% and 5–10 ml bupivacaine 0·25%. With serial blocks the patient may notice a gradual improvement. If no clinical or symptomatic improvement is noticed after two to three blocks this therapy should be stopped.

Diagnostic indications [13] include the differentiation of a variety of vasospastic diseases and to determine the advisability of a permanent blockade.

Therapeutic indications include (a) relief of vasospastic disorders of the upper extremity; (b) treatment of reflex sympathetic dystrophy or causalgia of the upper extremities; and (c) treatment of the early state of herpes zoster in the cervical area. The local anaesthetic may then be combined with a corticosteroid. The results of this technique remain empirical until controlled studies are performed [14].

Contraindications include impaired pulmonary function.

Complications and side effects include the following:

1 Horner's syndrome: ptosis, myosis and enophthalmus.
2 Phrenic nerve paresis.
3 Intravascular injection.
4 Recurrent laryngeal nerve block resulting in hoarseness and difficulty in swallowing.
5 Subjective feeling of dyspnoea.
6 Pneumothorax.
7 Intrathecal injection.
8 Inadvertent puncture of the oesophagus.

Using radiographic equipment, the incidence of complications decreases.

Reflex sympathetic dystrophy

Concerning reflex sympathetic dystrophy, when vasoconstriction predominates resulting in a cold and glistening extremity, the interruption of the sympathetic arc by blockade of the sympathetic efferent impulses to the limb may be helpful. The most commonly used techniques suitable to perform in day-care units are:

1 Regional intravenous sympathetic blockade with guanethidine or bretylium.
2 Upper extremity: cervical or stellate ganglion blockade.
3 Lower extremity: blockade of the lumbar sympathetic chain using local anaesthetics.

The stellate ganglion block is useful for diagnostic or prognostic purposes. The intravenous regional sympathetic technique has partially replaced the performance of a series of stellate ganglion blocks. To prevent major discomfort and pain for the patient if a series of stellate ganglion blocks are indicated, a permanent block should be considered. However, a destructive blockade with a neurolytic solution may cause a permanent Horner's syndrome.

Lumbar sympathectomy

The lumbar sympathetic ganglia lie along the anterior lateral surface of the vertebral bodies. Most of the sympathetic outflow to an extremity passes through L2, L3 and L4. There is no constant position for these ganglia and their positions may vary from side to side. The most important ganglion is found at the level L2. For applying a one-needle technique the L2 level is preferred.

The success rate of the blockade increases when a C-arm with image intensifier is available. After infiltration of the soft tissue with lidocaine 0·5–1%, 7–8 cm lateral to the spinous process of L2, insertion of the needle proceeds until it contacts the transverse process. A depth marker can be placed at 4·5–5 cm from the skin. The needle is then replaced by passing the transverse process at the lateral side of the vertebra.

Visualization by X-ray and the administration of radio-opaque dye is strongly recommended.

Lumbar sympathetic block is performed by injecting a local anaesthetic. If the patient shows clinical or symptomatic improvement a series of local anaesthetic blocks may be performed or a neurolytic solution may be injected.

Recommended drugs and dosage are 40–50 ml lidocaine 0·5%, or 5–7 ml per segment.

Side effects and complications include transient hypotension and inadvertent injections (subarachnoid or lumbar nerve block).

Diagnostic indications [15] include predicting the advisability of lumbar sympathectomy in vascular deficiencies of the lower extremity and differentiating varieties of vasospastic diseases.

Therapeutic indications include the relief of vasospastic diseases of the lower extremities and treatment of causalgia or reflex sympathetic dystrophy of the lower extremity.

Regional intravenous sympathetic blockade

In 1974 Hannington-Kiff [16] introduced the so-called regional intravenous sympathetic block with guanethidine to treat sympathetic reflex dystrophy. The technique of the regional intravenous blockade is analogous to the intravascular regional anaesthesia technique mentioned in Chapter 15. The local anaesthetic is replaced by a sympathetic blocking drug. An increasing duration of sympathetic blockade may be seen with a series of treatments.

Hannington-Kiff [16] administered guanethidine 20–30 mg with 500 U of heparin mixed in normal saline to make up a total volume of 25 ml for upper extremity blockade and 20–30 mg of guanethidine with 1000 U heparin and normal saline to make up a volume of 50 ml for lower extremity blockade.

The mean duration of the sympathetic blockade with guanethidine is 3–4 days [17]. Reserpine 1·25 mg in 50 ml normal saline showed no significant advantages over guanethidine [18]. Bretylium 1–1·25 mg kg^{-1} showed a duration of action of 2 weeks to 7 months; moreover its toxicity is minimal and this drug may be the first choice for regional intravenous sympathetic blockade [19, 20]. Adding lidocaine 0·5% to the injected solution the tourniquet time may be extended up to 20 min.

Indications include (a) sympathetic reflex dystrophy and causalgia; (b) diseases causing vasospasm in the extremities; and (c) improvement of blood flow and pain treatment in patients suffering from ischaemic extremities.

Contraindications for guanethidine are patients with phaeochromocytoma or those receiving momoamine oxidase inhibitors.

Complications and side effects of (a) guanethidine are postural hypotension and diarrhoea; and (b) bretylium are mild postural hypotension.

One important discharge criteria is the absence of postural hypotension.

Epidural or subarachnoid administration of opioids in patients suffering from cancer pain

In the terminal phase, patients with cancer pain who have either insufficient pain relief with high doses of morphine or side effects from systemic analgesics, may receive continuous epidural or intrathecal administration of morphine, which can be performed on an outpatient basis.

The number of patients, who receive spinal opioids for the management of cancer pain in the hospital or at home is increasing. Spinal analgesia may be attained either by intrathecal or by epidural administration of analgesics or local anaesthetics. Opioids may be administered as a bolus or by a continuous infusion using an external pump.

Continuous infusion with the possibility of administering 'top up' doses has to be preferred because the incidence of catheter occlusion is lower and single bolus injections may produce a 'peak and trough' drug effect.

The risk of infection can be minimized by tunnelling the catheter subcutaneously to the flank [21]. The advantages of using the intrathecal route of administration over the epidural are:

1 The intrathecal route is a direct one since there is no dura to be penetrated and the drug is deposited close to the opioid receptors [22].

2 Lower doses of opioids and local anaesthetics are necessary to attain analgesia with fewer side effects.

3 Better control over the route of administration: after aspiration cerebrospinal fluid confirms the correct position of the catheter tip.

4 In case of infection an early diagnosis and a better approach for treatment.

The epidural or intrathecal catheter has to be inserted in the operation room unit. The insertion and tunnelling of the catheter at home has to be avoided: being a foreign body, the incidence of infection of the catheter is partially determined by the sterile circumstances in which the procedure is performed. The catheter is connected to an external portable infusion pump, which may constantly deliver opioids or, if needed on demand. The proper dose of opioids should be titrated in the hospital. However, patients in the terminal stage of their life prefer to stay at home as much as possible. After an inadvertent dislocation of the catheter, replacement may be performed on an outpatient basis.

Regardless of the route of administration, pruritus [23], urinary retention [24], nausea or emesis may occur. After intrathecal insertion of the catheter postspinal headache, leakage of cerebrospinal fluid, meningitis or arachnoiditis also may occur.

The dosages must be individually titrated in order to obtain maximum pain relief with a minimum of side effects. The results of treatment with epidural and intrathecal opioids for pain relief in terminally ill patients are promising [25, 26].

Destructive techniques

Destructive blockades with neurolytic solutions

In day-care units the administration of neurolytic agents is only indicated for unilateral lumbar sympathectomy. The recommended dosage of the neurolytic solution is 2–3 ml phenol 1–2% for each segment. The possible side effect of postural hypotension following bilateral sympathectomy demands constant observation of the patient for more than 12 h.

Coeliac plexus blocks and bilateral sympathectomy should not be performed in day-care units: the patient has to be observed for more than 12 h.

Peripheral neurolytic blocks and stellate ganglion blocks with neurolytic agents should be avoided. Following peripheral neurolytic blocks, neuritis of the denervated nerve may occur, resulting in pain. The injection of a neurolytic solution into the stellate ganglion implies the permanent existence of Horner's syndrome. Also, damage to the brachial plexus with prolonged weakness and neuritis of the arm and involvement of the recurrent laryngeal nerve may occur. Performance of this procedure is not to be recommended, certainly not in a day-care unit since patients have to be observed for more than 12 h. A radiofrequency lesion of parts of the stellate ganglion has to be preferred because it is a more elegant and less destructive method.

Destructive blockades with radiofrequency lesions

Nervous tissue can withstand the effects of heat, up to 42·5°C. Letcher and Goldring [27] demonstrated that both radiofrequency current and heat selectively block the $A\delta$ and C-fibres before the α and β groups.

Thermocoagulation techniques with precisely controllable temperatures at the needle tip are possible. Using needles with small diameters the procedure is less painful for the patient and can be performed with local anaesthetics. For selective radiofrequency lesions a temperature of 50–70°C can be used for a period of 60–90 s. For all procedures an image intensifier is required.

Radiofrequency lesion of gasserian ganglion in patients suffering from trigeminal neuralgia

In patients suffering from trigeminal neuralgia, the lancinating pain triggered by non-painful stimuli may be treated by denervation of the affected part of the trigeminal division [28]. A radiofrequency lesion may be performed in the second or third division of the trigeminal ganglion without severe complications. A lesion in the first division may lead to anaesthesia of the cornea.

In the first part of this century, blocking the trigeminal ganglion with local anaesthetic was a common procedure. Eye surgery and ear, nose and throat operations were then performed using the trigeminal nerve blockade described by Härtel [29].

In 1973 Sweet and Wepsic [30] described the technique of selective thermocoagulation of parts of the trigeminal ganglion as follows. Under direct vision with the help of a C-arm with image intensifier, the anterolateral approach to the trigeminal ganglion is followed. After penetration of the skin 2·5–3 cm lateral to the labial commissure the operator places the index finger of one gloved hand in the patient's mouth, feeling the electrode as it is advanced just medial to the mandibular ramus. It is important to prevent penetration of the oral mucosa. The electrode is then directed in the coronal plane in the direction of the lateral border of the lacrimal caruncle. The electrode has to pass through the middle or medial third of the foramen ovale. A temperature of 60°C is sufficient to achieve adequate lesions. Administering electrical stimulation after proper placement of the needle, the affected area corresponding to the pain can be found. Thermocoagulation is often a painful procedure, and sedation may be helpful for the patient; however, localization of the proper position of the needle demands complete co-operation of the patient. Complications may include:

1 Injury to the internal carotid artery.

2 Inadvertent positioning of the needle followed by thermocoagulation.

3 The first division of the trigeminal ganglion should not be thermocoagulated. If the corneal reflex is absent, corneal ulcers may occur.

4 The effects of the blockade should be made known to the patient to prevent disappointment. A prognostic block may be performed but the extent of a block with local anaesthetic is greater than the effects of radiofrequency lesions. Patients are often suffering to such an extent that they accept the side effect of numbness of small parts in their face or mouth.

Radiofrequency lesions in the stellate ganglion

Following a radiofrequency lesion in the cervicothoracic sympathetic chain, Horner's syndrome is absent. After recovery, the patient may be discharged.

Percutaneous radiofrequency denervation of spinal facets [6]

In 1975 Shealy [31] described the percutaneous radiofrequency denervation of the spinal facets. The posterior facet syndrome can be treated by a percutaneous radiofrequency lesion of the nerve supplying the facet joint. The medial branch of the posterior primary ramus supplies both the lower portion of the joint capsule at this level and the upper portion of the capsule of the facet joint below [32]. To block a single facet joint, two nerves have to be localized, the one at this level and the one above.

At lumbar level the nerve can be reached from an introducing point 7 cm from the midline at the level of the appropriate transverse process [6]. The tip of the needle has to be placed into the groove between the transverse and the inferior facet joint. At the L5 level the distance from the midline should be 5 cm, otherwise the electrode may contact the iliac crest.

A prognostic block with local anaesthetic in a previous session is recommended. Moreover, electrical stimulation at a voltage below 1 V and a frequency of 50–100 Hz, should evoke a throbbing sensation. If the electrode is too close to the spinal root, severe radicular pain in the affected dermatome occurs with less than 1 V and dermatomal contractions may occur between 1 and 2 V using a frequency of 2 Hz. After administration of 1–2 ml lidocaine 1%, the thermolesion at a temperature of 80°C is made. For cervical facet denervation, the image intensifier has to be set at an angle of 45° to expose the vertebral foramen maximally and the needle must be placed immediately posterior to this vertebral foramen.

Percutaneous radiofrequency rhizotomy

In 1974 Uematsu *et al.* [33] described percutaneous radiofrequency rhizotomy. Back pain combined with radicular dermatomal pain may be treated with a percutaneous partial posterior rhizotomy. However, the efficacy of the technique according to Sluyter and Mehta has not been proven scientifically. The description of the technique is omitted here as the procedure has yet to be evaluated and it is definitely not a common routine procedure.

The radiofrequency lesions of the trigeminal ganglion are beneficial for the patient. However, their efficacy in relieving pain at lumbar and cervical level has not been proven scientifically. A prospective and long-term evaluation of these techniques is needed.

Discharge criteria and hospitalization

When discharging patients after blockades for pain relief, the same criteria as mentioned in Chapter 15 must be followed. Special attention should be paid to the effects and results of the prognostic and diagnostic blockades. After destructive blockades the anaesthetist should pay attention to the efficacy and side effects. Explanation of the procedure, the effects to be expected and open communication after a blockade are the most important factors for correct treatment of the patient.

References

1 Fordyce WE. *Behavioral Methods for Chronic Pain and Illness.* St Louis: CV Mosby, 1976.
2 Bonica JJ. Definitions and taxonomy of pain. In: Bonica JJ, ed. *The Management of Pain,* Vol. I, 2nd edn. Philadelphia: Lea & Febiger, 1990: 18.
3 Abrams SE. Pain—Acute and chronic. In: Barash PG, Cullen BF, Stoelting RK, eds. *Clinical Anesthesia.* Philadelphia: JB Lippincott, 1989: 1427–54.
4 Cyriax J. *Textbook of Orthopaedic Medicine,* Vol. 1, 7th edn. *Diagnosis of Soft Tissue Lesions.* London: Baillière Tindall, 1978: 240–54.
5 Churcher M. Peripheral nerve blocks in relief of intractable pain. In: Swerdlow M, ed. *Relief of Intractable Pain,* 2nd edn. London: Excerpta Medica, 1978: 99–120.
6 Sluyter E, Mehta M. Treatment of chronic back and neck pain by percutaneous thermal lesions. In: Lipton S, Miles J, eds. *Persistent Pain, Modern Methods of Treatment,* Vol. 3. London: Academic Press, 1981: 141–79.
7 Berger JJ, Perkins HM. Comparison of epidural methylprednisolone alone or combined with lidocaine for relieving postherpetic neuralgia. *Pain* 1990; S1–528 (suppl): S60.
8 Perkins HM, Hanlon PR. Epidural injection of local anesthetic and steroids for relief of pain secondary to herpes zoster. *Arch Surg* 1978; 113: 253–71.
9 Kepes ER, Duncalf D. Treatment of backache with spinal injections of local anesthetics, spinal and systemic steroids. A review. *Pain* 1985; 22: 33–47.
10 Quebec Task Force on Spinal Disorders. Magnitude of the problem. *Spine* 1987: 12 (suppl): S12–15.
11 Dougherty JH, Frazer RA. Complication following intraspinal injections of steroids. *J Neurosurg* 1978; 48: 1023–5.
12 Bernat JL, Sadowsky CH, Vincent FM. Sclerosing spinal pachymeningitis, a complication of intrathecal administration of Depomedrol of multiple sclerosis. *J Neurol Neurosurg Psychiat* 1976; 39: 1124–8.

13 Moore DC. *Regional Block*, 4th edn. Springfield IL: Charles C Thomas, 1973: 123–37.
14 Raj PP. Herpes zoster. In: *Abstract Manual International Pain Symposium Update*, 1992. The Southeastern Pain Institute at Georgia Baptist Medical Centre and School of Medicine, The Medical College of Georgia. Atlanta GA: Southern Pain Institute, 1992: 212–49.
15 Moore DC. *Regional Block*, 4th edn. Springfield IL: Charles C Thomas, 1973: 211–18.
16 Hannington-Kiff JG. Intravenous regional sympathetic block with guanethidine. *Lancet* 1974; i: 1019–20.
17 Driessen JJ, Werken C van der, Nicolai PA, Crul PF. Clinical effects of regional intravenous guanethidine (Ismelin) in reflex sympathetic dystrophy. *Acta Anaesth Scand* 1983; 27: 505–9.
18 Rocco AG, Kaul AF, Reisman J, Gallo JP, Lief PA. A comparison of regional intravenous guanethidine and reserpine in reflex sympathetic dystrophy: A controlled, randomized, double-blind crossover study. *Clin J Pain* 1989; 5: 205–9.
19 Ford SR, Forrest WH, Eltherington L. The treatment of reflex sympathetic dystrophy with intravenous regional bretylium. *Anesthesiology* 1988; 68: 137–40.
20 Hord AH, Rooks MD, Stephens BO, Rogers HG, Fleming LL. Intravenous regional bretylium and lidocaine for treatment of reflex sympathetic dystrophy: A randomized, double blind study. *Anesth Analg* 1992; 74: 818–21.
21 Cherry DA. Drug delivery systems for epidural administration of opioids. *Acta Anaesth Scand* 1987; 85 (suppl): 54–9.
22 Rawal N. Indications for the use of intraspinal opioids. In: Rawal N, Coombs DW, eds. *Spinal Narcotics*, Vol. 3, London: Kluwer Academic Publishers, 1990: 43–61.
23 Duffi BL. Itching as a side-effect of epidural morphine. *Anaesthesia* 1981; 36: 67.
24 Rawal N, Mollefors K, Axelsson K, Lingardh G, Widman B. An experimental study of urodynamic effects of epidural morphine and of naloxone reversal. *Anesth Analg* 1983; 62: 641–7.
25 Boersma FP, Blaak HB, Ten Kate-Ananis A, Zuurmond WWA, Lange JJ de. Technical complications and sequelae of long-term epidural cancer pain control: A review of 206 cases. *Pain Clin* 1993; 6: 121–7.
26 Sjöberg M, Appelgren L, Einarsson S *et al.* Long-term intrathecal morphine and bupivacaine in 'refractory' cancer pain. I. Results from the first series of 52 patients. *Acta Anaesth Scand* 1991; 35: 30–43.
27 Letcher FS, Goldring S. The effect of radiofrequency current and heat on peripheral nerve action potential in the cat. *J Neurosurg* 1968; 29: 42–7.
28 Wepsic JG. Neurosurgical treatment of chronic pain. *Int Anesth Clin* 1983; 21: 153–63.
29 Härtel F. *Die Lokalanaesthesie*. Stuttgart: Von Ferdinand Enke Verlag, 1916: 74–121.
30 Sweet WH, Wepsic JG. Controlled thermocoagulation of trigeminal ganglion and rootlets for differential destruction of pain fibres. Part I: Trigeminal neuralgia. *J Neurosurg* 1974; 39: 143–56.
31 Shealy CN. Percutaneous radiofrequency denervation of spinal facets. Treatment for chronic back pain and sciata. *J Neurosurg* 1975; 43: 448–51.
32 Bogduk N, Tynan W, Wilson AS. The nerve supply to the human lumbar intervertebral discs. *J Anat* 1981; 132: 39–56.
33 Uematsu S, Udvarhelyi GB, Benson DW, Siebens AA. Percutaneous radiofrequency rhizotomy. *Surg Neurol* 1974; 2: 319–25.

Chapter 10
The Future: the Effect of Minimally Invasive Therapy on Day-Case Anaesthesia

J. G. Whitwam

In a previous era practitioners of medicine divided into physicians or internists and surgeons. The former contemplated both the common and the esoteric while the latter, including obstetricians and gynaecologists, 'fixed things' and also performed most of the endoscopies and biopsies using little more than rigid hollow tubes with a light at the end, often as a service to the diagnostic efforts of their more reflective colleagues. The supporting team were the radiologists, who created pictures with X-rays, pathologists who had the last word in part on the living or wholly on the dead, and anaesthesiologists whose world divided into local and general although sometimes combining these for balanced anaesthesia which today is termed pre-emptive analgesia. General practitioners combined elements of many of these, deferring to institutions only when needs must. Professional associations easily reflected such clear divisions of duty.

At present this relatively clear-cut medical world is undergoing a major revolution, the roots of which started with the invention of the fibreoptic endoscope approximately 30 years ago, and more recently digital subtraction angiography (DSA) since these have made possible the visualization of organs, tissues and blood vessels without the need for direct surgical exposure. This has been the key to the increasing role of physicians and radiologists in interventional therapy and for example, DSA has been a major factor in the development of interventional radiology. Currently developments are continuing rapidly particularly in the increasing application of computers and equipment for DSA, ultrasound, computerized tomography (CT) and magnetic resonance imaging (MRI) systems.

In parallel are major developments in new therapeutic equipment including, for example, remote control instruments, lasers, angioplasty and drilling catheters, and local ultrasound scalpels to assist dissection and haemostasis. The stent is now an important therapeutic measure. There is no vessel or duct carrying blood, bile, secretions, urine or gas in which they are not being introduced, for example the urethra, bile ducts and blood vessels, including the coronary arteries and portocaval shunts.

This is the current state of development and the exploitation of new technology for interventional procedures is termed minimally invasive therapy (MIT), or alternatively minimal access surgery by some endoscopic surgeons.

Currently the driving forces are the technology, reduction in cosmetic injury and pain, shorter hospital stay or conversion of previously inpatient to day-case procedures, lower mortality and improved health economics since the results of well conducted clinical trials on large numbers of patients are now becoming available and indicate that many of the new procedures in expert hands are providing major benefits. Rapid osmosis of these new ideas and methods into social perception is inevitable. Although it is possible to make major savings in current account in relation to drugs, routine consumables, hotel charges and human resources, this is offset by high initial capital outlay for equipment and also the high cost of disposable operating instruments and catheters. The possibility of increasing the number of treatment episodes in a previously rationed health-care system without a major increase in current account is now an area of critical debate.

However, future developments continue apace both to improve the quality and range of surgery and training. Telepresence surgery, three-dimensional imaging and virtual reality systems are currently under active development. The biggest developments in the future will be in the field of robotics and computer control of surgical systems and teaching simulators. Already there has been a demonstration on international television of surgery being performed in an institution in Milan, Italy, on a live animal by a computer-controlled robot driven via a satellite link from a virtual reality model located in another institution in California, USA. To improve the accuracy of surgery both the surgically controlled robot and the robotically assisted surgeon are now possible.

Inevitably there is a downside. An overbureaucratic administration may be slow or incapable of changing from current to capital expenditure. 'Cowboys' who lack basic anatomical, pathological and physiological knowledge can set up as practitioners. Senior surgeons who wish to embrace these new techniques have a learning curve, but they also have the wisdom not to force the technology and, for example, will convert from a laparoscopic to an open cholecystectomy if prudent. The problem is more serious for inexperienced trainees, who feel under pressure to perform well and may be inadequately supervised. There is an urgent need to define those units which can provide teaching and a good apprenticeship. Alas the history of surgery and therapeutic procedures is littered with examples of new procedures or drugs which follow a pattern of development, and professional and public acceptance as a standard procedure, but finally properly conducted trials are performed leading to professional denunciation and discreditation.

The new technology blurs hitherto clear boundaries of specialization. Official bodies representing the health-care professions, who are charged with the maintenance of standards and the supervision and licensing of teaching cannot be expected to make enforceable recommendations which relate to the immediate cutting edge of the application of these new technologies, except in very general terms, and yet they are responsible for public safety.

The new techniques are now widely applicable throughout a whole range of clinical practice. Last chance procedures on critically ill patients are increasingly being performed in radiology departments and endoscopy units rather than conventional operating theatres.

Effect on anaesthesia

The implications of these new applications of technology for the speciality of anaesthesia and individual anaesthesiologists are wide ranging [1].

Risk analysis

Hitherto a typical national case mix for cold-booked surgery would be approximately 25% minor, 50% intermediate, about 20–25% major or major plus and up to 6% complex major (Fig. 10.1). In general the effect of MIT should be to reduce risk.

Classification of the type of procedure

The impact of MIT will be to alter the classification of a procedure, with a shift to the left (Fig. 10.1). For the treatment of any given pathological condition, the effect will be to reduce the procedural risk, shorten the period of hospital stay and increase the number of types of therapeutic episodes which can be managed on a day-case basis. Thus the move towards an expansion of day-case surgery will accelerate.

The new surgery

Although much of the application of new technology will be undertaken by surgeons using endoscopes, increasingly many other specialists are undertaking interventional procedures often on a day-case basis, e.g. radiologists (with interventional radiology), cardiologists (coronary angioplasty, closure of ductus arteriosus), gastroenterologists (ERPC), and rheumatologists (arthroscopy).

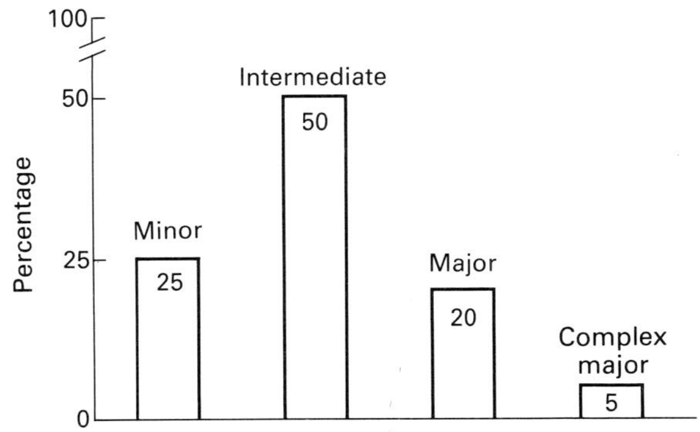

Fig. 10.1 Traditional type of conventional surgical case mix.

Location

An important consequence of the greater involvement of specialists other than surgeons, is to transfer work from conventional surgical areas to radiology departments and various clinics.

Anaesthesiologists and type of anaesthesia or sedation

A great deal of formal general anaesthesia will be replaced by monitored anaesthetic care (USA) or sedoanalgesia (UK). Most anaesthesiologists are already fully occupied and at present an increasing number of physicians without any formal anaesthetic training are practising sedation. The training of such staff in sedation comprises an apprenticeship with previous chiefs and presentations at meetings. In the future the number of administrations of intravenous anaesthetic drugs by non-anaesthetically trained doctors and dentists, for sedation, may exceed the episodes of those given by professional anaesthetists. A great deal of this work will be performed on day cases or outpatients.

Scanning units

However, at the other extreme the services of highly trained and experienced anaesthesiologists are required to supervise the general management and monitoring of critically ill patients whether undergoing last change procedures away from the normal operating theatre environment or investigations in scanning units. Clearly such environments require upgrading in terms of gas supplies, equipment and trained support for their increasing role in this vital aspect of clinical care. Although this is not strictly for ambulatory surgery such units could become increasingly involved in the management of patients who are not critically ill on a day-care basis.

Examples of clinical change

Three examples illustrate some changes in practice already introduced by using new technology.

Aortofemoral-popliteal vascular disease. Hitherto faced with a patient for conventional surgery the anaesthesiologist would be considering the patient's potential mortality, i.e. risk analysis, and booking either intensive care (ICU) or high dependency unit (HDU) facilities for postoperative care, i.e. risk management. Now with DSA, angioplasty catheters and lasers such patients can be managed with local infiltration of the groin and the introduction of catheters (3–7 Fogarty gauge or FG) into a femoral artery, using sedation. With good patient selection, providing their medical conditions are well controlled, an increasing number of these patients are being managed as day cases. The areas of critical debate are how much counselling and preparation are required, how long to retain the patient before discharge and arrangements for further care. The services of an anaesthesiologist may not be sought except for crisis management.

Cholecystectomy. This is still classified as a major procedure but when undertaken laparoscopically in competent hands, with conversion to an open procedure if necessary, which varies from 1–6% in different published series, there is a reduction in mortality, e.g. from around 2% for open procedures to less than 0·4%, and in some reports mortality has been negligible. In general the duration of surgery is not shortened, but the patient's postoperative course is simpler with discharge in less than 3–4 days and a return to work approximately 4 weeks earlier than for open procedures. In an increasing number of centres surgeons, on reviewing patients the day after surgery, can often find no reason for keeping many of them in hospital overnight. Hence an increasing number of selected patients are being managed as day-cases and laparoscopic cholecystectomy is now on the day-case agenda.

However, these new techniques may bring complications of their own. For example, laparoscopic surgery may be complicated by damage caused by the trochar to blood vessels or organs, leading to haemorrhage which may be concealed if either retroperitoneal or dispersed in the abdominal cavity by gas under pressure, and to the bowel, which if unsuspected can lead to subsequent peritonitis and septic shock. A high gas pressure in the abdomen, e.g. over 20–30 mmHg, will compromise venous return leading to a primary reduction in cardiac output with secondary autonomic effects leading, for example, to a rise in systemic vascular resistance and heart rate. Alternatively, the pressure may cause regurgitation of stomach contents with the risk of aspiration. Gas embolism is always a possibility. Finally the gas is dry and irritating and some workers feel that it should be humidified and introduced at body temperature to avoid cooling and pain. However, some others are reporting that the pressure delivery system may in fact warm the gas, with a compressive 'bicycle pump effect', so that additional warming may not be required.

Prostatectomy. This can now be performed without either general or regional anaesthesia. A technique using sedation with midazolam, local anaesthesia of the urethra with injection of local anaesthetic agents through needles introduced via an endoscope inside the prostate and bladder, combined with a non-steroidal analgesic drug, e.g. diclofenac (Voltarol), enables prostatectomy to be performed effectively with a very short hospital stay, and may not require formal hospital admission. The term sedoanalgesia has been applied to this technique. One of the team is dedicated to monitoring and acting as a 'minder' for the patients, but whenever possible an anaesthesiologist is to be preferred.

Anaesthesia versus sedation

The primary choice between anaesthesia and sedation often depends on the route of access (Table 10.1), although some patients, e.g. children and mentally disturbed patients, will always require general anaesthesia. By and large urological, gastrointestinal, many gynaecological, interventional radiological procedures, arthroscopy by rheumatologists and the activities of the cardiologists are performed using sedation and these practitioners often work as single-handed operator sedationists. They are generally inadequately trained and informed about the drugs they use and the life-threatening problems associated with the inadvertent induction of anaesthesia due to drug synergism.

Major laparoscopic surgery requires general anaesthesia and at a purely technical level one of the major problems is removal of the operating field from direct vision for all but the surgeon. Thus the anaesthesiologist is entirely dependent on monitors or the surgeon to indicate haemorrhage or other critical incidents, which in the abdomen may remain concealed. Whereas previously a single glance would lead to the ordering and administration of colloids or blood before there was any major change in the patient's condition, now, particularly in the presence of carbon dioxide under pressure, it can sometimes be difficult to interpret the data on the monitors in an immediate sense, so that volume replacement is initially delayed. Another problem is that an increasing number of patients are managed with a low level of ambient lighting, which again denies the anaesthetist immediate and continuous sight of the colour and skin condition of the patient, and which may, for example, delay the diagnosis of drug and transfusion reactions.

Table 10.1 Access routes for minimally invasive therapy

Orifices	Urethra
	Oropharynx
	  oesophagus
	  larynx, trachea, bronchi
	  maxillary sinuses
	Rectum
	Vagina

Intravascular	Arteries (e.g. femoral, brachial, radial) Veins (e.g. femoral, subclavian, jugular)
Coelomic cavities (endoscope plus gas)	Abdomen Thorax
Non-coelomic cavities	Joints (arthroscopy)
Tissue planes	Retroperitoneal (e.g. renal) Epidural space

Special ventilation systems

For endoscopic procedures involving, for example, laser surgery of the larynx and airways, the anaesthesiologist may require to practice total intravenous anaesthesia combined with either cricothyroid puncture and jet ventilation, and hence with systems with a high-frequency capability, or external cuirass ventilation using the newer higher frequency push–pull 'oscillatory' systems (see Chapter 18).

Personal and patient safety

The modern anaesthetist may require to take the necessary steps to avoid both personal and patient injury when lasers or other equipment is in use. The problems and necessary equipment for the practice of safe anaesthesia and continuous invasive monitoring in adults and children in MRI scanners, with high-intensity magnetic fields, must be clearly understood by those practising anaesthesia in these areas (see Chapter 22).

The new anaesthesiologist

The new generation of anaesthesiologists will be expected to provide a much wider range of techniques and services to facilitate the work of a much wider range of specialists and an example of the full menu expected from the modern anaesthesiologist is shown in Table 10.2.

Training

In the interests of procedural and public safety one of the major functions of at least some academic research units must be to develop and evaluate techniques for safe sedation and analgesia capable of extension, when necessary, for several hours and

Table 10.2 Menu of anaesthesia, sedation and sedoanalgesia

Monitored anaesthetic care (MAC)	
LA infiltration, regional anaesthesia limb and nerve conduction blocks	
Sedation	} or combinations
Patient-controlled sedation	
Central analgesia	
Sedoanalgesia—sedation plus LA and/or central analgesia	
GA	
Balanced anaesthesia—conduction block plus light GA	

GA, general anaesthesia; LA, local anaesthesia. MAC refers to general patient management in the UK (see Appendix 4).

which can be used by a wide range of practitioners. Another important role is the training of the 'minders' in monitoring, oxygen therapy, necessary emergency pharmacology and resuscitation.

The development of training systems based on virtual reality could have four principal functions: (a) for initial training; (b) to help the assessment of training and competence for certification; (c) to update anaesthesiologists and other practitioners, and for recertification; and (d) to assist the development of new techniques, procedures and the introduction of new drugs.

New anaesthetic agents

The development of short-acting, immediately reversible or less toxic anaesthetic agents, with low side effects and better drugs, for example for the relief of pain and the prevention of nausea and vomiting, have made significant improvements in the ease, comfort and safety of patient care and represent a major contribution by the pharmaceutical industry. Such developments have played a major role in procedural safety and the expansion of minimally invasive therapy and day-case surgery. With less pressure on recovery facilities and also a more rapid turnover of patients the reduction in unit costs combined with improvements in patient comfort may more than offset the increased costs of some of the newer anaesthetic agents and anti-emetic drugs.

Economics

Currently anaesthesiologists could suffer a serious loss of income with a move to sedation practice. However, if developments in computer-controlled anaesthesia parallel those in surgery then clearly this position would be reversed, since the analogy of the modern airline industry which still requires pilots must surely apply. However, at present in spite of the expansion of MIT and day-case surgery there is often little evidence of a reduction in inpatient time requiring the attention of anaesthesiologists.

Professional groupings

Inevitably a great many specialist groupings, national, regional and international have arisen for communication between physicians, surgeons and radiologists practising the new technologies which has led to several new journals. It is interesting that many of these follow conventional specialist groupings: for example, general surgeons have formed various associations for endoscopic surgery; orthopaedic surgeons for arthroscopy; radiologists those for interventional radiology; and gastroenterologists have also formed various endoscopic societies. However, one particular organization, the Society for Minimally Invasive Therapy (SMIT) is multidisciplinary and was formed in 1988. Among its primary aims are not only the rapid dissemination of information on new technology among all health-care workers, as opposed to its current application by limited conventional specialist groupings, but also to provide cross fertilization of ideas and applications between such groups. It also has the aim of acting as a forum for the meeting of those involved in the development of new technology and medical practitioners, so that its membership is open to all relevant disciplines, and those working in industry. It could provide an excellent vehicle for the discussion of physiology, pharmacology, and anaesthetic affairs including pain therapy and issues concerned with procedural safety. However, for the foreseeable future it seems likely that conventional historical groupings will continue to regulate standards of practice and education in the field for anaesthesia. Sedation practice at present is largely uncontrolled and unregulated and there are no recognized training centres except for specialists in anaesthesia.

Summary

Modern technology and the development of MIT is providing a much wider range of therapeutic options, reducing risk and allowing many more procedures to be undertaken as day-cases. Clearly complex health economic issues are involved but suffice it to say that the increase in day-case surgery is allowing the expansion of the number and type of therapeutic procedures without a commensurate increase in budgets. However, a switch from conventional anaesthesia to sedation practice, would imply a major reduction in income for anaesthesiologists since the fees for monitored anaesthetic care are much less than for formal anaesthesia. The question arises should anaesthesiologists, and for example a group responsible to them and in their department (e.g. anaesthetically trained nurses) undertake all sedation practice on day-cases wherever they are being managed? This would imply an increased role for groups of anaesthesiologists in both hospital and office practice as is increasingly the case in dental anaesthesia in the UK following the Poswillo report. Arguably developments in robotics could have major implications in the development of anaesthesia systems and demand a consistently higher standard of training for anaesthesiologists. If analogies are appropriate, not only should a day-case booking be like an airline reservation, i.e. never cancelled on the day, but also there are still two pilots supervising automatic 'fly by wire' aircraft. Much more initial training and subsequent revision and upgrading and recertification may be undertaken using virtual reality simulators.

Reference

1 Whitwam JG. Minimally invasive therapy—implications for anaesthesia. *Anaesthesia* 1993; 48: 937–9.

Part 2: Anaesthesia, Analgesia, Sedation

Adult anaesthesia

This section of the book contains the practical aspects of the subject, and also reference to the applied pharmacology of the benzodiazepines, particularly the importance of midazolam, its methods of administration and the newly developing techniques of patient controlled sedation, including theoretical aspects which may be useful to anyone planning to develop new systems for this purpose.

In Chapter 11 Drs Krzeminska and Fisher outline the principles involved in the provision of anaesthesia for adults in the day-case or outpatient setting. They do this against the background of having been involved in the commissioning of what is arguably one of the best purpose designed units in the UK at King's College Hospital, London. Because major laparoscopic surgery is now on the day-case agenda this book would not be complete without a discussion of this subject and Chapter 12 contains what is probably the most comprehensive review of the complications of laparoscopy to date.

This section also deals with the basics of anaesthesia in the specialist fields of ophthalmology (Chapter 13) and dentistry (Chapter 14). Dr Carr from London is well versed in the provision of both general and local anaesthesia in a new unit at Moorfields Hospital, London, while Dr Padfield practices outpatient dental anaesthesia in the traditional setting of a busy teaching hospital unit. In Chapter 15 Dr Zuurmond provides a comprehensive statement of the range of techniques for local anaesthesia which should be considered relevant for day-case patients.

Chapters 16 and 17 on sedation, sedoanalgesia and demand sedation contain a clear analysis of the pharmacological principles involved in the provision of sedation and sedoanalgesia. They provide a discussion of practical techniques, problems created by synergism and clear guidelines for dealing with such situations. Recent work from the USA is described showing that flumazenil reverses the depressant effects of midazolam on hypoxic-ventilatory drive restoring this to normal, hence laying the ghost of misinformation from the past that this single modality of action of midazolam was unique in not being reversed by flumazenil.

Professor Whitwam is a recognized international authority on this subject and this chapter will be of considerable interest for medical practitioners without formal training in anaesthesia who are obliged to provide sedation and/or analgesia, for example, gastroenterologists, interventional radiologists, cardiologists and rheumatologists.

Chapter 18 provides a brief description of the pros and cons of the various anaesthetic circuits that are in common use in anaesthetic practice. The authors discuss their relative merits and describe disposable, low-flow circle and Waters systems. This relatively brief discussion of anaesthetic circuits should provide the reader with a clear understanding of the choices involved. There then follows an outline of current techniques for ventilating patients undergoing endoscopic surgery on the airway since such patients are currently being managed as outpatients either for diagnostic procedures or for laser surgery of a limited extent. In Appendix 3 there is an outline of the physiological effects of high-frequency jet ventilation and the necessary monitoring for procedural safety. These techniques are now practised on a world-wide basis using total intravenous anaesthesia (TIVA). The final part is a brief outline of the principles of cuirass ventilation which although widely used during bronchoscopy many years ago fell into decline, but with more modern equipment it is undergoing a resurgence in some units performing endoscopic surgery on the upper airways.

Paediatric anaesthesia

There then follows a section on paediatric anaesthesia in three parts where Drs Lord and Morton discuss the problems peculiar to young children (Chapters 19–21), based on their considerable experience of this subject.

Since paediatric anaesthesia should always be the province of fully trained and arguably specialist anaesthetists, this section should be of interest to such specialists in that it presents a current overview of the subject based on experience in two busy centres. Dr Lord directs what is arguably one of the best organized paediatric day-case units in the UK. He is regarded as an expert in this field, particularly in relation to the psychological preparation of children for anaesthesia and surgery (Chapter 20). Dr Morton, of the Royal Hospital for Sick Children, Glasgow, is regarded as an authority in the field of local anaesthesia in children (Chapter 21). He gives a clear description of both theory and practice of local analgesia for children in the day-case setting.

Adult Anaesthesia

Chapter 11
Adult Day-Case Anaesthesia

A. P. Fisher and E. K. Krzeminska

The following description is based upon practice in the day surgery centre (DSC) of King's College Hospital, London. Differing local practices, circumstances and facilities may demand variations in the theme, but any protocol should ensure the safe and efficient selection, screening, treatment and discharge of informed, comfortable and hopefully satisfied patients. An overview of the preoperative processing of day patients through the system is provided in Fig. 11.1. An algorithm for medical selection and investigation is shown in Appendix A. Preoperative preparation for day surgery is reviewed by Goodwin and Ogg [1].

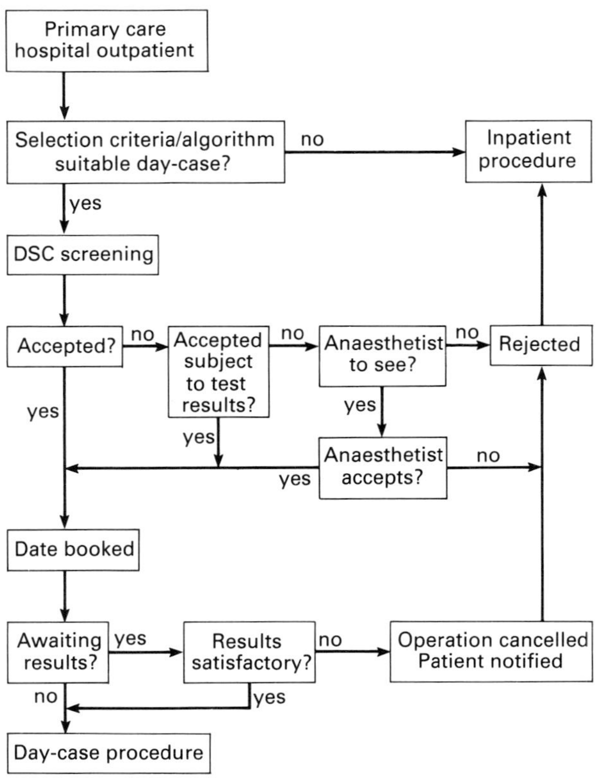

Fig. 11.1 Day-case processing flow chart.

Table 11.1 Selection criteria for day-case surgery

Surgery
Diagnostic-related group
Unlikely to cause
loss of independence or toilet function
severe morbidity, haemorrhage, pain, nausea, vomiting
Medical
ASA I, II or controlled III
Minimal investigation required
Anaesthetic
No adverse previous history, e.g. difficult intubation, delayed recovery, cardiac arrest
No personal or family history of a serious relevant inherited disorder, e.g. malignant hyperpyrexia and myopathies
Sociodomestic
Satisfactory home including telephone
24 h supervision by responsible adult
Transport—reasonable travelling time
Back-up arrangements—medical, nursing, communication
Medicolegal
Correct counselling and consent
Understanding by the patient of his or her responsibilities

Selection

Successful outcome in day surgery, in terms of a minimal incidence of complications and adverse postoperative symptomatology, along with maximum throughput of cases and patient satisfaction, is in large measure a function of selection. A high rate of complications, adverse symptomatology and poor throughput will impair the ability of the provider unit to compete effectively.

Selection begins in the surgical outpatient clinic, office or primary care system. Locally agreed guidelines for patient selection should be freely available. They should also undergo periodic review since criteria of suitability for treatment in any one-day surgery unit are likely to vary with local expertise, enthusiasm and experience coupled with practical, technical and pharmaceutical developments in surgery and anaesthesia. Acceptance of an individual patient not meeting the local criteria of suitability should be both uncommon and the subject of agreement between both anaesthetic and surgical staff and unit management. The latter because of possible knock-on effects on unit efficiency, admission and complication rates, and medicolegal issues.

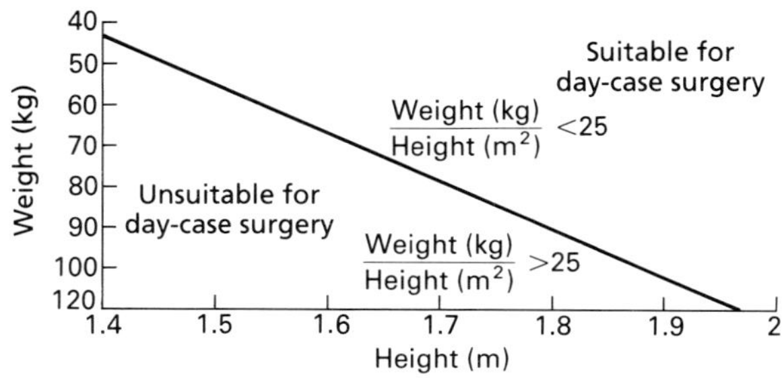

Fig. 11.2 Height-weight nomogram for day surgery selection. Adapted from Van Besouw and Williamson (D. J. Wilkinson, personal communication).

At the first outpatient clinic visit, an experienced surgeon should assess the patient against the day surgery unit's selection criteria of suitability for day care (Table 11.1).

Ideally this assessment will include height, weight and blood pressure measurements, and urine testing. A survey of the literature in 1985 by Van Besouw and Wilkinson (D. J. Wilkinson, personal communication) led to the construction of a height–weight nomogram which shows a reasonable threshold of height–weight combinations acceptable for day-case general anaesthesia. It is based primarily on the concept that weight (kg) divided by height^2 (m^2) should be less than 25 (Fig. 11.2). Arguably this is a better method of assessing obesity than the practice of most units which is to merely rely on the weight of the patient, with an arbitrary cut-off point.

Morbidly or grossly obese patients, or those falling only just on the wrong side of the line but with other complications, e.g. chronic obstructive pulmonary disease (COPD) or a history of gastro-oesophageal reflux, should not be selected for referral to the day-care unit. Routine urine dipstick testing is a cheap and easy means of detecting unsuspected diabetes or nephropathy in asymptomatic patients [2]. Unexplained proteinuria or glycosuria, or an unacceptably high blood pressure measurement in the clinic should lead to further outpatient investigation, whilst an elevated blood pressure of uncertain significance should be repeated later at the time of medical screening in the day surgery unit.

The patient also has responsibilities for their own welfare. An appreciation by the patient of the need for a responsible attitude to the postoperative period should be a part of the initial selection process. It is incumbent upon day surgery clinicians and nursing staff to ensure that the patient has received all the written and verbal information they need to behave safely and responsibly in the postoperative and preoperative periods.

Investigations

These should be initiated in the surgical outpatient clinic, in some circumstances supported by data from the primary care or other referral clinic with all results directed to the day surgery unit. Dresner and Soni [3] reviewed the role of routine preoperative tests and made the point that despite the routine ordering of many tests there is little evidence to support any usefulness of the results in terms of clinical management. For example, in a study of the results of screening tests in 200 ambulatory surgical patients, much of the high incidence of abnormality could have been predicted on the basis of history and examination, nor did the abnormal results influence patient outcome, calling into question the role of such screening [4].

They emphasized the importance of clinical assessment in screening patients and that such screening should specifically direct a requirement for tests which should not be performed, defensively or otherwise, as a routine. Indeed, despite their claimed importance in preoperative assessment, occasionally test results are only seen, reported or evaluated after surgery.

Wasted resource and unjustifiable physical insult to a patient by unnecessary investigation are reasons enough to restrict preoperative investigation of any patient to a minimum. Once ordered, examination of a test result should be mandatory since the performance of the test might medicolegally be assumed to indicate its relevance to the management of the case. The sometimes surprisingly difficult task, even in 1993, of retrieving and examining results prior to anaesthesia and surgery in some health-care units, might then interfere with the organizational logistics of an efficient, 'no on-the-day cancellation', day surgery service. This provides a secondary, but nevertheless pragmatic reason why investigation, particularly of day surgery patients, should be genuinely indicated.

What constitutes a genuine requirement for preoperative investigation? Investigations are required where there is known, or suspected, based upon history and examination, pathology which by its presence or treatment could be associated with derangement of the patient's physiological homeostasis and reserve, and *where the investigation is likely to add something to clinical assessment*. In such cases investigative confirmation of the existence and degree of pathology, if it cannot be adequately assessed clinically, leading to appropriate treatment to correct or reduce physiological derangement, helps in the assessment and reduction of risk of anaesthesia. In this respect measurement of *C-reactive protein* (CRP) or *serum amyloid A protein* (SAA) may be invaluable to assess the level of activity of intercurrent disease [5].

Haemoglobin estimation. Asymptomatic patients rarely yield abnormal results. For example, only 7 of 2117 patients undergoing maxillofacial and oral surgery were unpredictably found to have an Hb less than 10 g dl^{-1} [6]. These were all female and some would argue that Hb estimation is mandatory in all women of childbearing years because of the menstrual predisposition to anaemia. Clinical symptoms or signs of anaemia should be investigated.

Urine testing and blood chemistry. Fewer than 1% of patients under 40 years show abnormalities of blood biochemical values, leading to the assertion that routine urine testing is good enough in patients under 50 years old [7]. In a prospective study of 1062 surgical patients the incidence of blood biochemical analysis abnormalities was found to be 1·5% in the ASA I and 17% in the ASA II populations, rising to about 50%

Table 11.2 Indications for urea and electrolyte measurements. Adapted from Dresner and Soni [3]

ASA I	Only if clinically indicated
ASA II	Only if a clinical indication exists, e.g. diuretic therapy or grounds for suspecting renal impairment, e.g. long-standing diabetes
ASA III	All patients

Table 11.3 Indications for a preoperative electrocardiogram. Adapted from Dresner and Soni [3]

History suggesting heart disease, e.g. angina, myocardial infarction, breathlessness on exertion, hypertension, excessive fatigue during the working day, oedema, nocturnal dyspnoea, palpitations
Examination suggesting heart disease, e.g. cardiac enlargement, oedema, cyanosis, raised venous pressure, murmurs, disorder of rate or rhythm
Systemic disease known to be associated with cardiac involvement, e.g. hypertension, diabetes, rheumatic fever, family history of cardiomyopathy, endemic disorders or syndromes, e.g. acromegaly, Cushing's syndrome
Age—there are no hard and fast rules particularly if a portable monitor with ECG and SaO_2 functions is available

in ASA grade III patients or those on diuretics [8]. If testing is felt to be necessary then it should be focused on the higher risk groups (Table 11.2), bearing in mind that many of the usual 'abnormal' findings, e.g. glucose and urea, are unlikely to alter management in day surgery patients who have been clinically assessed as being in good health.

Electrocardiogram (ECG). The increasing prevalence of ECG abnormalities with age, more so in men than women, is largely predictable in individual patients on the basis of history and examination. Unless ECG testing is focused on those who clinically are likely to show abnormalities the routine preoperative ECG is an inefficient investigation [9]. However, the presence of a modern portable monitor for the measurement of blood pressure, heart rate, SaO_2 and a display of a routine ECG in the assessment unit resolves this problem, provided that hard copy is not required. Based upon a review of the routine ECG by Goldberger and O'Konski [10] Dresner and Soni [3] drew up indications for a full preanaesthetic ECG assessment which has been modified and adopted for day surgery patients (Table 11.3).

Chest X-ray examination. Reports of the utility of preoperative chest X-rays by the Royal College of Radiologists [11] and Tape and Mushlin [12] indicates the higher yield of abnormal results by selecting a higher risk population for investigation (Table 11.4)

Table 11.4 Indications for a preoperative chest X-ray. Adapted from Dresner and Soni [3]

History suggestive of active lung disease
Asthma
Haemoptysis
Pleural pain
Cough—recent, or change in type of cough, e.g. in patients with chronic bronchitis
Hoarseness—recent, not resolving
Systemic disturbance, e.g. breathlessness, fever, sweating
Physical signs of lung disease
Low SaO_2, an assessment monitor (or cyanosis)
Clinical chest examination
Symptoms and signs of heart or pulmonary disease

There is no indication for routine preoperative chest X-rays for baseline assessment or in the elderly in the absence of a suitable clinical history.

but casts doubt on any value of the findings in terms of altered clinical management. In the context of day surgery and anaesthesia it is probably reasonable to suggest that if a chest X-ray is requested on the basis that it is really likely to affect a clinically based management plan, then the patient is probably inappropriately selected for day surgery.

Conclusions. A retrospective study [13] of 325 patients who had preadmission testing prior to ambulatory surgery discovered at least one laboratory abnormality in 84% of the patients, an abnormal ECG in 24% and an abnormal chest X-ray in 19%. Of the abnormal laboratory results, 96% were ignored by the attending physicians and only 1% of patients potentially benefited from preadmission testing. It was concluded that investigation should be selective, based upon history and clinical examination.

In the context of a carefully selected day surgery population, given the weight of the available evidence, investigations along guidelines such as those shown in the algorithm in Appendix A should suffice. This type of algorithm now forms the basis of an increasing number of computerized assessment programs for which software is available. A display of a visual questionnaire on the computer screen allows self-assessment by the patient although arguably a simple hard copy will suffice (see Appendix B). However, after completion of the questionnaire a nurse or physician can work through risk factors and recommend investigations with the patient on a computer screen with the results immediately to hand for recording or reports.

It is emphasized that these are only guidelines. The principle of aiming investigations at those patients where abnormalities are more likely to be found should always be applied. Whilst the clinical judgement of the individual anaesthetist remains the final responsibility for anaesthetizing the patient, it is important that a local consensus view is reached about which investigations are or are not necessary if

Table 11.5 Objectives of day surgery centre visit by patient for assessment and booking*

Familiarization of patient with location of unit
Verification of appropriate patient selection (Table 11.1)
Verification of recommended investigation (Appendix A)
Detailed nurse administered screening, questionnaire and guidelines (Appendices B and C)
Referral of difficult assessment to anaesthesiologist
Discussion and counselling of the patient for the forthcoming investigation, procedures and treatment
Provision of written information and instructions regarding the procedure (Appendix D)
Fixing a date for the procedure (this is normally within 4–6 weeks of any laboratory investigation). If there is a long delay, for example due to a significant waiting list, reassessment may be required

* While each unit may write its own information booklet, most follow the recommendations of their national societies where these exist. The most recent guidelines for patients are from the American Society of Anesthiologists and are probably, from the patient's point of view, the best of their type.

patients are to be presented appropriately investigated to the day surgery centre (DSC) and not cancelled on the day. Such consensus is more likely to be forthcoming amongst senior anaesthetists, which is an important reason for the continuous presence of senior anaesthetists in the day surgery setting.

DSC booking visit

If deemed suitable for day-case management the clinician refers the patient to the DSC along with details of the planned procedure, any relevant investigations now requested or already done (e.g. sickle screen) with results if available. The patient proceeds from the clinic, if necessary via the pathology block for blood test(s) and/or the cardiac department for ECG, to the DSC for the screening and booking visit.

Whilst outpatient selection of suitable patients is successful in most cases, in a busy surgical clinic there may often be little time for thorough exploration of, for example, the sociodomestic issues pertinent to day care. Similarly, medical issues may only be briefly touched upon. For such reasons and where, as at King's College Hospital, potential DSC patients originate from a wide variety of surgical disciplines and clinics staffed by different and changing personnel, it is necessary for patients to travel a 'final common pathway' if a series of important clinical objectives are to be attained in a standardized, reproducible, quality assured fashion and the DSC is to be able to organize the utilization of its facilities by patients and clinical staff in an efficient manner. This 'path' is the DSC screening and booking visit where the objectives are as listed in Table 11.5. These activities are performed by DSC nurses supported by clerical and administrative staff.

In taking charge of the attainment of these objectives motivated and experienced day unit nursing staff protect the unit from inappropriate use and minimize the chances of on-the-day-cancellations, an unacceptable event. A patient who has satisfied the day surgery centre based screening is then given a date for operation and written information (both general and procedure-specific) to reinforce what has already been discussed with the nurse. Appendix D indicates the general information which should be imparted to patients who are to undergo day-case general anaesthesia. Where an investigation result is required, the patient is advised that the date given is subject to satisfactory test results. If the nurse requires referral to an anaesthetist, no date is given until the patient has been seen by a senior anaesthetist.

Of particular importance to anaesthetists, who are not usually in a position to see day patients before the morning of the operative day, is the efficacy of the nurse administered and guided questionnaire (see Appendix B), and medical screening procedures ensuring that unsuitable patients are not booked into the unit. The success or otherwise of this aspect of the unit's organization is in large measure dependent upon the enthusiasm with which all the staff support and monitor its development and practice. It is in everyone's interests to ensure success. Of help in this regard is the development with the DSC nurses, based upon the Royal College of Surgeons of England model of supportive guidelines [14] (see Appendix C) in the use of the medical questionnaire which are intended to help the nurse decide upon the significance of positive responses to the questions.

Preoperative management

On the operation day a number of admission checks need to be made (Table 11.6.) Omission of formal assessment by an anaesthetist at a preadmission visit was found to have no deleterious effect upon preoperative anxiety in a study of 63 women undergoing ambulatory minor gynaecological surgery [15] and Arellano *et al.* [16] found that the best timing of a preoperative visit for reduction of anxiety was immediately prior to surgery.

Table 11.6 Final checks on day of procedure

Has the patient:
Had serious health problem since booking?
Arranged a responsible companion for 24 h?
Taken any medicines or drugs?
Is the patient:
Ill in any way today?
Appropriately fasted?
Pregnant?

A survey of 124 preoperative patients revealed that the three most stressful preoperative experiences were waiting to go into the operating theatre, denture removal and fluid deprivation [17]. Even in the best organized day surgery units patients cannot yet walk into theatre from the street. Good unit organization and the keeping of staggered appointments may go some way towards minimizing on-the-day preoperative waiting, but if operating slots in day surgery theatres are not to be left unused then it seems inevitable that there must be some degree of waiting. Dentures can certainly be left in place until induction of anaesthesia and there are arguments for and against removing them [18, 19]. Ultimately, the decision to proceed lies with the individual anaesthetist on the day, since legally he or she will be held responsible.

Fluids

There is accumulating evidence that allowing oral fluids up to 2 h before elective surgery enhances preoperative comfort without compromising perioperative safety in healthy, unpremedicated patients [20, 21]. A review of the evidence for and against preoperative starvation found no adverse effect on gastric contents or postoperative nausea in patients allowed to drink until 2 h preoperatively [22].

A Canadian teaching hospital modified its guidelines in 1988 to recommend a 3 h fast period for elective surgical patients. The change was reportedly well received and a follow-up study of day-case patients confirmed no difference in gastric fluid volume or pH between those patients allowed to drink and those who fasted from midnight [23, 24].

Goodwin *et al.* [25] reported upon the symptomatic benefit of 150 ml of oral fluid 1·5–2 h preoperatively without adverse effect in 50 patients compared with a midnight fast control group.

Premedication

In seeking to allow rapid recovery and early return to 'street-fitness' it is common practice to avoid sedative premedication in day case anaesthesia. Nevertheless certain patients do benefit from the administration of a variety of drugs in advance of transfer to the anaesthetic room or operating theatre (Table 11.7).

Children, and some adults, appreciate the application of a eutectic mixture of local anaesthetics (EMLA) cream prior to establishing venous access. Anxiolytic agents may benefit some adult patients, whilst for some children sedative premedication is of value. In attempting to provide pre-emptive analgesia, non-steroidal anti-inflammatory drugs may be given in advance of surgery but these can cause a variety of serious complications in susceptible patients (see Chapter 2). Drugs which reduce gastric volume and increase gastric pH should be considered for patients with symptomatic reflux from hiatus hernia, and in patients presenting for second trimester terminations of pregnancy.

Table 11.7 Considerations in premedication

Counselling of the patient
Eutectic mixture of local anaesthetic (EMLA) cream
Benzodiazepines
β adrenergic blockers
α_2 adrenergic agonists
Non-steroidal anti-inflammatory drugs unless contraindicated (see Chapter 2)
Aspiration prophylaxis
Opioids only if necessary

Whilst many fears may be allayed by careful explanation preoperatively, some patients feel better as a result of anxiolytic premedication. A 'premed' is expected by many patients and this should be discussed during the counselling process.

Anxiolytics. Of the benzodiazepines, midazolam has been found to be as effective as temazepam [26], and its short terminal half-life of 1·75 h makes it preferable. Yet despite apparently good recovery, psychomotor function was still depressed with both agents at 4 h [27]. However, in another study of 75 patients including a placebo group both drugs were found to be equally effective with no recovery delay [28].

In children Weldon *et al.* [29] found 0·5 mg kg^{-1} midazolam orally to be maximally effective at 30 min with no recovery delay by comparison with placebo. They found no further benefit with adjunctive atropine or pethidine. Parnis *et al.* [30] in a study of 200 children showed that whilst oral midazolam was an effective premedicant, the use of both diazepam and midazolam was associated with longer stays in the recovery room; this however was not associated with an increased length of stay. Parnis showed also that a high proportion of unsedated children were calm at induction of anaesthesia; many, if not most, children do not require sedative or anxiolytic premedication.

Opioids. Long-acting opioid premedication is not usually employed because of its potential undesirable side effects. In a study of 150 adults undergoing a variety of day-surgical procedures Shafer *et al.* [31] found intramuscular midazolam to be an effective anxiolytic which did not prolong discharge time; in the same study it was shown that intravenous fentanyl and oxymorphone were also effective and reduced both the dose of induction agent required and the incidence of respiratory problems, e.g. coughing. Oxycodone, moreover, was associated with a lower incidence of postoperative pain at home. However, both opioids were associated with a high incidence of nausea and vomiting. By contrast, intramuscular alfentanil was found to be well tolerated and caused less lasting sedation than midazolam [32]. Oral transmucosal fentanyl has been found to produce effective short-lasting sedation in children and to facilitate inhalational induction. However, a high incidence of postoperative nausea and vomiting was reported and this was not significantly reduced by the prophylactic use of droperidol [33].

Other premedicants. In an effort to avoid the sedation associated with conventional anxiolytic agents and the side effects of opioids, β-blockers have been evaluated. Dyck and Chung [34] showed no difference between the anxiolytic effects of propranolol, diazepam and placebo. More recently, MacKenzie [35] has used the short-acting β-blocker timolol with good effect and no significant haemodynamic disturbance.

The α_2 agonists are currently arousing interest as premedicants. Whilst clonidine has been found to compare favourably with diazepam in producing sedation, reducing anxiety and improving cardiovascular stability in elderly patients undergoing general anaesthesia [36], the shorter-acting dexmedetomidine may prove of value in the day surgical setting. Several potentially useful effects have been reported, e.g. reduction in the minimal alveolar concentration (MAC) of volatile agents, attenuation of haemodynamic response to intubation, reduction of postoperative nausea and fatigue following minor gynaecological surgery and a reduction in postoperative opioid requirement [37].

Gastric acid aspiration prophylaxis. A certain proportion of patients presenting for day-case surgery are considered to be at risk of aspiration of gastric contents, notably those with symptomatic reflux, known hiatus hernia and patients in the second trimester of pregnancy. Histamine receptor (H_2) antagonists, as used prophylactically in obstetric anaesthetic practice, may be prescribed, with or without metoclopramide. Susceptible patients identified at the time of screening may be given an oral H_2 antagonist to take at home on the evening before surgery and/or early on the day of admission. The effect of ranitidine, famotidine and the gastric parietal cell proton pump blocker omeprazole were compared with placebo by Escolano *et al.* [38]. Both H_2 antagonists and omeprazole in a single oral dose produced significant increase in gastric pH and reduction in gastric fluid volume, but omeprazole may need to be administered in two doses for maximal effect (see also Chapter 2).

Other considerations

In the DSC of King's College Hospital a patient is provided with both an easy chair and a 'King's trolley' which serves as bed, trolley and operating table. As an operating table it raises, lowers, tilts head up or head down, and will take leg stirrups, arm boards, and infusion stands. This purpose-designed trolley obviates the need for patient transfers from bed to trolley, trolley to operating table, operating table to trolley, and finally trolley to bed. A variety of such equipment is now available with some degree of customization on request to the manufacturers.

It is not within the remit of this chapter to debate the place of the anaesthetic room in modern anaesthetic practice [39]. Soni and Thomas [40] could not demonstrate any difference in anxiety in patients admitted directly to operating theatre or anaesthetic room. In King's DSC these rooms have been retained as 'holding' and 'anaesthetic preparation' rooms where the blood pressure cuffs, ECG leads and an intravenous cannula are placed prior to induction of anaesthesia. With the exit of the previous patient to recovery the next patient is then immediately ready for induction of anaesthesia which for adults generally takes place in the operating theatre. The patient is thus monitored from the induction of anaesthesia onwards without discontinuity or trolley to table transfer. Arguably this is an important consideration in procedural safety.

Anaesthetic technique

There can be little dispute about the need to utilize anaesthetic techniques which provide rapid recovery, good postoperative analgesia and minimal adverse symptomatology of which postoperative pain, nausea and vomiting are the most serious. These objectives are generating much research in this field.

It is impossible to be dogmatic about which anaesthetic technique should be used for which operation. The introduction of new agents (propofol, alfentanil, mivacurium and desflurane), the laryngeal mask, improvements in monitoring, record keeping, in risk analysis and procedural safety, together with the increasing application of minimally invasive therapy, are all contributing to the development of day-case anaesthesia. The anaesthesiologist must rapidly accept new ideas and changed practices. To do otherwise is to withdraw from peer and public credibility.

Propofol has established its place in day-case anaesthesia on the basis of improved recovery characteristics. A comparative study of propofol, thiopentone, methohexitone and etomidate showed more rapid recovery with propofol and led to a change in clinical practice in one very important internationally established day-case unit [41]. Comparison of thiopentone with propofol in another study in which patients were followed for 48 h found that patients given propofol were fit for discharge sooner and perceived greater postoperative wellbeing than patients who received thiopentone [42]. The merits of propofol are discussed in some detail in Chapter 2.

Newer inhalational agents. The relative merits of desflurane and sevoflurane together with the current status of halothane, enflurane and isoflurane are reviewed in Chapter 2.

Airway management—laryngeal mask airway (LMA). Because of the different natures of outpatient and inpatient surgery, the LMA is likely to have a much more prominent place in the context of day-case anaesthesia where it may increasingly usurp the place of the traditional face mask. Such use has been reported to cause a reduction in episodes of desaturation, and increased eficiency by freeing the anaesthetist's hands

[43]. It also reduces the anatomical deadspace and by ensuring a sealed or leak-free airway it allows the accurate measurement of the end tidal carbon dioxide concentration thereby completing full minimal monitoring during anaesthesia. Two recent editorials review the place of the LMA in anaesthetic practice [44, 45]. The latter indicates those circumstances in which the authors feel that the LMA is appropriate or inappropriate and makes reference to reports of pulmonary aspiration with the LMA [46]. This implies that the conventional cuffed tracheal tube should be used in patients with a high risk of aspiration of stomach contents, e.g. emergency procedures, oesophageal reflux or pregnancy. One study has shown that gynaecological laparoscopy in procedures of short duration and in suitably selected patients may be safely performed in spontaneously breathing patients in whom the airway is maintained with a laryngeal mask [47].

Barker *et al.* [48] reported a study in which 56 patients with no recognizable risk factors for regurgitation each swallowed a gelatine capsule containing methylene blue 10 min before induction of anaesthesia. None of the 28 patients in whom general anaesthesia was administered via a face mask and Guedel airway, but seven (25%) in a LMA group, were found to have regurgitated dye. The suggestion that this finding in the LMA group might indicate a lowering of lower oesophageal sphincter (LOS) tone by the presence of the LMA in the pharynx seems to have been confirmed by a subsequently reported study [49]. This would further strengthen the case for the continued use of conventional tracheal tubes in patients at high risk of aspiration of stomach contents.

Looking at airway protection from above rather than below, John *et al.* [50] found that blue dye placed in the pharynx above a laryngeal mask did not contaminate the airway in a group of 64 patients, suggesting protection for oral and ear, nose and throat (ENT) surgery. A subsequent study has also demonstrated successful use of a reinforced LMA in adenotonsillectomy as an alternative to tracheal intubation, with protection of the larynx from blood-soiling and easier postoperative airway management by comparison with extubation and use of a Guedel airway [51].

Where intubation is preferred, in a study of 100 adults undergoing dental extraction in whom either alfentanil or suxamethonium were used as adjuncts to propofol prior to intubation, smaller incidences of postoperative myalgia and sore throat were found in the alfentanil group but not without some intubation failures and less good intubating conditions [52]. Such manoeuvres intended to improve patients' postoperative well-being highlight the need for experienced anaesthetists in day surgery.

Circuits—Humphrey ADE circuit. During inhalational day-case anaesthesia of short to medium duration the cost and antipollution benefits of low flow circle absorbers are less than for procedures of longer duration. By combining the efficiencies of the Mapleson A and D configurations for spontaneous and controlled ventilation respectively, the Humphrey ADE breathing system provides a cost-effective means of reducing expenditure on expensive volatile agents when used as an alternative to the Bain circuit in spontaneously breathing patients and, by a single lever movement, the convenience of immediate transition to a ventilated Mapleson D/E configuration. The system provides a lightweight, easily scavenged breathing circuit applicable to both adults and children [53–55]. The ADE system is conveniently used, as in King's DSC, in conjunction with a Nuffield 200 ventilator with both adult and paediatric valves. The relative merits of the various anaesthetic circuits in common use are reviewed in Chapter 18.

Monitoring

There being no such thing as a minor anaesthetic, monitoring in the day-case setting should be as comprehensive as it should be in an inpatient setting, and in accordance with generally accepted minimal monitoring standards [56, 57]. The more invasive forms of monitoring are unlikely to be necessary in day case patients and surgery. Monitoring in the King's College Hospital DSC consists of pulse oximetry, ECG, non-invasive blood pressure, inspiratory and expiratory fractional concentrations of oxygen, carbon dioxide and volatile agent. Temperature probes are not routinely placed but are immediately available.

The use of recovery room patient monitors which will accept the theatre monitoring leads already attached to the patient means that on transfer to the recovery area there is only minimal discontinuity in patient monitoring. ECG, blood pressure and SaO_2 are routinely monitored during recovery. A 'tram' system with portable monitors allows total continuity of monitoring. Alternatively each patient can be attached to a portable fully comprehensive monitor from the preinduction period until the patient leaves the recovery room. Such systems are referred to as 'seamless' monitoring.

Recovery

Many patients emerging from well-conducted anaesthesia appropriate for day-case surgery will open their eyes whilst still fully monitored by the anaesthetist in the operating theatre. Others may take a few minutes to awaken. Either way, a short period in a designated, fully equipped recovery area staffed by trained personnel, in close proximity to the anaesthetist, allows safe completion of awakening, establishment of 'ward fitness', immediate identification and treatment of any adverse postoperative symptoms, and ordered, informed transfer of the care of the postoperative patient to the ward nursing staff.

Discharge

There is no test available which is either clinically practical or allows the setting of a 'pass mark' for safe discharge home. Discharge is allowed by the DSC nursing staff

Table 11.8 Discharge criteria after general anaesthesia/sedation. A patient who has undergone a procedure involving the administration of general anaesthetic or sedative drugs must fulfil the following criteria before being allowed home

Walks without difficulty
Pain/nausea adequately controlled
No suspected haemorrhage or visceral leak (e.g. laparoscopic procedures)
Not vomiting/tolerating oral fluids
Has passed urine (where relevant)
Responsible adult companion present
Patient and companion reminded of 24 h restrictions
Discharge reminder sheet issued
Suitable transport available

Table 11.9 Discharge reminders

Now that you are going home we wish to remind you that after a general anaesthetic or sedation there is a period in which your judgement, performance and reaction time are impaired, even though you may feel quite normal again. It is therefore very important that:

1 Until you feel perfectly well again, or while you are taking strong painkillers, and in any case for at least 24 (preferably 48) h after your anaesthetic or sedation, you should not drink alcohol, drive a car, ride a bicycle, operate machinery, use a cooker, do anything potentially dangerous to yourself or others, or make important decisions

2 You should remain in the care of a responsible adult for 24 h after your operation

3 You should take painkillers or further sedatives only on the advice of a doctor

when a number of simple clinical and social criteria are met (Table 11.8). Nor is it possible to advise individual patients as to when exactly they will be able to undertake their usual activities safely once more, as people differ in their recovery characteristics.

The patient should be discharged with verbal and written reminders (Table 11.9) about restrictions on activities and also information on operation-specific aftercare. Emphasis should be laid on the need for a responsible attitude to the recovery period, in particular that the full range of skilled activities of daily life, e.g. driving, should not be resumed until the patient feels perfectly well again, is not taking painkillers or anti-emetics which may affect mental acuity or reaction times, and in any case not before 24 h have elapsed since anaesthesia.

Postoperative analgesia

Good postoperative analgesia is a prime requisite for day surgery. Pain varies in nature and intensity according to the operative site and surgical technique. Increasingly invasive procedures are being undertaken as day surgical procedures, for example laparoscopic cholecystectomy, prostatectomy, thyroidectomy.

The drugs available for postoperative analgesia include simple analgesics, non-steroidal anti-inflammatory drugs (NSAIDs), opioids and local anaesthetics. Often a combination of techniques provides 'balanced analgesia' directed at pain of multiple pathophysiology. The concept of 'pre-emptive analgesia', discussed recently by Bush [58], which has been in use for many years, is particularly relevant in day surgery because of the need to discharge the patient home comfortably and without drug-induced side effects.

Opioids

The ideal analgesic for use in day surgery would combine potent peroperative action with a long duration of effect sufficient to provide adequate postoperative analgesia but without side effects which might delay discharge.

The administration of powerful, long-acting opioids in the day-surgery setting, with the side-effects of sedation, nausea, vomiting, pruritus and respiratory depression, may make the patient feel ill, delay discharge and even necessitate overnight admission [59]. In seeking to minimize adverse postoperative side effects whilst maximizing the peroperative analgesic effect, short-acting opioids such as fentanyl and alfentanil are therefore often employed since they have durations of action which mirror the duration of many day surgical procedures. The shorter half-life of alfentanil (1·5 vs. 3 h) makes it the more desirable opioid for use in day surgery. Alfentanil may be given as an infusion with a reduction in both dose requirement and recovery time [60].

This peroperative analgesia strategy is at the cost of potentially inadequate postoperative pain relief, although alfentanil may be self-administered by the patient using a patient controlled analgesia device in the immediate postoperative period [61]. The provision of postoperative analgesia usually demands alternative analgesic drugs or procedures.

Minor analgesics

Simple oral analgesics such as paracetamol and aspirin, used alone or in combination with the 'milder' opioids such as dextropropoxyphene and codeine, may suffice to provide good postoperative analgesia for many operations.

NSAIDs

NSAIDs are used increasingly to provide postoperative analgesia, without the side effects of opioids [62], having been shown to reduce the postoperative opioid requirements following a variety of surgical procedures [63–66] and to be effective adjuvants to simple oral analgesics after minor surgery [67].

Table 11.10 Options for postoperative analgesia

Pre-emptive analgesia
Local anaesthetics
Simple analgesics
Non-steroidal anti-inflammatory drugs
Opioids only if necessary

These drugs act by inhibiting prostaglandin synthesis and hence the formation of mediators involved in initiating pain perception. It has been shown that they are more effective when administered preoperatively [68–70] presumably because the presence of drug levels in the tissues preoperatively reduces the inflammatory response mediated by arachidonic acid and thus dampens the effect of a nociceptive stimulus [71]. Moreover, the duration of action of NSAIDs far exceeds that of the short-acting opioids, lasting well into the discharge period.

Commonly used NSAIDs in day surgery are aspirin, diclofenac, indomethacin and naproxen, although others are being evaluated. Piroxicam is now available in oral, injectable and rectal formulations. Ketorolac (30 mg i.v.) has a ceiling effect equivalent to 10 mg of morphine with a delay of approximately 40 min to peak effect, without the side effects associated with opioids [72]. In a comparison of preoperative administration of ketorolac, fentanyl and a new partial μ agonist dezocine (available in the USA), ketorolac produced better analgesia than fentanyl, without the nausea and vomiting associated with the other two drugs [73].

NSAIDs are not without side effects which are generally less distressing than those of opioids, and are less likely to be troublesome when used short term as in association with day surgery. However, they can cause serious side effects in susceptible patients including anaphylaxis, bronchospasm, renal failure and loss of platelet function (see Chapter 2) (Table 11.10).

Local anaesthetics

Topical application of local anaesthetic preparations may provide good analgesia following minor surgery. Tree-Trakarn *et al.* [74] reported that the analgesic effect following circumcision of lignocaine gel, ointment and spray was comparable to that produced by dorsal nerve block of the penis in children and adults. EMLA (a 5% eutectic mixture of lignocaine and prilocaine) has been used to provide surface analgesia in circumcision but with a short-lived effect for 45 min by comparison with 4–6 h analgesia after dorsal nerve block [75]. In adults, bupivacaine instillation was found to be as effective as inguinal field block in providing postoperative analgesia following herniorrhaphy [76] thereby providing genuine pre-emptive analgesia [58].

Wound infiltration and field block are widely employed to ensure good immediate postoperative analgesia, bupivacaine being the agent of choice because of its longer duration of action compared with other local anaesthetics. Infiltration has been shown to be more effective when performed preincisionally [77], presumably by blocking the initiation of impulse transmission in pain pathways. By contrast Dierking *et al.* [78] could find no evidence that preincisional inguinal field block provided better postoperative analgesia than postclosure block in a double-blind, randomized study of 32 patients undergoing inguinal herniorrhaphy.

Instillation of local anaesthetic subdiaphragmatically after laparoscopy has been used to reduce shoulder pain [79]. Bilateral rectus sheath block can reduce significantly postoperative pain after diagnostic laparoscopy [80], whilst for the more painful procedure of laparoscopic sterilization Smith *et al.* [81] successfully employed bilateral mesosalpinx block.

Joint infiltration with local anaesthetic has provided effective pain relief after orthopaedic surgery [82]. Intra-articular bupivacaine has been found to permit earlier mobilization and lesser analgesic requirement in day-case arthroscopy [83]. Whilst the evidence for peripheral opioid receptors in humans remains inconclusive, in animals opioids have been shown to have peripheral antinociceptive actions [84], and intra-articular morphine (1 mg) has been shown to produce naloxone-reversible analgesia in arthroscopic knee surgery [85], although another study disputes its efficacy by comparison with bupivacaine [86].

Specific nerve and plexus blocks may be used as appropriate to provide both operative and postoperative analgesia for a variety of procedures, e.g. ankle block for foot surgery, brachial plexus block for upper limb procedures.

Regional techniques such as spinal and epidural blocks are however probably least utilized in the day-case setting since their advantages, e.g. no loss of consciousness if used alone for anaesthesia, avoidance of complications of general anaesthesia, and extension of analgesia into the postoperative period, are generally perceived to be outweighed by their potential complications, e.g. excessive motor and sensory blockade, spinal headache and urinary retention, which increase patient discomfort and may delay or prevent discharge.

Despite these considerations, caudal block has been shown to provide effective analgesia in children and adults undergoing perirectal surgery and circumcision, and a postdischarge survey carried out in 102 patients following either general or spinal anaesthesia for day-surgical transurethral resection of the prostate (TURP), showed a significant incidence of nausea and vomiting in the general anaesthesia group, yet a low incidence of headache in the spinal group [87]. Bupivacaine used spinally produces prolonged side effects as well as analgesia. Shorter-acting agents such as hyperbaric 5% lignocaine, isobaric 2% lignocaine and more recently hypobaric 0·5% lignocaine

[88] have been used, the latter producing discharge times 205 ($\pm$45) min after the block was performed.

The guiding principle should be to employ the simplest effective block in preference to one with more widespread effects. The use of local anaesthetic blockade in conjunction with other forms of analgesia, may reduce the requirement for the latter, thus minimizing the risk of their side effects [89]. In addition some surgery may be performed solely with the use of regional techniques [90] (Chapter 15).

Patients should be warned that local anaesthetic effects will wear off after a few hours and that they may then need to take oral analgesics or use analgesic suppositories. An adequate supply with instructions as to use, including the advice that painkillers should be taken sooner rather than later if pain is worsening, should be provided prior to discharge home.

Postoperative nausea and vomiting (PONV)

Not only is this an unpleasant experience for the patient, it prolongs the duration of recovery and increases costs per patient [91]. For a review of PONV in day-case surgery see Wetchler [92]. Potential factors in the genesis of PONV are listed in Table 11.11.

Table 11.11 Potential factors in the genesis of postoperative nausea and vomiting (PONV)

Patient
Age
Sex
Obesity
History of motion sickness
History of PONV
Phase of menstrual cycle
Delayed gastric emptying
Anxiety
Operation
Nature/site
Duration
Anaesthetic
Seniority of anaesthetist
Premedication
Induction/maintenance agents
Reversal of relaxation
Postoperative pain
Opioid analgesics
Movement

Patient factors

There are several possible patient factors in the aetiology of PONV that have to be taken into account in making a preanaesthetic assessment whilst realizing that some of these factors are only indefinitely implicated (for review see Lerman [93]) and some (age, sex, obesity, history of motion sickness, history of PONV) are in any case not amenable to preoperative manipulation.

There are several studies reported in the literature which suggest that histories of motion sickness or previous PONV indicate susceptibility to PONV [94, 95].

There is a higher incidence of PONV in females and it is suggested that this relates to the varying serum concentrations of female sex hormones during the menstrual cycle; whilst efforts could be made to reduce it by timing day surgical interventions with the menstrual cycle, it remains unclear when would be the best time. Thus Beattie *et al.* [96] found post laparoscopy nausea and vomiting to be worst in the luteal phase while Honkavaara *et al.* [97] found the menstrual period as the time of greatest risk.

Whilst anxiety is thought to delay preoperative gastric emptying and is associated with air-swallowing which might induce gastrointestinal distension which would be aggravated by the use of nitrous oxide and its diffusion into the gas spaces, the importance of anxiety in predisposing to PONV is unclear. Nevertheless, it would be prudent, if prescribing premedication in the day-case context, to avoid drugs (e.g. opioids) which delay gastric emptying or cause nausea and vomiting.

Surgical factors

Variations in propensity to PONV with the site and nature of surgery are well established but neither is it the purpose of this chapter to review, nor can the anaesthetist influence, these variables.

The literature is inconclusive concerning any relationship between an increasing duration of surgery with a rising incidence of PONV. Performance of day-case surgery by experienced anaesthetic and surgical personnel should minimize any surgical contribution to PONV that may exist.

Anaesthetic factors

For review see Rabey and Smith [98] and Kapur [99] who review the causes and consequences of postoperative nausea with special regard to day-cases, and suggest treatments, with emphasis on the newer 5-hydroxytryptamine (HT_3) antagonists.

Seniority of anaesthetist. It has been long recognized that patients anaesthetized by more experienced anaesthetists suffer less PONV. It has been suggested that this may relate to maintenance at a deeper level of anaesthesia by less experienced anaesthetists but a more specific mechanism has been identified by Hovorka *et al.* [100] who reported that the incidence of PONV in women is greater after manual ventilation of the lungs by inexperienced compared with more experienced anaesthetists. This could be a function of GI distension by the delivered gases.

Pain and opioid drugs. The relative contributory roles to PONV of both pain and associated opioid analgesic treatment have been examined.

Jakobsson *et al.* [101] recorded that PONV is increased by pain whilst in another study [102] in day-case patients undergoing knee arthroscopy there was no difference in the proportions of patients with or without pain who experienced PONV. Although Andersen and Krohg [103] record that nausea associated with the pain of abdominal surgery was reduced by opioid administration, Lerman [93] expresses the more generally held belief that opioids are associated with more PONV than they relieve.

However, the greater incidence of PONV in patients given opioids has long been recognized [104]. More recently, in the retrospective analysis of data from a multicentre study of 17 201 patients reported by Forrest *et al.* [105], substitution of fentanyl for a volatile agent was associated with significant increase in the incidence of PONV.

Benzodiazepines. There is currently no evidence to support the concept that anxiolytic premedication with benzodiazepines is associated with a reduction in the incidence of PONV.

Induction/maintenance agents. The study by Forrest *et al.* [105] showed no difference between the commonly used volatile agents (halothane, enflurane and isoflurane) in the incidence of PONV.

In seeking to maximize the quality of recovery of day-case patients there is much interest in the use of propofol which is generally believed to be associated with less PONV. For example, Watcha *et al.* [106] found that, in children undergoing day-case strabismus surgery, maintenance of anaesthesia by propofol infusion was associated with a lower incidence of PONV than when anaesthesia was maintained with inhalational agents [106]. Kortilla *et al.* [107] also found a relatively low incidence when using propofol.

It has been suggested that propofol has anti-emetic properties [108, 109], while others suggest that not only does it reduce the need for anti-emetic medication but that it also reduces unplanned hospital admission due to nausea and vomiting [110].

Nitrous oxide. Ranta *et al.* [111] suggest that in major surgery it is possible that stronger nauseogenic factors override any beneficial effect on the incidence of PONV deriving from the omission of nitrous oxide, but which could become apparent in more minor day-case surgery.

However, while at least three studies associate the use of nitrous oxide with PONV in gynaecological laparoscopy [112, 113] or minor gynaecological procedures [114], another two failed to demonstrate any link [115, 116].

Reversal of neuromuscular blockade. Antagonism of neuromuscular block with neostigmine and atropine is associated with increased emesis, suggesting that neostigmine has an emetic property [117].

Postoperative fluids. Lerman [93] draws attention to the fact that the long recognized provocation of episodes of PONV by the first fluid intake after anaesthesia and surgery is at odds with the insistence upon tolerance of oral fluids before hospital or day-unit discharge. It has been suggested that elective restriction of postoperative oral fluids may delay and reduce the incidence of PONV. In a study involving postoperative children when fluids were offered only when the child requested, predischarge episodes of PONV and times to discharge were both reduced, however, after including postdischarge episodes there was no overall reduction in the incidence of PONV [118]. Should future studies confirm this effect of postoperative fluid restriction on the pattern of PONV, it might alter the oral fluid and discharge policies, and postoperative advice of day units. If longer periods of postoperative fluid restriction are proposed then it might also become increasingly important to accept the current move towards shorter preoperative starvation and to examine the potential values of peroperative intravenous fluid administration in this respect.

Treatment

Gastric suction. There is disagreement in the literature as to the effectiveness of gastric suction in minimizing PONV. Two recent reports indicate it to be particularly effective in association with gynaecological laparoscopy [119, 120].

Transdermal scopolamine. Whilst Bailey *et al.* [121] found transdermal hyoscine to be effective in reducing nausea and vomiting in women undergoing day-case laparoscopy and its efficacy has been reported after major gynaecological surgery and papaveretum [122] analgesia, there are a number of publications which fail to support the role of hyoscine administered in this way as an effective antiemetic [123, 124]. Overall it seems that transdermal hyoscine, particularly if applied several hours before surgery does have some effect in preventing PONV but that clarification of its role in the antiemetic armamentarium, and any specific relevance to day-case anaesthesia, is still required.

Metoclopramide and droperidol. For a thorough review of the literature on anti-emetic drugs in the management of PONV the reader is referred to Rowbotham [125] who concludes that whilst metoclopramide is a popular anti-emetic its performance in well-controlled clinical trials is disappointing and there seems to be no indication for its intravenous administration at induction of anaesthesia for the prevention of PONV. The literature indicates that droperidol is a more effective anti-emetic drug. Studies testifying to the efficacy of low dose (20 $\mu g\ kg^{-1}$ or 0·625–1·25 mg) droperidol demonstrate either no prolongation [126] or a reduction [127] in the length of stay after outpatient laparoscopy under general anaesthesia. Poler *et al.* [128] concluded that droperidol 20 μg kg^{-1} was an acceptable compromise between decreased emetic sequelae and increased postoperative sedation. Doses above about 1·25 mg are associated with increasingly obvious drowsiness. Delayed side effects in day-case patients after droperidol administration, such as anxiety and restlessness at home, e.g. 23% of women given droperidol 1·25 mg in one study [129], require further assessment, particularly in terms of their significance to the patient.

Acupuncture. Dundee *et al.* have shown that either manual needling [130] or electric current via an acupuncture needle [131] at the P6 acupuncture point results in a significant reduction in PONV. Acupuncture anti-emesis is reviewed by Dundee and McMillan [132].

Ondansetron. A number of papers testify to the postoperative anti-emetic efficacy of ondansetron in placebo-controlled studies [132–136]. More recently a double-blind trial in patients undergoing general anaesthesia for dilatation and curettage has reported ondansetron to be significantly more effective than either metoclopramide or droperidol in preventing postoperative vomiting [137]. No doubt further reports will establish whether this new class of anti-emetic drug, a $5HT_3$ selective serotonin antagonist, is set to become the 'magic bullet' of PONV. There are now several $5HT_3$ antagonist 'me too' drugs from different companies which have different pharmacokinetic properties and are currently undergoing clinical trials.

Intraoperative fluid therapy. At least two studies suggest that intravenous fluid therapy is of benefit in reducing postoperative emetic symptomatology in minor or day-case surgery [138, 139]. However, a more recent study in a rather small number of patients failed to demonstrate any obvious benefit [140]. Clearly the definitive answer to the question lies in the need for further research in this area. Possibly a reduction in preoperative nil-by-mouth time (see Preoperative fluid management above) in the context of short duration, minor to intermediate, day-case surgery will be found to have an effect upon any contribution of oral fluid deprivation to the incidence of PONV.

Ephedrine. Rothenberg *et al.* [141] found that the administration of ephedrine 0·5 mg kg^{-1} i.m. before termination of anaesthesia was as effective as droperidol 0·04 mg kg^{-1} i.m. and significantly more effective than a placebo in reducing PONV. In a subsequent paper the same group reported that the ephedrine treated patients were less sedated and could be discharged home earlier than the droperidol treated patients [142]. By contrast, Poler and White [143] found that ephedrine 25 mg i.m. did not decrease emetic sequelae.

On the basis that aerospace research has demonstrated the superior efficacy of a combination of a sympathomimetic and an anticholinergic drug in preventing motion

Table 11.12 Suggested measures to reduce PONV

Avoid
Hypoxaemia, opioids, nitrous oxide, uneven anaesthesia
Sudden excessive movements which will stimulate the vestibular mechanism
Prolonged preoperative starvation and fluid deprivation
Delays and situations likely to cause stress and anxiety
Employ, use, create or consider
Counselling
Friendly cheerful staff
Welcoming, orderly, calm, efficient environment
Local anaesthesia whenever possible
Propofol
Light stable general anaesthesia
Ondansetron or other anti-emetic $5HT_3$ antagonist when indicated
Pre-emptive analgesia, ideally with local anaesthesia
Preoperative oral fluids up to 3 h, and light foods up to 4 h before induction of anaesthesia
Perioperative fluids i.v. to delay the need for oral fluid in the early postoperative period

sickness Garbin and Bogetz [144] have made a preliminary examination of the efficacy in preventing PONV of ephedrine and hydroxyzine versus ephedrine alone, with encouraging results.

With the variety of patient, surgical and anaesthetic factors which have a bearing on the incidence of PONV it is not surprising that it is impossible to discern from the literature any one answer to the problem. Blanket prophylactic pharmacological anti-emetics for all day-case patients are unnecessary and therefore arguably unjustified. At present it seems that one rational approach an individual anaesthetist can make to the problem of PONV in day-case patients lies in audit to recognize problem groups in their own practice and the preoperative identification of patients with a history of motion sickness or previous PONV, or excessive preoperative anxiety. A range of manoeuvres and techniques which are associated with the lowest incidence of PONV can be selected, particularly for high-risk patients (Table 11.12). Continuing audit should then facilitate the progressive improvement of the anaesthetist's practice with regard to the minimization of PONV.

Audit

It is essential that an adequate resource for audit is identified in the planning of a new unit (Table 11.13). Any shortfall in the provision of the means (financial, clerical, computing) by which efficient and informative audit may be conducted will hinder the evolution of procedures and protocols designed to maximize unit efficiency and patient satisfaction whilst minimizing clinical complications and eliminating procedural and administrative inadequacies. Within the available resource it is clearly the re-

Table 11.13 Audit. Some areas of anaesthetic interest

Referral patterns
Patient satisfaction
Patient demography
Case mix
On-the-day cancellations
Anaesthetic techniques
Duration of events
Time to recovery and discharge
Postoperative morbidity
Hospital admissions and reasons
Equipment service record
Research interests

sponsibility of an individual day-case unit to decide upon its own style, means and foci of audit, but amongst the more obvious areas requiring examination are the following. Is the referral pattern correct? Are patients being selected appropriately by surgeons? Is preoperative investigation effective? Are patients being appropriately investigated (e.g. sickle screening) in outpatients before referral to the day unit? What is the incidence of on-the-day-cancellations? Are the selection and screening procedures adequate? How effective are anaesthetic techniques in the unit in minimizing adverse postoperative symptomatology? Are postoperative questionnaires (Audit Commission; procedure specific; anaesthetist specific) being used to capture relevant data? What is the incidence of hospital admission? What are the associations with hospital admission? Are there associations with particular procedures, surgeons and anaesthetists or even the day of the week or timing of the procedure? Which grade of surgeon and anaesthetist performs the procedure and who is in charge in the unit each day? Are any particular surgeons or anaesthetists associated with bad selection, morbidity or delays?

The future

The success of day surgery will depend on public perception of, and demand for, a high quality, desirable service. Anaesthetists figure prominently in the provision of such a service which demands meticulous attention to detail in both organizational and clinical terms. Assessment of the degree to which their efforts meet with success requires continuous provider and patient evaluation of the service. The establishment of the machinery by which such audit is conducted must be given some priority when establishing a new service.

The ceiling of application of day-case surgery is unlikely to lie with the specialty of anaesthesia. The pharmaceutical and technological industries will continue to search for and provide better drugs and drug delivery systems. For example, where short duration neuromuscular blockade is required for procedures lasting a few minutes only, and in a day surgery context where rapid sequence induction and intubation should be irrelevant, mivacurium may become widely used as a means of avoiding both the myalgic consequences of suxamethonium administration and the need for neostigmine reversal, with its possible emetic effect, of longer acting neuromuscular blocking drugs.

It is already quite possible to anaesthetize patients for several hours and discharge them on the same day. Future agents may further facilitate the conduct of longer day-stay general anaesthetics if day-stay compatible surgical procedures are developed which demand more time than anaesthetists are currently prepared to offer their surgical colleagues.

However, more expensive agents and techniques threaten to put a ceiling on the degree of day-case anaesthetic excellence which might otherwise be achieved. In some quarters the use of propofol infusions has already been challenged on cost grounds. It is vital that continuing research effort is able to generate the data from which to ascertain the nature of, and confirm cost-benefit arguments to support the use of, the best day-case anaesthetic techniques.

Appendix A: Medical selection and investigation algorithm

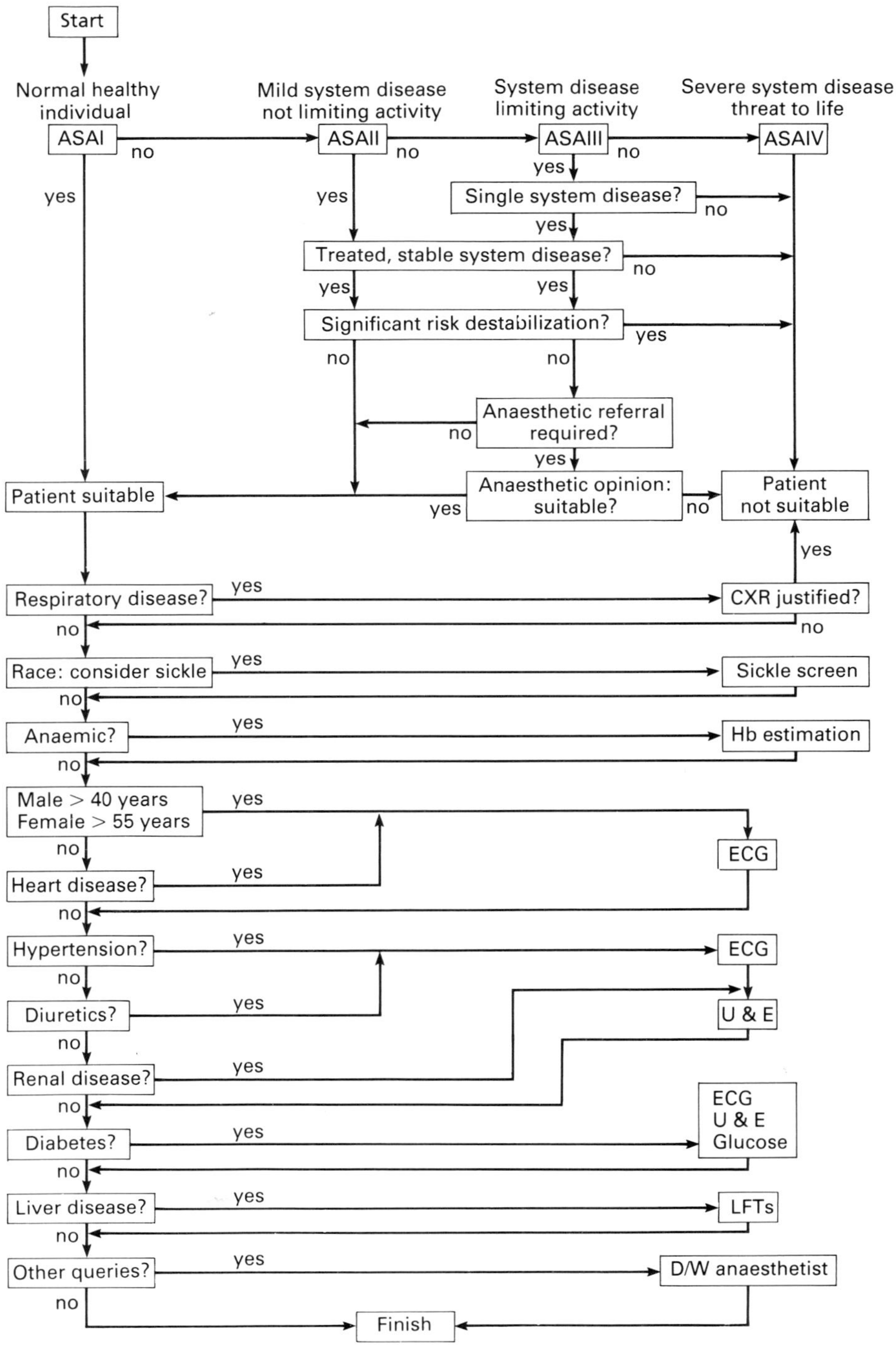

Appendix B: Day surgery medical screening questionnaire

1	Have you had an operation before?	Yes/No
2	Have you had any problems with anaesthetics?	Yes/No
3	Have any of your relations had problems with anaesthetics?	Yes/No
4	Are you taking any medicines (tablets, patches, inhalers, injections)?	Yes/No
5	Are you taking steroid tablets currently/recently?	Yes/No
6	Have you any allergies (drugs, plasters, etc.)?	Yes/No
7	Have you had serious illnesses in the past?	Yes/No
8	Do you have high blood pressure?	Yes/No
9	Do you get chest pains, indigestion or heartburn?	Yes/No
10	Do you have blackouts or faint easily?	Yes/No
11	Do you get breathless easily?	Yes/No
12	Do you have asthma or bronchitis?	Yes/No
13	Do you smoke?	Yes/No
14	Have you ever had a convulsion or a fit?	Yes/No
15	Do you have arthritis?	Yes/No
16	Do you have muscle disease?	Yes/No
17	Do you have anaemia or other blood disorder?	Yes/No
18	Do you know your sickle status (if relevant)?	Yes/No
19	Do you bleed badly or bruise without cause?	Yes/No
20	Have you been jaundiced (turned yellow)?	Yes/No
21	Do you drink alcohol?	Yes/No
22	Do you have kidney disease?	Yes/No
23	Do you have diabetes (sugar in the urine)?	Yes/No
24	Do you have a hiatus hernia?	Yes/No
25	Do you get heartburn or tummy acid in the throat?	Yes/No
26	Do you have crowns, loose or artificial teeth?	Yes/No
27	Do you have contact lenses or hearing aid?	Yes/No
28	If female, are you/could you be pregnant?	Yes/No
29	If female, are you taking an oral contraceptive pill?	Yes/No

If YES to any of the above, please refer to Appendix C.

Appendix C: Medical screening questionnaire guidance notes

	Action
1 List operations. If you suspect any of these may affect suitability for day-case surgery	Anaesthetist
2 Record problem (see 3)	
3 If a personal or family history of malignant hyperpyrexia	Reject and see anaesthetist
If a personal or family history of Scoline (suxamethonium) sensitivity	Anaesthetist
If other significant problems, or if in doubt as to suitability for day-case surgery	Anaesthetist
4 List medications. Advise on continuation of essential medications on operation day	
if on insulin	Anaesthetist
if on anticoagulants	Reject
5 If on systemic steroids currently or within recent months	Anaesthetist
6 List allergies	Inform anaesthetist
7 List serious illnesses. If you suspect any of these may affect suitability for day-case	Anaesthetist
If history of murmur, consider antibiotic cover	Inform anaesthetist
8 If blood pressure > 160/100 (or > 180/100 for > 60 years old) then repeat measurement later. If remains greater	Reject
9 If pain due to hiatus hernia/reflux oesophagitis reliably diagnosed, consider gastric acid aspiration prophylaxis	Inform anaesthetist
Otherwise, if pain occurring at rest or walking on the flat	Reject
If definite or possible history of heart attack within last 6 months	Reject
If pain normally well controlled, occurring only exceptionally	Needs electrocardiogram
10 Record what causes fainting or blackout. If on exercise, or patient > 60 years old	Reject
11 If breathless lying flat, at rest, walking on flat or after one flight of stairs	Reject
If activities of daily living severely limited	Reject
12 If severely limits activities of daily living	Reject
13 Discourage smoking, certainly until operation	
14 If epileptic, well controlled on medication	Accept
If fit within last year, or with anaesthesia	Reject
15 If severely disabled	Reject
If neck involved	Anaesthetist

Continued on p. 194.

Appendix C *Contd.*

		Action
16	If severely limits activities of daily living	Reject
	If myasthenia gravis or myotonic dystrophy	Reject
	If family history of cataracts	Reject
17	If recently anaemic If suspect anaemia (pallor, diet, menorraghia, haematuria)	Needs full blood count
	If Hb < 10 g dl^{-1} and symptomatic cardiovascular or renal disease	Reject
	If Hb < 10 g dl^{-1}	Anaesthetist
18	Record sickle status	
	If high risk race unaware of sickle status	Needs sickle test
	If negative	Accept
	If positive, sickle trait (Hb SA)	Accept
	If positive, sickle disease (Hb SS) or Hb SC	Reject
19	If haemophiliac	Reject
	If requiring hospital treatment	Reject
	If bruising without known cause If excessive bleeding after tooth extraction If family history of bleeding/bruising	Needs clotting screen and platelet count
	If abnormal result	Reject
20	If jaundice due to gallstones or hepatitis A	Accept
	If possibly due to hepatitis B	Needs hepatitis B test
	If hepatitis B positive	Inform anaesthetist
21	Record weekly alcohol consumption in units: 1 unit = half pint beer/1 glass wine/1 measure spirit. 'Safe' weekly intake = 21 units (male), 14 units (female) with 2–3 alcohol free days per week.	Inform anaesthetist
	Advise patient if drinking above 'safe' limit.	
	If drinking excessively	Needs liver function test
22	If dialysis dependent	Reject
	If chronic kidney disease	Needs urine and electrolyte tests
	If abnormal	Anaesthetist
23	If poorly controlled (random blood sugar or BM Stix > 17 mmol l^{-1}, or positive urinalysis)	Reject
	Diet-controlled	Accept
	Controlled non-insulin dependent on tablets	Anaesthetist
	If insulin dependent	Anaesthetist
24 25	Consider preoperative gastric acid aspiration prophylaxis	Anaesthetist
26	Indicate crowns, caps, bridgework, etc.	Inform anaesthetist
27	Record any appliances, prostheses	Inform anaesthetist
28	If not for termination	Surgeon
29	If oestrogen containing pill and 'demobilizing' or venous operation on leg(s)	Surgeon

Appendix D: General anaesthesia—information for patients

- You should have nothing to eat or drink from midnight before a morning operation
- You may have a light breakfast not later than 7.00 am before an afternoon operation
- If you usually take tablets in the morning please ask a member of staff what you should do on the morning of your operation
- After a general anaesthetic there is a period in which your judgement and reactions might not be as good as usual, without you realizing it. It is very important that for as long as you may feel less than perfectly well, or are taking painkillers, and in any case for at least 24 h after your anaesthetic, that you:
  do not drink alcohol
  do not take sleeping tablets
  do not drive a car or ride a bicycle
  do not operate machinery or use a cooker
  do not make important decisions
  do not sign legal documents
  do not do anything which might become dangerous to yourself or others
- You must arrange for a responsible adult to collect you from the Day Surgery Centre and look after you for at least 24 h after your operation
- Some patients experience one or more temporary after-effects of a general anaesthetic such as:
  loss of appetite
  tiredness or fatigue
  dizziness or faintness
  headache
  nausea
  sore throat
  muscle pain
  tenderness at injection site
  These effects are usually minor and wear off within a day or two. If you are worried about how you feel then you should ring the Day Surgery Centre or your GP

References

1 Goodwin APL, Ogg TW. Preoperative preparation for day surgery. *Br J Hosp Med* 1992; 47: 197–201.
2 Morgan AG. Is routine urine testing in outpatient clinics useful? *Br Med J* 1988; 297: 1173.
3 Dresner M, Soni N. Preoperative assessment. *Curr Op Anaesth* 1989; 2: 701–8.
4 Johnson H Jr, Knee-Ioli S, Butler TA, Munoz E, Wise L. Are routine preoperative laboratory screening tests necessary to evaluate ambulatory surgical patients? *Surgery* 1988; 104: 639–45.
5 Whitwam JG. C-reactive and serum amyloid A acute phase proteins in procedural risk assessment and management. *Curr Op Anaesth* 1993; 6 (*suppl* 1): S1–S8.
6 Walton GM. The cost benefit of routine pre-operative Hb investigations for oral surgery. *Br Dent J* 1988; 165: 406–7.

7 Campbell IT, Gosling P. Preoperative biochemical screening: routine urine testing is good enough in patients under 50. *Br Med J* 1988; 2: 803–4.
8 McCleane GJ. Urea and electrolyte measurement in preoperative surgical patients. *Anaesthesia* 1988; 43: 413–15.
9 Rabkin SW, Horne JM. Preoperative electrocardiography: Effect of new abnormalities on clinical decisions. *Canad Med Ass J* 1983; 128: 146–7.
10 Goldberger AL, O'Konski M. Utility of the routine electrocardiogram before surgery and on general hospital admission. *Ann Intern Med* 1986; 105: 552–7.
11 Royal College Working Party on the Effective Use of Diagnostic Radiology. Preoperative chest radiology. National study by the Royal College of Radiologists. *Lancet* 1979; ii: 83–6.
12 Tape TG, Mushlin AI. The utility of routine chest radiographs. *Ann Int Med* 1986; 104: 663–70.
13 Golub R, Cantu R, Sorrento JJ, Stein HD. Efficacy of preadmission testing in ambulatory surgical patients. *Am J Surg* 1992; 163; 565–70.
14 Commission on the Provision of Surgical Services. *Guidelines for Day Care Surgery*, revised edn. London: Royal College of Surgeons of England, 1992.
15 Twersky RS, Lebovits AH, Lewis M, Frank D. Early anesthesia evaluation of the ambulatory surgical patient: does it really help? *J Clin Anesth* 1992; 4: 204–7.
16 Arellano R, Cruise C, Chung F. Timing of the anesthetist's preoperative outpatient interview. *Anesth Analg* 1989; 68: 645–8.
17 Cobley M, Dunne JA, Sanders LD. Stressful pre-operative preparation procedures. *Anaesthesia* 1991; 46: 1019–22.
18 Brighouse D. Pre-operative removal of dentures (Letter). *Anaesthesia* 1991; 46: 992.
19 Harrison JC, Horton WA. Pre-operative removal of dentures (Letter). *Anaesthesia* 1991; 46: 992.
20 Strunin L: How long should patients fast before surgery? Time for new guidelines (Editorial). *Br J Anaesth* 1993; 70: 1–3.
21 Phillips S, Hutchinson S, Davidson T. Preoperative drinking does not affect gastric contents. *Br J Anaesth* 1993; 70: 6–9.
22 Read MS, Vaughan RS: Allowing pre-operative patients to drink: effects on patient's safety and comfort of unlimited oral water until 2 hours before anaesthesia. *Acta Anaesth Scand* 1991; 35: 591–5.
23 The shortened fluid fast and the Canadian Anaesthetists' Society new guidelines for fasting in elective/surgical patients. *Can J Anaesth* 1990; 37: 905–6.
24 Scarr M, Maltby JR, Jani K, Sutherland LR. Volume and acidity of residual gastric fluid after oral fluid ingestion before elective ambulatory surgery. *Canad Med Ass J* 1989; 14: 1151–4.
25 Goodwin APL, Rowe WL, Ogg TW, Samaan A. Oral fluids prior to day surgery. *Anaesthesia* 1991; 46: 1066–8.
26 Beechey APG, Eltringham RJ, Studd C. Temazepam as premedication in day surgery. *Anaesthesia* 1981; 36: 10–15.
27 Nightingale JJ, Norman J. A comparison of midazolam and temazepam for premedication of day case patients. *Anaesthesia* 1988; 43: 111–13.
28 Turner GA, Paech M. A comparison of oral midazolam solution with temazepam as a day case premedicant. *Anaesth Intens Care* 1991; 19: 365–8.
29 Weldon BC, Watcha MF, White PF. Oral midazolam in children: effect of time and adjunctive therapy. *Anesth Analg* 1992; 75: 51–5.
30 Parnis SJ, Foate JA, van der Walt JH, Short T, Crowe CE. Oral midazolam is an effective premedication for children having day-stay anaesthesia. *Anaesth Intens Care* 1992; 20: 9–14.
31 Shafer A, White PF, Urquhart ML, Doze VA. Outpatient premedication: Use of midazolam and opioid analgesics. *Anesthesiology* 1989; 71: 495–501.
32 Virkkila ME, Ali-Melkkia TM, Kanto JH. Premedication for outpatient cataract surgery: a

comparative study of intramuscular alfentanil, midazolam and placebo. *Acta Anaesth Scand* 1992; 36: 559–63.
33 Friesen RH, Lockhart CH. Oral transmucosal fentanyl citrate for preanaesthetic medication of paediatric day surgery patients with and without droperidol as prophylactic antiemetic. *Anesthesiology* 1992; 76: 46–51.
34 Dyck JB, Chung F. A comparison of propranolol and diazepam for preoperative anxiolysis. *Can J Anaesth* 1991; 38: 704–9.
35 MacKenzie JW. A novel approach to anxiolytic premedication for daycase patients. *J Roy Soc Med* 1991; 84: 646–9.
36 Kumar A, Bose S, Bhattacharya A, Tandon OP, Kundra P. Oral clonidine premedication in elderly patients undergoing intraocular surgery. *Acta Anaesth Scand* 1992; 36: 159–64.
37 Peden CJ, Prys-Roberts C. Dexmedetomidine—a powerful new adjunct to anaesthesia (editorial II). *Br J Anaesth* 1992; 68: 123–5.
38 Escolano F, Castano J, Lopez R, Bisbe E, Alcon A. Effects of omeprazole, ranitidine, famotidine and placebo on gastric secretion in patients undergoing elective surgery. *Br J Anaesth* 1992; 69: 404–6.
39 Meyer-Witting M, Wilkinson DJ. A safe haven or a dangerous place—should we keep the anaesthetic room? (Editorial). *Anaesthesia* 1992; 47: 1021–2.
40 Soni JC, Thomas DA. Comparison of anxiety before induction of anaesthesia in the anaesthetic room or operating theatre. *Anaesthesia* 1989; 44: 651–5.
41 Heath PJ, Kennedy DJ, Ogg TW, Dunling C, Gilks WR. Which intravenous induction agent for day-surgery? A comparison of propofol, thiopentone, methohexitone and etomidate. *Anaesthesia* 1988; 43: 365–8.
42 Millar JM, Jewkes CF. Recovery and morbidity after daycase anaesthesia. A comparison of propofol with thiopentone-enflurane with and without alfentanil. *Anaesthesia* 1988; 43: 738–43.
43 Smith I, White PF. Use of the laryngeal mask airway as an alternative to a face mask during outpatient arthroscopy. *Anesthesiology* 1992; 77: 850–5.
44 Wilson IG. The laryngeal mask airway in paediatric practice (Editorial). *Br J Anaesth* 1993; 70: 124–5.
45 Fisher JA, Ananthanaryan C, Edelist G. Role of the laryngeal mask in airway management (Editorial). *Can J Anaesth* 1992; 39: 1–3.
46 Nanji GM, Maltby JR. Vomiting and aspiration pneumonitis with the laryngeal mask airway. *Can J Anaesth* 1992; 39: 69–70.
47 Goodwin APL, Rowe WL, Ogg TW. Day case laparoscopy. A comparison of two anaesthetic techniques using the laryngeal mask during spontaneous breathing. *Anaesthesia* 1992; 47: 892–5.
48 Barker P, Langton JA, Murphy PJ, Rowbotham DJ. Regurgitation of gastric contents during general anaesthesia using the laryngeal mask airway. *Br J Anaesth* 1992; 69: 314–15.
49 Rabey PG, Murphy PJ, Langton JA, Barker P, Rowbotham DJ. Effect of the laryngeal mask airway on lower oesophageal sphincter pressure in patients during general anaesthesia. *Br J Anaesth* 1992; 69: 346–8.
50 John RE, Hill S, Hughes TJ. Airway protection by the laryngeal mask. *Anaesthesia* 1991; 46: 366–7.
51 Williams PJ, Bailey PM. Comparison of the reinforced laryngeal mask airway and tracheal intubation for adenotonsillectomy. *Br J Anaesth* 1993; 70: 30–3.
52 Alcock R, Peachey T, Lynch M, McEwan T. Comparison of alfentanil with suxamethonium in facilitating nasotracheal intubation in day-case anaesthesia. *Br J Anaesth* 1993; 70: 34–7.
53 Dixon J, Chakrabarti MK, Morgan M. An assessment of the Humphrey ADE anaesthetic system

in the Mapleson A mode during spontaneous ventilation. *Anaesthesia* 1984; 39: 593–6.
54 Shulman MS, Brodsky JB. The ADE system—a new anesthetic breathing system. *Anesth Analg* 1984; 63: 273.
55 Orlikowski CEP, Ewart MC, Bingham RM. The Humphrey ADE system; evaluation in paediatric use. *Br J Anaesth* 1991; 66: 253–7.
56 Association of Anaesthetists. *Recommendations for Standards of Monitoring During Anaesthesia and Recovery*. London: Association of Anaesthetists of Great Britain and Ireland, 1988.
57 Eichhorn JH, Cooper JB, Cullen DJ, Maier WR, Philip JH, Seeman RG. Standards for patient monitoring during anesthesia at Harvard Medical School. *J Am Med Ass* 1986; 256: 1017–20.
58 Bush D. Pre-emptive analgesia (Editorial). *Br Med J* 1993; 306: 285–6.
59 White PF, Shafer A. Nausea and vomiting: cause and prophylaxis. *Sem Anaesth* 1987; 6: 300–8.
60 White PF, Coe V, Shafer A, Sung ML. Comparison of alfentanil with fentanyl for outpatient anesthesia. *Anesthesiology* 1986; 64: 100–6.
61 Zelcer J, White PF, Chester S, Paull JD, Molnar R. Intraoperative patient-controlled analgesia: An alternative to physician administration during outpatient monitored anesthesia care. *Anesth Analg* 1992; 75: 41–4.
62 Postoperative pain relief and non-opioid analgesics (Editorial). *Lancet* 1991; 337: 524–6.
63 Derbyshire DR, Richardson J. Voltarol (Diclofenac) as perioperative analgesic supplement. *Br J Anaesth* 1987; 59: 1327P–8.
64 Reasbeck PG, Rice ML, Reasbeck JC. Double-blind controlled trial of indomethacin as an adjunct to narcotic analgesia after major abdominal surgery. *Lancet* 1982; ii: 115–18.
65 Hodsman NBA, Burns J, Blyth A, Kenny GNC, McArdle CS, Rotman H. The morphine-sparing effect of diclofenac sodium following abdominal surgery. *Anaesthesia* 1987; 42: 1005–8.
66 McLoughlin C, McKinney MS, Fee JPH, Boules Z. Diclofenac for day-case arthroscopy; comparison with standard opioid therapy. *Br J Anaesth* 1990; 65: 620–3.
67 Matthews RW, Scully CM, Levers BGH. The efficacy of diclofenac sodium (Voltarol) with and without paracetamol in the control of postsurgical dental pain. *Br Dent J* 1984; 157: 357–9.
68 Campbell WI. Analgesic side-effects and minor surgery; which analgesic for minor and day-case surgery. *Br J Anaesth* 1990; 64: 617–20.
69 Comfort V, Code WE, Rooney ME, Yip RW. Naproxen premedication reduces postoperative tubal ligation pain. *Can J Anaesth* 1992; 39: 349–52.
70 Baer GA, Rorarius MGF, Kolehmainen S, Seun S. The effect of paracetamol or diclofenac administered before operation on postoperative pain and behaviour after adenoidectomy in small children. *Anaesthesia* 1992; 47: 1078–80.
71 Wall PD. The prevention of postoperative pain. *Pain* 1988; 33: 289–90.
72 O'Hara DA, Fragen RJ, Kinzer M, Pemberton D. Ketorolac trometamine as compared with morphine sulphate for the treatment of postoperative pain. *Clin Pharmacol Ther* 1987; 41: 556–661.
73 Ding Y, White PF. Comparative effects of ketorolac, dezocine and fentanyl as adjuvants during outpatient anaesthesia. *Anesth Analg* 1992; 75: 566–71.
74 Tree-Trakarn T, Pirayavaraporn S, Lertakyamanee J. Topical analgesia for relief of post-circumcision pain. *Anesthesiology* 1987; 667: 395–9.
75 Lee JJ. EMLA for postoperative analgesia for daycase circumcision in children: a comparison with dorsal nerve of penis block. *Anaesthesia* 1992; 47: 1081–3.
76 Spittal MJ, Hunter SJ. A comparison of bupivacaine instillation and inguinal field block for control of pain after herniorrhaphy. *Ann Roy Coll Surg Engl* 1992; 74: 85–8.
77 Ejlersen E, Andersen HB, Eliasen K, Mogensen T. A comparison between preincisional and postincisional lidocaine infiltration and postoperative pain. *Anesth Analg* 1992; 74: 495–8.
78 Dierking GW, Dahl JB, Kanstrup J, Dahl A, Kehlet H. Effect of pre- vs. postoperative inguinal field

block on postoperative pain after herniorrhaphy. *Br J Anaesth* 1992; 68: 344–8.
79 Narchi P, Benhamou D, Fernandez H. Intraperitoneal local anaesthetic for shoulder pain after day-case laparoscopy. *Lancet* 1991; 338: 1569–70.
80 Smith BE, Suchak M, Siggins D, Challands J. Rectus sheath block for diagnostic laparoscopy. *Anaesthesia* 1988; 43: 947–8.
81 Smith BE, MacPherson GH, de Jonge M, Griffiths JM. Rectus sheath and mesosalpinx block for laparoscopic sterilisation. *Anaesthesia* 1991; 46: 875–7.
82 Chirwa SS, Macleod BA, Day B. Intraarticular bupivacaine after arthroscopic meniscectomy: a randomised double-blind controlled study. *Arthroscopy* 1989; 5: 33–5.
83 Smith I, van Hemelrijck J, White PF, Shively R. Effects of local anaesthesia on recovery after outpatient arthroscopy. *Anesth Analg* 1991; 73: 536–9.
84 Stein C. Peripheral mechanisms of opioid analgesia. *Anesth Analg* 1993; 76: 182–91.
85 Stein C, Comisel K, Haimeri E *et al.* Analgesic effect of intraarticular morphine after arthroscopic knee surgery. *N Engl J Med* 1991; 325: 1123–6.
86 Heard SO, Edwards WT, Ferrari D *et al.* Analgesic effect of intraarticular bupivacaine or morphine after arthroscopic knee surgery: a randomised prospective double-blind study. *Anesth Analg* 1992; 74: 822–6.
87 Fancourt-Smith PF, Merrick P. Anaesthesia for outpatient TURP. *Can J Anaesth* 1992; 39: 893–6.
88 Bodily MN, Carpenter RL, Owens BD. Lidocaine 0·5% spinal anaesthesia; a hypobaric solution for short-stay perirectal surgery. *Can J Anaesth* 1992; 39: 770–3.
89 Baker AB. Analgesia for day surgery. *Med J Austr* 1992; 156: 274–80.
90 Philip BK. Regional anaesthesia for ambulatory surgery. *Can J Anaesth* 1992; 39: R3–6.
91 Metter SE, Kitz DS, Young ML, Baldeck AM, Apfelbaum JL, Lecky JH. Nausea and vomiting after outpatient laparoscopy: Incidence, impact on recovery room stay and cost. *Anesth Analg* 1987; 66: S116.
92 Wetchler BV. Postoperative nausea and vomiting in day-case surgery. *Br J Anaesth* 1992; 69 (suppl 1): 33S–9.
93 Lerman J. Surgical and patient factors involved in postoperative nausea and vomiting. *Br J Anaesth* 1992; 69 (suppl 1): 24S–32.
94 Muir JJ, Warner MA, Offord KP, Buck CF, Harper JV, Kunkel SE. Role of nitrous oxide and other factors in postoperative nausea and vomiting: a randomised and blinded prospective study. *Anesthesiology* 1987; 66: 513–18.
95 Kamath B, Curran J, Hawkey C *et al.* Anaesthesia, movement and emesis. *Br J Anaesth* 1990; 64: 728–30.
96 Beattie WS, Lindblad T, Buckley DN, Forrest JB. The incidence of postoperative nausea and vomiting in women undergoing laparoscopy is influenced by the day of the menstrual cycle. *Can J Anaesth* 1991; 38: 298–302.
97 Honkavaara P, Lehtinen A-M, Hovorka J, Korttila K. Nausea and vomiting after gynaecological laparoscopy depends upon the phase of the menstrual cycle. *Can J Anaesth* 1991; 38: 876–9.
98 Rabey PG, Smith G. Anaesthetic factors contributing to postoperative nausea and vomiting. *Br J Anaesth* 1992; 69 (suppl 1): 40S–45S.
99 Kapur PA. The big 'little' problem (Editorial). *Anesth Analg* 1991; 73: 243–5.
100 Hovorka J, Korttila K, Erkola O. The experience of the person ventilating the lungs does influence postoperative nausea and vomiting. *Acta Anaesth Scand* 1990; 34: 203–5.
101 Jakobsson J, Davidson S, Andreen M, Westgreen M. Opioid supplementation to propofol anaesthesia for outpatient abortion: A comparison between alfentanil, fentanyl and placebo. *Acta Anaesth Scand* 1991; 35: 767–70.
102 Parnass SM, McCarthy RJ, Ivankovich AD. The role of pain as a cause of postoperative

nausea/vomiting after outpatient anesthesia. *Anesth Analg* 1992; 74: S233.
103 Andersen R, Krohg K. Pain as a major cause of postoperative nausea. *Canad Anaesth Soc J* 1976; 23: 366–9.
104 Riding JE. Post-operative vomiting. *Proc Roy Soc Med* 1960; 53: 671–7.
105 Forrest JB, Cahalan MK, Rehder K *et al.* Multicenter study of general anesthesia. II. Results. *Anesthesiology* 1990; 72: 262–8.
106 Watcha MF, Simeon RM, White PF, Stevens JL. Effect of propofol on the incidence of postoperative vomiting after strabismus surgery in pediatric outpatients. *Anesthesiology* 1991; 75: 204–9.
107 Korttila K, Ostman P, Faure E *et al.* Randomized comparison of recovery after propofol-nitrous oxide versus thiopentone-isoflurane-nitrous oxide anaesthesia in patients undergoing ambulatory surgery. *Acta Anaesth Scand* 1990; 34: 400–3.
108 McCollum JSC, Milligan KR, Dundee JW. The antiemetic action of propofol. *Anaesthesia* 1988; 43: 239–40.
109 Borgeat A, Wilder-Smith OHG, Saiah M, Rifat K. Subhypnotic doses of propofol possess direct antiemetic properties. *Anesth Analg* 1992; 74: 359–41.
110 Raftery S, Sherry E. Total intravenous anaesthesia with propofol and alfentanil protects against postoperative nausea and vomiting. *Can J Anaesth* 1992; 39: 37–40.
111 Ranta P, Nuutinen L, Laitinen J. The role of nitrous oxide in postoperative nausea and recovery in patients undergoing upper abdominal surgery. *Acta Anaesth Scand* 1991; 35: 339–41.
112 Lonie DS, Harper NJN. Nitrous oxide anaesthesia and vomiting. *Anaesthesia* 1986; 41: 703–7.
113 Felts JA, Poler M, Spitznagel EL. Nitrous oxide, nausea, and vomiting after outpatient gynecologic surgery. *J Clin Anesth* 1990; 2: 168–71.
114 Melnick BM, Johnson LS. Effects of eliminating nitrous oxide in outpatient anaesthesia. *Anesthesiology* 1987; 67: 982–4.
115 Hovorka J, Korttila K, Erkola O. Nitrous oxide does not increase nausea and vomiting following gynaecological laparoscopy. *Can J Anaesth* 1989; 36: 145–8.
116 Sengupta P, Plantevin OM. Nitrous oxide and day-case laparoscopy: Effects on nausea, vomiting and return to normal activity. *Br J Anaesth* 1988; 60: 570–3.
117 King MJ, Milazkiewicz R, Carli F, Deacock AR. Influence of neostigmine on postoperative vomiting. *Br J Anaesth* 1988; 61: 403–6.
118 Schreiner MS, Nicolson SC, Martin T, Whitney L. Should children drink before discharge from day surgery? *Anesthesiology* 1992; 76: 528–33.
119 Kraynack BJ, Bates MF, Gintautas J. Antiemetic efficacy of ranitidine, metoclopramide and gastric suctioning in outpatient laparoscopy. *Anesth Analg* 1990; 70: S213.
120 McCarroll SM, Mori S, Bras PJ, Saunder PR. The effect of gastric intubation and removal of gastric contents on the incidence of postoperative nausea and vomiting. *Anesth Analg* 1990; 70: S262.
121 Bailey PL, Steisand JB, Pace NL *et al.* Transdermal scopolamine reduces nausea and vomiting after outpatient laparoscopy. *Anesthesiology* 1990; 72: 977–80.
122 Uppington J, Dunnet J, Blogg CE. Transdermal hyoscine and postoperative nausea and vomiting. *Anaesthesia* 1986; 41: 16–20.
123 Aronson JK, Sear JW. Transdermal hyoscine (scopolamine) and postoperative vomiting. *Anaesthesia* 1986; 41: 1–3.
124 Tigerstedt I, Salmela L, Aromaa U. Double-blind comparison of transdermal scopolamine, droperidol and placebo against postoperative nausea and vomiting. *Acta Anaesth Scand* 1988; 32: 454–7.
125 Rowbotham DJ. Current management of postoperative nausea and vomiting. *Br J Anaesth* 1992; 69 (suppl 1): 46S–59S.
126 Pandit SK, Kothary SP, Pandit UA, Randel G, Levy L. Dose-response study of droperidol and metoclopramide as antiemetics for outpatient anesthesia. *Anesth Analg* 1989; 68: 798–802.

127 Wetchler BV, Collins IS, Jacob L. Antiemetic effects of droperidol on the ambulatory surgery patient. *Anesth Rev* 1982; 9: 23–6.

128 Poler SM, White PF, Margrabe D, Krause B. Nausea and vomiting in outpatients: Use of droperidol prophylaxis. *Anesthesiology* 1989; 71: A134.

129 Melnick B, Sawyer R, Karambelkar D, Phitayakorn P, Uy NT, Patel R. Delayed side effects of droperidol after ambulatory general anesthesia. *Anesth Analg* 1989; 69: 748–51.

130 Dundee JW, Chestnutt WN, Ghaly RG, Lynas AG. Traditional Chinese acupuncture: A potentially useful antiemetic? *Br Med J* 1986; 293: 583–4.

131 Ghaly RG, Fitzpatrick KTJ, Dundee JW. Antiemetic studies with traditional Chinese acupuncture. *Anaesthesia* 1987; 42: 1108–10.

132 Dundee JW, McMillan CM. Positive evidence for P6 acupuncture antiemesis. *Postgrad Med J* 1991; 67: 417–22.

133 Wetchler BV, Sung YF, Duncalf D, Joslyn AF. Ondansetron decreases emetic symptoms following outpatient laparoscopy. *Anesthesiology* 1990; 73: A36.

134 Kovac A, McKenzie R, O'Connor *et al.* Prophylactic intravenous ondansetron in female outpatients undergoing gynecologic surgery: A muticenter dose-comparison study. *Eur J Anaesth* 1992; 9 (suppl 6): 39–50.

135 Larijani GE, Gratz I, Afshar M, Minassian S. Treatment of postoperative nausea and vomiting with ondansetron: A randomized, double-blind comparison with placebo. *Anesth Analg* 1991; 73: 246–9.

136 Mingus M, Scuderi P, Wetchler B *et al.* In: *Ondansetron Effectively Treats Postoperative Nausea and Vomiting Following Ambulatory Surgery.* 10th World Congress of Anaesthesiologists 1992; A502.

137 Alon E, Himmelseher S. Ondansetron in the treatment of postoperative vomiting: A randomized, double-blind comparison with droperidol and metoclopramide. *Anesth Analg* 1992; 75: 561–5.

138 Keane PW, Murray PF. Intravenous fluids in minor surgery: Their effect on recovery from anaesthesia. *Anaesthesia* 1986; 41: 635–7.

139 Cook R, Anderson S, Riseborough M, Blogg CE. Intravenous fluid load and recovery: A double-blind comparison in gynaecological patients who had day-case laparoscopy. *Anaesthesia* 1990; 45: 826–30.

140 Ooi LG, Goldhill DR, Griffiths A, Smith C. I.V. fluids and minor gynaecological surgery: Effect on recovery from anaesthesia. *Br J Anaesth* 1992; 68: 576–9.

141 Rothenberg D, Parnass S, Newman L, Litwack K, Ivankovich A. Ephedrine minimises postoperative nausea and vomiting in outpatients. *Anesthesiology* 1989; 71: A322.

142 Rothenberg DM, Parnass SM, Litwack K, McCarthy RJ, Newman LM. Efficacy of ephedrine in the prevention of postoperative nausea and vomiting. *Anesth Analg* 1991; 72: 58–61.

143 Poler SM, White PF. Does ephedrine decrease nausea and vomiting after outpatient anesthesia? *Anesthesiology* 1989; 71: A995.

144 Garbin GS, Bogetz MS. Efficacy of ephedrine and hydroxyzine in preventing postoperative nausea and vomiting (Abstract). *Anesthesiology* 1992; 77: A3.

Chapter 12
Laparoscopy and its Complications

A. M. Skelly and J. G. Whitwam

Laparoscopy is an endoscopic procedure using a fibreoptic visual system, for which three-dimensional imaging techniques are now available. It allows inspection of the interior of the abdominal or thoracic cavities using a 'telescope' passed through a trocar introduced using a small incision.

The initial trocar is inserted blindly through the abdominal wall. To minimize the risk of intra-abdominal damage and to obtain clear visualization of the abdominal contents a pneumoperitoneum is induced, usually by insufflating carbon dioxide (CO_2) into the peritoneum through a Verres needle. Other gases have been used including nitrous oxide (N_2O), air, nitrogen and helium. Diathermy is used during laparoscopy for other than diagnostic procedures and CO_2 is usually preferred as the insufflatory gas because it does not support combustion and is readily available at low cost.

Although gynaecologists have utilized the laparoscopy both diagnostically and therapeutically for several decades, laparoscopic surgery has only recently gained acceptance in the wider surgical community.

Hitherto diagnostic gynaecological cases predominated in this specialty, but in recent years gynaecological surgical procedures increasingly are being performed on a one day basis, e.g. female sterilization, ovarian cyst drainage, oöcyte collection.

However, in the last 5–6 years there has been an unprecedented increase in the range and numbers of laparoscopic procedures to treat conditions which were previously managed with conventional open surgery using only scalpels, forceps, diathermy, sutures and ligatures and possibly staples, without assisted vision or magnification.

This revolution is being made possible by advances in technology and laparoscopic surgery and provides major advantages for patients, for example in the reduction in cosmetic injury and pain, a much shorter period of hospitalization, reduced mortality, with a much earlier return to full activity and work. The surgeon can benefit from the use of image enhancement and in the future from robotic-assisted equipment. There are major areas of critical debate, in risk analysis and health economics and all these issues are amply demonstrated in the operation of cholecystectomy where an increasing number of selected patients are being managed as day cases, albeit by the best surgeons with a very thorough predischarge review and evaluation.

Many more surgeons are planning to increase the range and number of operations being performed laparoscopically as day-cases. However, the enthusiasm for the new

Table 12.1 Complications of laparoscopy

Gas insufflation
Changes in cardiovascular and respiratory function
Cardiac dysrryhthmias
Misplacement of insufflating gas
Hypothermia
Trauma by Verres needle or trocar
Haemorrhage
Bowel/other visceral damage
General complications
Anaesthesia
Gastric aspiration
Nerve injury
Postoperative pain
Conversion to laparotomy

technologies and minimally invasive surgery must be tempered by the occurrence of a number of potentially serious complications, most of which occur during the creation of the initial pneumoperitoneum and, in particular, during the insertion of the Verres needle and the principal trocar [1]. Unfortunately others are due to poor surgery.

The complications of laparoscopy will be discussed with respect to gas introduction, trocar insertion and the general factors relating to the procedure such as anaesthesia, positioning of the patient and postoperative problems, which assume more significance in day surgery (Table 12.1).

Complications resulting from gas insufflation

Changes in cardiovascular and respiratory function

It is important to recognize that the intra-abdominal insufflation of gas will lead to changes in haemodynamic and pulmonary function in all patients [2]. A minor increase in intra-abdominal pressure may initially cause an increase in central venous pressure (CVP), heart rate, mean arterial blood pressure and cardiac output. However an increase in pressure above 25 cmH_2O can lead to a reduction in CVP and cardiac output [3–6] due to compression of the inferior vena cava (IVC) and a reduction in venous return. These higher pressures are undesirable and do not lead to improved visualization.

In general, pressures up to 10–15 mmHg are well tolerated but intra-abdominal pressures above 30 mmHg put a severe stress on the ability of the cardiovascular system to compensate. The situation is complex.

Mechanically the problem starts with compression of structures, including the IVC in the abdomen and a rise in intrathoracic pressure during mechanical ventilation due to 'splinting' of the diaphragm, which causes a reduction in venous return, CVP and hence cardiac output. This is the primary change.

Everything that follows is a combination of the response to these primary mechanical events and also the direct effects of carbon dioxide absorption on the circulation. With the reduction in venous return and a fall in cardiac output, baroreflex-mediated compensation with increased sympathetic outflow and a reduction in vagal activity will occur causing increased myocardial contractility, a rise in heart rate, an increase in systemic vascular resistance, with appropriate changes in derived variables, all of which are predictable. The end tidal carbon dioxide concentration increases progressively with time [7, 8] which may cause a further increase in efferent sympathetic activity and an increase in plasma catecholamine concentrations. This will further increase the contractility of the heart and increase the systemic arterial pressure [9].

The result is that the patient's condition appears to be satisfactory [6–8] with a normal or elevated blood pressure, albeit with a tachycardia. Therefore decompensation when it occurs may be sudden and unexpected and could, for example, be precipitated by concealed or unmeasured haemorrhage during laparoscopic procedures. Recent work presented at the inaugural meeting of the newly formed European Association for Endoscopic Surgery (EAES) on the effects of laparoscopic cholecystectomy on cardiac patients, of New York Heart Association (NYHA) grades I, II and III, suggests that even relatively sick cardiac patients tolerate the procedure remarkably well. However, on investigation they show haemodynamic changes indicating a degree of compensation suggesting that there is a possibility of acute decompensation which could be precipitated, for example, by concealed haemorrhage. It is suggested that intraperitoneal pressures should be kept below 10 mmHg in these patients, and haemorrhage and hypoxaemia should be avoided.

Pneumoperitoneum with either carbon dioxide or nitrous oxide has been shown to cause a reduction in tidal volume and minute ventilation as well as an increase in respiratory rate in spontaneously breathing patients. This is due to elevation of the diaphragm, i.e. 'splinting' which can also cause basal atelectasis with a right to left shunt and ventilation-perfusion mismatch [10, 11]. In addition pulmonary function is impaired by the use of the Trendelenburg position, which is used to assist the visualization of pelvic structures. The combination of impaired ventilation and reduced cardiac output may cause a reduction in arterial oxygen saturation [12]. Furthermore, when carbon dioxide is used for insufflation, significant absorption of carbon dioxide occurs from the peritoneum causing a rise in arterial $P\text{CO}_2$ within 15 min [13] but the peak $P\text{aCO}_2$ concentration may not occur until after the end of the procedure.

The incidence of hypercarbia and hypoxaemia can be reduced by using general anaesthesia with controlled ventilation. However, the use of intermittent positive pressure ventilation may contribute to the reduction in cardiac output and hypotension since, as explained above, any increase in the mean intrathoracic pressure will further impair venous return.

Nevertheless there is some evidence that muscle relaxation and controlled ventilation are associated with reduced postoperative morbidity compared with spontaneous ventilation in intubated patients [14]. An increase in airway pressure in the presence of muscle relaxation, has been shown to reflect the reduction in thoracic compliance associated with the raised intra-abdominal pressure [12]. Monitoring of airway pressure can thus be used to aid in the assessment of the optimum amount of insufflated gas. However, direct monitoring of intraperitoneal pressure should be mandatory.

Cardiac arrhythmias

Cardiac arrhythmias are common during laparoscopy. In one study [15], 47% of patients developed arrhythmias of which 30% were associated with bradycardia. The latter may progress to asystole and several cases have been described in the literature [16]. Possible causes for such arrhythmias during laparoscopy include hypercapnia and hypoxaemia from hypoventilation during anaesthesia, with a decreased cardiac output and consequent lowered coronary artery perfusion, secondary to elevated intra-abdominal pressure, and also to a profound vagal reflex response to the peritoneal distension [17]. The vagal response may have become more noticeable since the introduction of the newer muscle relaxants, vecuronium and atracurium, with their lack of vagolytic activity. As a result the routine use of anticholinergic agents, such as atropine, has been suggested when using these agents [18], and this would appear to be sound advice particularly when using anaesthesia based on propofol and opioids.

Inadvertent misplacement of the insufflating gas

The most common pneumoperitoneal complication is inadvertent gas insufflation in the omentum which is usually without serious consequences [2]. Subcutaneous emphysema has been reported, especially with higher abdominal pressures or insufflator malfunction, when the gas escapes at the needle or trocar site and dissects subcutaneously, occasionally reaching massive proportions [19].

Pneumomediastinum alone or in association with a pneumothorax, in one case bilateral, has been reported as well as pneumopericardium [20–22].

Preperitoneal gas insufflation dissects the peritoneum from the abdominal wall. If extensive it can preclude successful endoscopy. However, laparoscopy can usually be performed without difficulty once the gas is released and/or absorbed.

Almost all of these complications of the pneumoperitoneum are due to improper needle position. They occur in less than 1% of cases. More rarely, cases of gas embolism also occur [23–25] which can cause significant morbidity and may have a fatal outcome. The gas enters the circulation and travels to the right atrium where it tends to mix with the blood present and forms a foam which in sufficient quantity may cause outlet obstruction of the pulmonary artery. Signs include a fall in the end tidal carbon dioxide concentration, which can detect as little as 0·25–0·5 ml kg^{-1} min^{-1} of gas entrainment into the venous circulation [26]. In addition a fall in arterial oxygen saturation, SaO_2 and electrocardiogram (ECG) changes compatible with right heart strain may be noticed. Additionally, a 'mill wheel' cardiac murmur may be heard on auscultation. A protocol for the emergency management of gas embolism should be developed for every operating suite where laparoscopy is performed, which should include a head down position and the application of positive end expiratory pressure (PEEP), aspiration of the contents of the right side of the heart and main pulmonary artery and also the possibility of left ventricular aspiration, i.e. in addition to other routine measures such as oxygen therapy and the use of cardiac and circulatory support drugs if indicated.

Hypothermia

The range and duration of operative laparoscopic techniques are increasing. This expansion exposes patients to increased operating time, larger volumes of carbon dioxide for the maintenance of a pneumoperitoneum, and higher gas flow rates. The gas used is provided from cylinders or pipelines and is routinely delivered unwarmed and dry. This causes a reduction in the core temperature of the patient which has been evaluated and found to be 0·3 °C for each 50 l of carbon dioxide delivered [27]. Warming of the carbon dioxide to a temperature of approximately 30°C prior to abdominal delivery has therefore been suggested and shown to be of value [28].

Traumatic complications of needle/trocar insertion

Haemorrhage

Bleeding can occur from three sites:

1 From the anterior abdominal wall at the trocar insertion site. This will normally stop with compression but may cause a large haematoma of the abdominal wall.

2 Bleeding may occur due to tearing of adhesions which are stretched by the expanding pneumoperitoneum.

3 Bleeding from trauma to major intra-abdominal vessels. A review of 15 cases of major vessel injury [29] revealed that most (85%) were caused by the pneumoperitoneum needle. Characteristically the terminal aorta and its major branches are injured although iliac vein damage is well documented [30].

Haemorrhage is arguably the most important single cause of death and major central nervous system morbidity due to laparoscopy. The increased intra-abdominal pressure caused by insufflation and retroperitoneal haematoma formation may tamponade even a large vessel injury [31]. This means that significant vascular damage may go unnoticed at the time of laparoscopy. Additionally, a fall in end tidal carbon dioxide concentration due to low blood flow secondary to haemorrhage may be misinterpreted as gas embolism or as a reduction in blood flow due to mechanical effects of the pneumoperitoneum on cardiac output as discussed above.

When the pressure gradients return to normal at the end of the procedure, the gas having been let out of the abdominal cavity, bleeding may restart and progress slowly or quickly into the retroperitoneal space or intraperitoneally, eventually leading to hypovolaemic shock. The situation may be compounded by delay in performing a laparotomy due to the false sense of security regarding vessel injury resulting from the fact that no intraperitoneal blood was seen during laparoscopy.

In the review mentioned above [29], most of the lesions could be treated by simple suture. Recovery was the rule but two of the 15 patients died. The experience of the surgeon and correct technique are important factors in the prevention of this potentially lethal complication which is probably under reported.

Bowel/other visceral damage

Bowel damage can take either of two different forms:

1 The Verres needle or trocar can directly puncture the intestine and the laparoscopy can even be introduced into its lumen. Intestinal perforation usually involves the colon and less commonly the small intestine [2]. The bowel is normally relatively mobile within the abdominal cavity and most reported cases are related to the presence of adhesions fixing a loop or loops of bowel, or to an inadequate pneumoperitoneum. A recent review of 4532 outpatient laparoscopic procedures using the classical umbilical site for trocar insertion, revealed four patients with bowel injury [32].

2 More worrying for day-case laparoscopy is the possibility of grazing the bowel with the Verres needle or trocar leading to damage of the serosa or deeper layers of the bowel wall. This could remain unseen if the affected piece of bowel moves, or is pushed, out of view. Delayed peritonitis or abscess formation may occur after the patient has returned home and such patients can develop septic shock, the treatment of which is likely to be delayed due to the circumstances. Additionally, adhesions may form between damaged loops of bowel which may make further surgery more difficult or may even cause intestinal obstruction.

Other intra-abdominal structures which may be damaged include the bladder, which is normally emptied by catheterization immediately prior to Verres needle insertion to minimize the risk, the ureter, which is rarely damaged and the diagnosis usually made radiologically in the postoperative period [33], and the liver.

General complications associated with laparoscopy

Anaesthesia

The anaesthetist must use a technique which not only allows for optimal surgical conditions but also provides intraoperative patient comfort and safety, and a rapid postoperative recovery.

Any of the complications of general anaesthesia, e.g. anaphylaxis, may occur. Additionally, since many anaesthetists favour controlled ventilation facilitated by muscle relaxation, as discussed earlier, difficulties may occur with intubation or with reversal of the muscle relaxant used, particularly since many of these procedures are of short duration and relaxants with short duration of action should be preferred.

Gastric aspiration

It has been assumed that the combination of Trendelenburg position and pneumoperitoneum must predispose to passive regurgitation, particularly in the relatively obese [34]. However, the incidence appears to be low [35] and there is a report that lower oesophageal sphincter (LOS) tone, which is capable of a rapid adaptive response to increases in intragastric pressure [36], increases in response to peritoneal insufflation during laparoscopy [37]. This would tend to maintain the barrier pressure, i.e. the LOS pressure minus the intragastric pressure, which prevents gastro-oesophageal reflux.

One study investigating the frequency of regurgitation during laparoscopy [35] found an incidence of less than 2% although this may be an overestimate as all patients in this study were given atropine 0·6 mg i.v. at induction, a drug known to markedly reduce the LOS tone. Preoperative metoclopramide (10 mg orally or i.v.) may increase the tone of the LOS and promote gastric emptying thus decreasing the incidence of regurgitation and aspiration. If the patient has a history of oesophageal reflux there is a case for preoperative preparation of the patient with ranitidine or omeprazole to reduce gastric acidity and hence minimize the potential consequences of inadvertant pulmonary aspiration of gastric contents. In addition a rapid sequence induction of anaesthesia should be used to reduce the risk of such aspiration.

Nerve injury

Nerve damage can be caused by lack of care when positioning patients for laparoscopy, particularly in gynaecological surgery. The common peroneal nerve is at risk of compression against the fibula when the patients legs are positioned inside the supporting poles. Femoral neuropathy has been reported [38] after laparoscopy as a result of extreme flexion, abduction and lateral rotation of the hip joint. Brachial plexus injury can also occur from traction during head down tilt.

Postoperative pain

A certain number of patients will complain of shoulder tip pain following laparoscopy. This referred pain is due to the presence of intraperitoneal gas which causes diaphragmatic irritation. Some surgeons believe that this is particularly true if the gas is dry and dirty and/or contains debris from excessive use of diathermy, although there is no direct evidence for this view. The incidence of this pain, which causes delay in discharge of patients from day units, can be minimized by evacuating as much gas as possible from the peritoneum through the trocar at the end of the procedure. However, other surgeons hold the view that no matter how much effort is made to evacuate all the gas, the problem can remain due to back leak of air before final removal of the canulae. Again this is anecdotal.

Conversion to laparotomy

It is important to realize that 3–5% of all laparoscopic procedures require conversion to an open laparotomy [39], either because of inability to perform the operation laparoscopically or because of a complication. The incidence is obviously much lower in diagnostic day-cases but will probably increase as more complicated procedures are performed.

Conclusions

Laparoscopy is a remarkably safe procedure especially considering that many of these procedures are performed in training programmes by relatively inexperienced surgeons. A review [2] of a number of series totalling more than 200 000 laparoscopies for all types of surgery both inpatient and day-case suggests that a serious complication resulting in surgical intervention can be expected in 1 in 660 cases, whilst the risk of death is 1 in 2000. A review of gynaecological laparoscopies [40] gave the incidence of death as 1 in 12 500 and the risk of major complication as 1 in 3300 for diagnostic laparoscopy and 1 in 2500 for sterilization.

Enthusiasm for this method of surgery must be tempered with care in its practice if complication rates are to be maintained at an acceptable level and the procedure is to earn a permanent place in the therapeutic menu, particularly for day-case procedures.

References

1 Oshinsky GS, Smith AD. Laparoscopic needles and trocars: an overview of designs and complications. *Laparoendosc Surg* 1992; 2: 117–25.
2 Nord HJ. Complications of laparoscopy. *Endoscopy* 1992; 24: 693–700.
3 Smith I, Benzie RJ, Corgon NL, Kelman GR, Swapp GH. Cardiovascular effect of peritoneal insufflation of carbon dioxide for laparoscopy. *Br Med J* 1971; iii: 410–11.
4 Kelman GR, Swapp GH, Smith I, Benzie RJ, Gordon NL. Cardiac output and arterial blood gas tension during laparoscopy. *Br J Anaesth* 1972; 44: 1155–62.

5 Motew M, Invankovich AD, Bieniarz J, Albrecht RF, Zahed B, Slommegna A. Cardiovascular effect and acid base and blood gas changes during laparoscopy. *Am J Obstet Gynaecol* 1973; 115: 1002–12.

6 Cunningham AJ, Turner J, Rosenraum S, Rafferty T. Transoesophageal echocardiographic assessment of haemodynamic function during laparoscopic cholecystectomy. *Br J Anaesth* 1993; 70: 621–5.

7 Liu SY, Leighton T, Davis I, Klein S, Lippman M, Bongard F. Prospective analysis of cardiopulmonary responses to laparoscopic cholecystectomy. *J Laparoendosc Surg* 1991; 1: 241–6.

8 Wittgen CM, Andrus CH, Fitzgerald SD, Baudendistal LJ, Dahms TE, Kaminski DL. Analysis of the haemodynamic and ventilatory effects of laparoscopic cholecystectomy. *Arch Surg* 1991; 126: 997–1001.

9 Rasmussen JP, Dauchot PJ, De Palma RG *et al*. Cardiac function and hypercarbia. *Arch Surg* 1978; 113: 1196–200.

10 Brown DR, Fishburne JI, Robertson VO, Hulka JF. Ventilatory and blood gas changes during laparoscopy with local anaesthesia. *Am J Obstet Gynaecol* 1976; 124: 741.

11 Brady C, Harkleroad L, Pierson WP. Alterations in oxygen saturation and ventilation after intravenous sedation for peritoneoscopy. *Arch Intern Med* 1989; 149: 1029–32.

12 Lew JK, Gin T, Oh TE. Anaesthetic problems during laparoscopic cholecystectomy. *Anaesth Intens Care* 1992; 20: 91–2.

13 Leighton T, Pianim N, Lui SY, Kono M, Klein S, Bongard F. Effectors of hypercarbia during experimental pneumoperitoneum. *Am Surg* 1992; 58: 717–21.

14 Skacel M, Sengupta P, Plantevin OM. Morbidity after day case laparoscopy: a comparison of two techniques of tracheal anaesthesia. *Anaesthesia* 1986; 41: 537–41.

15 Myles PS. Bradyarrhythmias and laparoscopy: a prospective study of heart rate changes with laparoscopy. *Aust NZ J Obstet Gynaecol* 1991; 31: 171–3.

16 Shifren JL, Aldestein L, Finkler NJ. Asystolic cardiac arrest: a rare complication of laparoscopy. *Obstet Gynaecol* 1992; 79: 840–1.

17 Harris MNE. Cardiac arrhythmias during anaesthesia for laparoscopy. *Br J Anaesth* 1984; 56: 1213–16.

18 Doyle DJ, Mark PW. Laparoscopy and vagal arrest (Letter). *Anaesthesia* 1989; 44: 448.

19 Kalhan SB, Reaney JA, Collins RL. Pneumomediastinum and subcutaneous emphysema during laparoscopy. *Cleve Clin J Med* 1990; 57: 639–42.

20 Shah P, Ramakantan R. Pneumoperitoneum and pneumomediastinum: unusual complications of laparoscopy. *J Postgrad Med* 1990; 36: 31–2.

21 Knos GB, Sung YF, Toledo A. Pneumopericardium associated with laparoscopy. *J Clin Anaesth* 1991; 3: 56–9.

22 Pascual JB, Barranda MM, Tarrero M, Gutierrez FM, Garrido IM, Errasti CA. Subcutaneous emphysema, pneumomediastinum, bilateral pneumothorax and pneumopericardium after laparoscopy. *Endoscopy* 1990; 22: 59.

23 Duncan C. Carbon dioxide embolism during laparoscopy: a case report. *American Association of Nurse Anesthetists Journal* 1992; 69: 139–44.

24 Au-Yeung P. Gas embolism during attempted laparoscopic vagotomy (Letter). *Anaesthesia* 1992; 47: 817.

25 Bradfield ST. Gas embolism during laparoscopy (Letter). *Anaesth Intens Care* 1991; 19: 474.

26 Kirby RR. Respiratory system. In: Gravenstein N, ed. *Manual of Complications during Anaesthesia*. Philadelphia: JB Lippincott, 1991: 302–52.

27 Ott DE. Laparoscopic hypothermia. *J Laparoendosc Surgery* 1991; 1: 137.

28 Ott DE. Correction of laparoscopic insufflation hypothermia. *J Laparoendosc Surgery* 1991; 1: 183–6.
29 Baadsgaard SE, Bille S, Eggeblad K. Major vascular injury during gynaecological laparoscopy. Report of a case and review of published cases. *Acta Obstet Gynaecol Scand* 1989; 68: 283–5.
30 Evans RM, Hulbert JC, Reddy PK. Complications of laparoscopy. *Semin Urol* 1992; 10: 164–8.
31 Reich H. Pelvic side wall dissection. *Clin Obstet Gynaecol* 1991; 34: 412–22.
32 Kaali SG, Barad DH. Incidence of bowel injury due to dense adhesions at the site of direct trocar insertion. *J Reprod Med* 1992; 3: 617–18.
33 Gomel V, James C. Intraoperative management of ureteral injury during operative laparoscopy. *Fertil Steril* 1991; 55: 416–19.
34 Lamberty JM. Gynaecological laparoscopy. *Br J Anaesth* 1985; 57: 718.
35 Duffy BL. Regurgitation during pelvic laparoscopy. *Br J Anaesth* 1979; 51: 1089–90.
36 Smith G, Dalling R, Williams TIR. Gastro-oesophageal pressure gradient changes produced by induction of anaesthesia and suxamethonium. *Br J Anaesth* 1978; 50: 1137–41.
37 Jones MJ, Mitchell RW, Hindocha N. Effect of increased intra-abdominal pressure during laparoscopy on the lower oesophageal sphincter. *Anaesth Analg* 1989; 68: 63–5.
38 Heshlag A, Loy RA, Lavy G, DeCherney AH. Femoral neuropathy after laparoscopy. A case report. *J Reprod Med* 1990; 35: 575–6.
39 Hanley ES. Anaesthesia for laparoscopic surgery. *Surg Clin N Am* 1992; 72: 1013–19.
40 Chamberlain G, Brown JC. Gynaecological laparoscopy. *The report of a working of the confidential enquiry into gynaecological laparoscopy*. London: Royal College of Obstetricians and Gynaecologists, 1978.

Chapter 13
Ophthalmic Day-Case Anaesthesia

C. Carr

In recent years there has been an increasing trend towards day-case surgery in many surgical specialities [1]. Although this has primarily been in response to economic pressures it is now becoming obvious that there are other advantages in performing suitable surgery on a day-case basis [2, 3]. Many patients find it less disrupting to their lives to be in and out of hospital on the same day. In a self-contained day surgery unit cancellation of elective surgery due to emergency admissions does not occur.

The Guidelines for day-case surgery published by the Royal College of Surgeons of England in 1985 recommended only strabismus surgery in children and various simple ophthalmic plastic procedures as suitable for day-case treatment [4]. Day-case surgery for intraocular procedures was thought unlikely to become widespread due to the high levels of pre- and postoperative care required in the community.

The postoperative complications of raised intraocular pressure, iris prolapse and endophthalmitis following cataract extraction have been considerably reduced by advances in techniques of surgery and anaesthesia [5]. Numerous reports of successful management of routine intraocular surgery on a day-case basis have now been published [6–9]. It has even been suggested that selected cases of vitreoretinal surgery could be performed as day-cases [10, 11].

The revised edition of Guidelines for Day Case Surgery (1992) now includes intraocular surgery in its list of appropriate ophthalmic operations [12] (Table 13.1).

Current practice

Age-related cataract constitutes the main surgical workload of ophthalmic services and the bulk of ophthalmic waiting lists in the UK [13]. There is inevitably pressure on the surgeon to provide the most beneficial, efficient and cost-effective procedure available. A variety of operative and anaesthetic techniques exist. Current ophthalmic literature suggests an increased interest in the use of local anaesthesia [14, 15], day-case surgery [6–8] and phacoemulsification [16], for cataract surgery.

In the USA virtually all cataract extractions are performed under local anaesthesia and the hospital stay rarely exceeds 2 h [17].

Surveys in the UK reveal that the operation of choice in age-related cataract is extracapsular cataract extraction with posterior chamber lens implant [13, 18, 19]. Only 8% of cases in the National Cataract Surgery Survey were treated on a day-care

Table 13.1 Appropriate ophthalmic operations for day-case surgery

Adults	Cataract surgery Corneal transplant surgery Procedures on the eyelid or tarsal plate Operations on the lacrymal apparatus Correction of strabismus
Children	Correction of strabismus Examination under anaesthetic for conditions such as buphthalmos, retinoblastoma Electrodiagnostic tests

basis. Of these, 95% were performed under local anaesthesia. Of the inpatient group 42% were performed under local anaesthesia. The most popular technique for local anaesthesia is retrobulbar injection with a facial nerve block, although there is increasing use of peribulbar infiltration. The majority of local blocks are performed by the operating surgeon.

Selection of patients for ophthalmic day-case surgery

In ophthalmology a distinction should be made between outpatient surgery and day-case surgery [20] (Appendix 1).

Outpatient surgery includes simple operations that do not carry the risk of serious postoperative complications, for example, eyelid cysts, minor plastic surgery of the eyelids, removal of corneal graft sutures, cryotherapy, electrolysis of eyelid lesions and laser therapy. These patients are not admitted to hospital and remain ambulant in their own clothes.

Day-case surgery is reserved for more complex procedures when the patient is formally admitted to hospital for the day of operation. They may be given a hospital bed or a reclining chair, and local or general anaesthesia used. The most common forms of eye surgery performed as day-case procedures are cataract extraction and strabismus correction.

Selection criteria must be agreed on and adhered to locally to prevent unnecessary cancellations and unexpected inpatient admissions. The selection of patients for local or general anaesthesia is a separate issue as all ophthalmic surgical procedures suitable for day-case can be equally well performed under either form of anaesthesia.

Selection criteria fall into three main categories, surgical, medical and social (Table 13.2).

Table 13.2 Selection of patients for ophthalmic day-case surgery

Surgical criteria	Routine surgery anticipated Minor postoperative complications Mild or no postoperative pain Surgery of short duration (30–60 min)
Medical criteria	American Society of Anesthesiologists [21] (ASA) class I (fit and healthy) ASA class II (mild treated systemic disease such as mild hypertension, mild asthma, non-insulin dependent diabetic) ASA class III is acceptable if the underlying medical condition is well controlled No history of anaesthetic problems Patient must not be grossly obese Age limit, often limited to 1–70 years but will depend on interaction of other factors such as health and social circumstances
Social criteria	Distance and ease of travel to hospital Responsible adult escort available Responsible adult supervision on postoperative night Registered with a general medical practitioner

The population presenting for day-case ophthalmic surgery will present particular problems within each of these categories and a carefully structured assessment protocol to make sure these are picked up and dealt with is necessary. Assessment will involve teamwork and should take place in several structured stages. Many of the patients will be elderly and have poor vision, and communication may be slow and difficult. It is vital that time is taken to ensure that the patient and their escort understand what is going to happen and also what is expected of them. Many day-case units have leaflets explaining these details but elderly patients for cataract extraction may not be able to read them [22].

Assessment of patients can take place at three stages, at the initial surgical clinic visit, at a preoperative assessment clinic and on the day of operation. Co-ordination and documentation of these assessments is usually the responsibility of the nursing staff of the day-case unit.

Initial clinic visit

It is the responsibility of the surgeon listing the patient for surgery in the clinic to determine whether the patient is willing and suitable for day-case surgery. Many of the patients for routine cataract extraction will have medical problems such as untreated hypertension that will require liaison with their general medical practitioner to ensure correct diagnosis and treatment and a chance to render them fit for surgery and anaesthesia.

Table 13.3 Routine investigations for ophthalmic day-case surgery

Weight
Blood pressure
Urinalysis
Peak flow rate
Biometry in cataract patients

The form of anaesthesia should also be considered and discussed with the patient at this time. The choice between local and general anaesthesia will depend on many factors but the contraindications to local anaesthesia must be taken into account to avoid disaster. It is at this point that liaison with the anaesthetic staff could take place to determine the best form of anaesthesia for a particular patient. Day-case ophthalmic surgery on children will usually require general anaesthesia.

Patients fulfilling the admission criteria should be seen by staff from the day-case unit and preferably visit the unit itself as they leave the clinic. This allows the day-unit staff to confirm the patient's suitability for day-case surgery and to acquaint the patient with the procedures.

All patients for intraocular surgery or for any operation requiring general anaesthesia should attend an assessment clinic on the unit a few weeks before the intended date of operation but not sufficiently far ahead to invalidate immediate relevance of the clinical assessment, for example the results of blood tests. In the absence of renal impairment or anaemia 4 weeks is accepted as the upper limit of delay in many units.

Assessment clinic

A full medical history, including current medication and allergies is taken by the staff of the day-case unit. A standard tick sheet, filled in by the nursing staff is the best way of accomplishing this as most of them will be unable to fill in a form themselves. There are various examples of such forms in the literature.

Routine investigations should be performed in all adult patients whether their operation is to be performed under local or general anaesthesia (Table 13.3).

Special investigations should only be ordered when indicated (Table 13.4).

Referral to the patient's general medical practitioner or to the anaesthetic staff may be necessary at this stage for the management of uncontrolled medical conditions, or assessment of suitability for local or general anaesthesia.

The day-ward staff should also undertake a social assessment. Patients for cataract extraction will be expected to attend on the day following surgery for slit-lamp examination, and will need transport for this. Problems with travel or home support can readily be solved with hostel accommodation on the night after surgery. It is important to remember that patients selected for hostel stay must be able to care for

Table 13.4 Special investigations for ophthalmic day-case surgery

Haemoglobin for all women, men over 60 years and those with signs of anaemia
Sickledex test and haemoglobin electrophoresis testing if sickle disease is indicated
ECG for patients over 60 years and those with signs or symptoms of cardiovascular disease, e.g. hypertension, abnormal cardiac rhythm, symptoms or signs suggestive of myocardial ischaemia or coronary thrombosis
Urea, creatinine and electrolytes in patients over 60 years, those with renal disease and those taking cardiac, renal or steroid drugs
Blood sugar estimation in diabetics and those receiving steroids
Chest X-ray in those with a history or signs of chronic lung disease or suggestion of malignancy or tuberculosis or a low preoperative SaO_2

themselves on the postoperative night. For example, they must have adequate vision in the eye not subject to surgery. The patient and escort must be fully informed about what to expect on admission and given written and verbal instructions for the day of surgery. Of particular importance is the length of time the patient should starve for and what medication they should continue to take. The form of anaesthesia should be carefully discussed as patients may not understand what is involved with a local or a general anaesthetic. If necessary tuition about the instillation of eye drops is given at this stage.

Patients having minor surgery under local anaesthesia can be admitted and checked in the day-care unit on the day of operation.

Day of operation

On the day of operation the ophthalmic patient is admitted to the day-care ward. Those for general anaesthesia should be scheduled for the morning or early afternoon, those for local anaesthesia can be scheduled for the afternoon. The day-ward staff take routine observations of pulse, blood pressure and temperature and check that the patient is appropriately starved and that an escort is available.

The surgeon checks the operation to be performed, that the correct eye is marked if appropriate and that the consent form is signed.

The anaesthetist checks the patient's current health and medication and that the patient is appropriately listed for local or general anaesthesia. Premedication may be prescribed if necessary.

Anaesthesia for ophthalmic day-case surgery

The form of the anaesthesia will depend on the surgeon, the patient, the anaesthetist and the operation. In most instances children will require general anaesthesia, and the majority of strabismus operations in adults are also performed under general anaesthesia. For uncomplicated cataract extraction performed on a day-care basis, either local or general anaesthesia may be used.

Ophthalmic day-case anaesthesia in children

The ophthalmic operations performed on a day-care basis in children have particular concerns for the anaesthetist. For example, gaining the co-operation of a young child without premedication, the presence of parents at induction, and choice of anaesthetic technique to ensure rapid recovery with as few sequelae as possible (see Chapters 19 and 20).

In ophthalmic procedures the child's head must be held still, often under an operating microscope which means the airway must be secured. This is usually achieved by intubation although the laryngeal mask airway can provide satisfactory conditions. During surgery the anaesthetist is remote from the child and full monitoring and secure intravenous access are vital.

Correction of strabismus

This is one of the most common eye operations performed in children, the majority of whom are healthy and suitable for day-care treatment. There are particular problems involved with strabismus surgery of which the anaesthetist must be fully aware (Table 13.5).

The oculocardiac reflex. This is a vagally induced bradycardia following traction of the extraocular muscles, or pressure on other orbital structures [23]. Prophylaxis with atropine (0·02 mg kg^{-1}) or glycopyrrolate (0·01 mg kg^{-1}) administered intravenously at the induction of anaesthesia is usual [24] since their administration intramuscularly or orally as premedication is ineffective in this respect. Treatment of the reflex should it occur depends on the severity. If extreme bradycardia occurs the surgeon should stop eye manipulation immediately and when the heart rate returns to normal a small dose of atropine (0·01 mg kg^{-1}) i.v. is given before resuming surgery.

Malignant hyperthermia. Malignant hyperthermia is an inherited predisposition to a hypermetabolic state involving calcium in muscle tissue. This state is triggered by

Table 13.5 Special concerns with strabismus surgery in children

Postoperative eyepatches—child education and awareness
Oculocardiac reflex—prophylaxis and treatment
Malignant hyperthermia
Forced duction testing and suxamethonium
Postoperative vomiting—prophylaxis

stress and exposure to certain anaesthetics including halothane and suxamethonium. It is reported to occur more frequently in children undergoing strabismus surgery [25]. During anaesthesia often the first signs are a rise in heart rate and the end distal carbon dioxide concentration. The management of this condition is outlined in Appendix 2.

Masseter muscle spasm or jaw rigidity may herald the onset of malignant hyperthermia so that the operative procedure should be abandoned and the child carefully monitored. However, if no other symptoms follow treatment with dantrolene is not usually necessary [26].

Postoperative vomiting. Vomiting after eye muscle surgery occurs frequently. Prophylactic administration of intravenous droperidol (0·075 mg kg^{-1}) at induction or 30 min before the end of surgery is very effective in reducing the frequency and severity of vomiting [27]. Ondansetron and other $5HT_3$ antagonists are proving highly successful in the management of nausea and vomiting (see Chapters 2 and 3).

Examination under anaesthesia (EUA)

EUA in ophthalmic surgery is performed for a wide variety of reasons in children and may proceed to surgery that requires the child to remain in hospital postoperatively. Conditions that may be treated on a day-care basis are retinoblastoma and congenital glaucoma.

Retinoblastoma is inherited by dominant genes with partial penetrance and the children of a known case must be examined at frequent intervals for the appearance of the tumour. This is performed from the first week of life, initially every month and then at longer intervals up to the age of 6 years. The anaesthetist is faced with frequently repeated anaesthetics in a child whose co-operation may deteriorate. Use of the eutectic mixture of local anaesthetics (EMLA) and intravenous induction is ideal, although inhalation induction may be necessary, when halothane should be avoided. The airway is best secured by intubation or a laryngeal mask airway as the child's head will be remote from the anaesthetist.

Congenital glaucoma presents at birth or in the first year of life. The child will have to be examined at frequent intervals to check intraocular pressure, corneal diameter, optic disc and drainage angle of the anterior chamber. This takes about 30 min. Intravenous or intramuscular ketamine is often used to avoid the lowering of intraocular pressure by inhalation anaesthetics. If it is necessary to proceed to goniotomy the anaesthetic must be converted to endotracheal anaesthesia as unacceptable eye movement occurs with ketamine alone.

Electrodiagnostic procedures on children are usually performed in the anaesthetic room, in the dark, with bulky machinery. The anaesthetist will need to secure the airway with an endotracheal tube or laryngeal mask airway. Full monitoring will be necessary.

Miscellaneous procedures. Probing and syringing of the tear duct is usually performed on a day-care basis. Although this may be a very rapid procedure that does not require complete immobility of the head, the possible flow of saline into the airway usually necessitates the use of an endotracheal tube and a throat pack.

Incision and curretage of a mebonian cyst is a rapid procedure and intubation is not necessary.

Ophthalmic day-case anaesthesia in adults

Until recently general anaesthesia was regarded by most ophthalmic surgeons as the ideal for intraocular surgery [14]. Ocular akinesis is guaranteed and intraocular pressure may be controlled by hyperventilation of the patient.

In selected patients however, local anaesthesia can also provide good operating conditions. Traditionally this has been a retrobulbar block combined with a facial nerve block administered by the surgeon [18]. On occasion serious side effects have occurred such as globe perforation [28], or direct spread of local anaesthetic agents to the central nervous system [29, 30]. There has been a move to alternative techniques and to the involvement of the anaesthetist [17]. This allows the anaesthetist to be involved in the choice of anaesthetic, the preparation and counselling of the patient, and monitoring during the procedure and treatment of any complications [31].

General anaesthesia for ophthalmic day-case surgery

Strabismus surgery

Although adult eye muscle surgery may be performed under local anaesthesia it is usually necessary to use general anaesthesia. In cases of trauma or previous surgery deep dissection in the orbit is required and general anaesthesia is more pleasant for the patient.

Apart from the usual considerations of day-case anaesthesia special concerns in strabismus surgery in adults are much as in children.

The airway must be secured by a tracheal tube or laryngeal mask airway. Suxamethonium is usually avoided as the surgeon may wish to perform traction tests on the extraocular muscles to assess elasticity and location of mechanical restrictions. This means a non-depolarizing muscle relaxant and controlled ventilation must be used if the anaesthetist uses an endotracheal tube. Avoidance of muscle relaxants is possible if a laryngeal mask airway is used. This is put in place following induction of anaesthesia with alfentanyl (10 $\mu g\ kg^{-1}$) and propofol (1–2 $mg\ kg^{-1}$). The patient can then be allowed to breathe spontaneously.

The oculocardiac reflex is a problem in adults as well as children and similar prophylaxis with intravenous atropine (0·02 $mg\ kg^{-1}$) or glycopyrrolate (0·01 $mg\ kg^{-1}$) may be given at induction of anaesthesia.

Nausea and vomiting are reduced by intraoperative use of droperidol (0·075 $mg\ kg^{-1}$) as in children.

Postoperative pain is relieved by simple analgesics such as paracetamol. Non-steroidal anti-inflammatory drugs such as diclofenac or ketorolac may be given by suppository or intramuscular injection.

Cataract surgery

General anaesthesia for routine day-case cataract extraction is indicated in those patients who would prefer it, and those who would be unable to lie flat and still on the operating table. It should be avoided if there is a risk of morbidity or mortality from the anaesthetic itself. This would mainly be in the case of respiratory problems, either airway difficulties such as a known difficult intubation, or respiratory failure which could occur with obstructive airways disease or musculoskeletal diseases. Cardiovascular problems including ischaemic heart disease or cardiac arrythmias may well be better managed under general anaesthesia provided the condition is medically controlled. Adverse reactions to anaesthetic agents as in malignant hyperthermia or allergy would be relative contraindications to general anaesthesia.

Cataract surgery does not cause much surgical stimulation of the patient. This means light anaesthesia with paralysis and ventilation can be used to provide an immobile eye and controlled intraocular pressure. This is usually accomplished by securing the airway with an endotracheal tube. It is important to prevent coughing and straining which will cause a rise in intraocular pressure. This is done with an intravenous induction with thiopentone (3–5 $mg\ kg^{-1}$) or propofol (1–2 $mg\ kg^{-1}$) and a muscle relaxant, either vercuronium (0·1 $mg\ kg^{-1}$) or atracurium (0·5 $mg\ kg^{-1}$). Autonomic reflex response to intubation may be obtunded with the short-acting opiate alfentanil (10 $\mu g\ kg^{-1}$) or with a second small dose of the induction agent immediately prior to intubation. Anaesthesia may be maintained with positive pressure ventilation with oxygen, nitrous oxide and an inhalational agent.

Alternative techniques using laryngeal mask airways instead of tracheal tubes have been described [32, 33]. Total intravenous anaesthesia with propofol and alfentanil infusions have also been described and are used with muscle relaxants and positive pressure ventilation to provide desirable operating conditions.

A smooth emergence from anaesthesia, avoiding coughing and straining, with careful attention to airway maintenance and removal of secretions will prevent a rise in intraocular pressure.

Full monitoring in accordance with published recommendations [34] should be used throughout the procedure. This is particularly important as the anaesthetist is remote from the patient who is fully draped, with the head held immobile under the operating microscope, and immediate access is undesirable and difficult.

Local anaesthesia for ophthalmic day-case surgery

Local anaesthesia for cataract extraction is indicated in the routine uncomplicated case. It should be seen as an alternative method of anaesthesia for the more fit and healthy and not as a means of operating on those unfit for general anaesthesia [17]. It is a prerequisite for local anaesthesia for cataract surgery that the patient can lie still and flat comfortably. If they are unable to do this or have other contraindications to local anaesthesia, such as an inability to co-operate or a language difficulty, general anaesthesia will be necessary (Table 13.6).

Retrobulbar anaesthesia

Retrobulbar anaesthesia is still widely used [18]. It was first performed in 1884 using cocaine [35]. The technique involves the introduction of a needle percutaneously from an inferotemporal entry point aiming for the apex of the orbit. A small volume (2 ml) of local anaesthetic is deposited within the extraocular muscle cone. To prevent contraction of the orbicularis oculi muscle a facial nerve block must also be performed. Onset of the block is rapid.

Table 13.6 Contraindications to ophthalmic local anaesthesia

Patient refusal
Unable to co-operate due to dementia, deafness, language barrier
Unable to lie still due to uncontrolled cough or tremor
Unable to lie flat, breathless at rest due to respiratory or cardiac disease
Unstable medical condition—cardiac ischaemia or arrythmias
Coagulation defect
Allergy to local anaesthetic

Table 13.7 Local complications of ophthalmic local anaesthesia

Retrobulbar haemorrhage
Globe perforation
Central retinal artery embolism
Optic nerve damage
Periorbital ecchymosis
Extraocular muscle paresis

Table 13.8 Systemic complications of ophthalmic local anaesthesia

Subarachnoid injection of local anaesthetic
cranial nerve block
respiratory arrest
cardiac arrest
Intravascular injection of local anaesthetic—grand mal seizures
Exacerbation of pre-existing medical condition

Rare but serious complications have occurred. Local complications such as retrobulbar haemorrhage, globe perforation, and optic nerve damage [36] are well documented (Table 13.7). Systemic complications are due to spread of the local anaesthetic along the dural sheath of the optic nerve to the brain stem, or to direct intravascular injection. This causes a variety of symptoms from drowsiness, blindness of the contralateral eye, convulsions, loss of consciousness and cardiopulmonary arrest [37, 38] (Table 13.8).

Peribulbar anaesthesia

Peribulbar anaesthesia was first described in 1986 [39] and is a technique designed to provide good operating conditions while avoiding the rare but potentially life-threatening complications of retrobulbar anaesthesia [40]. It is well accepted by the patient as there is little discomfort during insertion of the block and a facial nerve block is not necessary. Large volumes of local anaesthetic are placed outside the muscle cone with the needle tip no further back than the equator of the eye. The local anaesthetic spreads to the apex and all compartments of the orbit through the network of orbital connective tissue. Onset of the block is relatively slow compared to a retrobulbar block and a pressure device of some sort is required to reduce the intraocular pressure.

Subconjunctival anaesthesia

A technique described for cataract surgery in which superior bulbar subconjunctival infiltration is used together with a facial nerve block. A superior rectus suture is used to steady the globe during surgery [41].

Sub-Tenon's infiltration

This is a technique that seeks to avoid all the complications of a sharp needle being passed into the orbit. A blunt cannula is passed through the conjunctiva, under Tenon's capsule and local anaesthetic infiltrated directly posterior to the globe [42].

Management of patients under local anaesthesia for ophthalmic day-case surgery

Traditionally the operating surgeon has inserted the local anaesthetic block and then operated on the patient without the assistance of an anaesthetist. However, the potentially life-threatening complications that may arise have led to the recommendation that an anaesthetist should be present for resuscitation should this be required, and to arrange for the monitoring of the patient's general condition throughout the operation [34].

All patients undergoing ophthalmic local anaesthesia should have intravenous access secured prior to administration of the block. This is then readily available for resuscitation or on occasion for sedation.

It is important to make the patients comfortable on the operating table and to provide a means of communication should they become distressed during the procedure. Monitoring consists of, arterial oxygen saturation (SaO_2), electrocardiogram (ECG) and non-invasive blood pressure measurement, although this is not measured automatically at frequent intervals due to patient discomfort during infiltration of the blood pressure cuff. All these measures apply to any sedative or sedoanalgesic practice (see Chapter 16).

Sedation for ophthalmic local anaesthesia

The ideal patient undergoing ophthalmic surgery is conscious, co-operative and pain free. This should be achieved by making sure the patient is well prepared and counselled prior to local anaesthesia and surgery. Despite this some patients are very anxious during the procedure and may become restless. This can be helped to a certain extent by light sedation, either using premedication with oral temazepam or the administration of midazolam or propofol intravenously during surgery. However, the patient's response to a predetermined dose of sedative is unpredictable. Oversedation may occur with upper airway obstruction and loss of the patient's co-operation while undersedation may leave the patient restless [43].

These problems may be overcome by using patient controlled sedation techniques where the patient determines their own level of sedation. This has been shown to be effective during day-case dental surgery [44].

Conclusion

Day-case ophthalmic surgery is gaining in popularity particularly for cataract extraction. Many units are publishing success stories in managing their ophthalmic patients on this basis and there is no doubt that it is popular with the patients [45]. The current debate concerning the relative merits of local and general anaesthesia in the UK must be resolved at local level depending on the resources available. There is evidence to show that local anaesthesia may have a beneficial effect in preventing the hormonal, metabolic and cardiovascular changes that occur with general anaesthesia [46]. However, studies show no evidence of long-term postoperative cognitive dysfunction in patients undergoing cataract surgery under general anaesthesia compared to local anaesthesia, despite marked fluctuations in pulse and blood pressure and episodes of oxygen desaturation [47]. If the anaesthetist is involved in the administration of local anaesthesia as recommended [31] perhaps the choice of anaesthesia could be made by the patients. A new approach to demand sedation where the patient is in total control and determines both the initial level of sedation and its subsequent maintenance is currently under investigation [48].

References

1 Ogg TW, Obey PA. The workload of a purpose built day surgical unit. *Ann Roy Coll Surg* 1987; 69: 110–12.

2 Audit Commission. *A Short Cut to Better Services—Day Surgery in England and Wales*. London: HMSO, 1991.

3 NHS Management Executive Value for Money Unit. *Day Surgery—Making it Happen*. London: HMSO, 1991.

4 Commission on the Provision of Surgical Services. *Guidelines for Day Case Surgery*. London: Royal College of Surgeons of England, 1985.

5 Acheson JF, McHugh JD, Falcon MG. Changing patterns of early complications in cataract surgery with new techniques: A surgical audit. *Br J Ophthalmol* 1988; 72: 481–4.

6 Watts MT, Pearce JL. Day-case cataract surgery. *Br J Ophthalmol* 1988; 72: 897–9.

7 Strong NP, Wigmore W *et al.* Daycase cataract surgery. *Br J Ophthalmol* 1991; 75: 731–3.

8 Strong NP, Wigmore W *et al.* Ophthalmic day case surgery: the role of the dedicated day case unit. *Health Trends* 1992; 24: 148–50.

9 Eason J, Seward H, Mount A. Daycare cataract surgery—Croyden experience. *J One-Day Surg* 1993; 2: 9–12.

10 Leaver P. Prospects for day-case vitreoretinal surgery (Editorial). *Br J Ophthalmol* 1992; 76: 65.

11 Cannon CS, Gross JG *et al.* Evaluation of outpatient experience with vitreoretinal surgery. *Br J Ophthalmol* 1992; 76: 68–71.

12 Commission on the Provision of Surgical Services. *Guidelines for Day Case Surgery*, revised edn. London: Royal College of Surgeons of England, 1992.

13 Courtney P. The national cataract surgery survey: 1. Method and descriptive features. *Eye* 1992; 6: 487–92.

14 Steele A. Local anaesthesia for cataract surgery (Editorial). *Br J Ophthalmol* 1990; 74: 195.

15 Smith R. An adjunct to local anaesthesia (Editorial). *Br J Ophthalmol* 1991; 75: 129.

16 Hattenhauer JM. To phaco or not. *Arch Ophthalmol* 1991; 109: 315.

17 Rubin AP. Anaesthesia for cataract surgery—time for a change? *Anaesthesia* 1990; 45: 717–18.

18 Hodgkins PR, Luff AJ *et al.* Current practice of cataract extraction and anaesthesia. *Br J Ophthalmol* 1992; 76: 323–6.

19 Steele A. Cataract management (Editorial). *Br J Ophthalmol* 1992; 76: 321.

20 College of Ophthalmologists advice on day case surgery in ophthalmology. *J One-Day Surg* 1993; 2: 14.

21 American Society of Anesthesiologists. New classification of physical status. *Anesthesiology* 1963; 24: 111.

22 Baskerville PA, Heddle RM, Jarrett PEM. Preparation for surgery: information tapes for the patient. *Practitioner* 1985; 229: 677–8.

23 Bosomworth PP, Ziegler CH, Jacoby J. The oculocardiac reflex in eye muscle surgery. *Anesthesiology* 1958; 19: 7–10.

24 Meyer EF, Tomeldon SA. Glycopyrrolate compared with atropine in the prevention of the oculocardiac reflex during eye muscle surgery. *Anesthesiology* 1979; 51: 350–2.

25 Beasley H. Hyperthermia associated with ophthalmic surgery. *Am J Ophthalmol* 1974; 77: 76.

26 Carroll JB. Increased incidence of masseter spasm in children with strabismus anesthetized with halothane and succinylcholine. *Anesthesiology* 1987; 67: 559–61.

27 Lerman J, Eustis S, Smith DR. Effect of droperidol pretreatment on postanesthetic vomiting in children undergoing strabismus surgery. *Anesthesiology* 1986; 65: 322–5.

28 Feibel RM. Current concepts in retrobulbar anaesthesia. *Ophthalmology* 1985; 30: 102–10.

29 Nicoll JMV, Arharya PA *et al.* Central nervous system complications after 6000 retrobulbar blocks. *J Anaesth Analg* 1987; 66.

30 Chang JL, Gonzales-Abola E *et al.* Brain stem anaesthesia following retrobulbar block. *Anaesthesiology* 1984; 61: 789–90.

31 *Report of the Joint Working Party on Anaesthesia in Ophthalmic Surgery.* London: Royal College of Anaesthetists and College of Ophthalmologists, 1993.

32 Holden R, Morsman CDG *et al.* Intra-ocular pressure changes using the laryngeal mask airway and tracheal tube. *Anaesthesia* 1991; 46: 922–4.

33 Akhtar TM, McMurray P *et al.* A comparison of laryngeal mask airway with tracheal tube for intra-ocular ophthalmic surgery. *Anaesthesia* 1992; 47: 668–71.

34 *Recommendations for Standards of Monitoring during Anaesthesia and Recovery.* London: The Association of Anaesthetists of Great Britain and Ireland, 1988.

35 Knapp H. On cocaine and its uses in ophthalmic surgery. *Arch Ophthalmol* 1884; 13: 402–48.

36 Morgan CM, Schatz H *et al.* Ocular complications associated with retrobulbar injections. *Ophthalmology* 1988; 95: 660–5.

37 Meyers EF, Ramirez RC, Boniuk I. Gran mal seizures after retrobulbar block. *Arch Ophthalmol* 1978; 96: 847.

38 Javitt JC, Addiego R *et al.* Brain stem anaesthesia after retrobulbar block. *Ophthalmology* 1987; 94: 718–24.

39 Davis DB II, Mandel MR. Posterior peribulbar anaesthesia—an alternative to retrobulbar anaesthesia. *J Cataract Refract Surg* 1986; 12: 182–4.

40 Wang HS. Peribulbar anaesthesia for ophthalmic procedures. *J Cataract Refract Surg* 1988; 14: 441–3.

41 Redmond RM, Dallas NL. Extracapsular cataract extraction under local anaesthesia without retrobulbar injection. *Br J Ophthalmol* 1990; 74: 203–4.

42 Stevens JD. A new local anaesthesia technique for cataract extraction by one quadrant sub-Tenon's infiltration. *Br J Ophthalmol* 1992; 76: 670–4.

43 Salmon JF, Mets B *et al.* Intravenous sedation for ocular surgery under local anaesthesia. *Br J Ophthalmol* 1992; 76: 598–601.

44 Osborne GA, Rudkin GE *et al.* Intra-operative patient-controlled sedation. Comparison of patient-controlled sedation with anaesthetist administered midazolam and fentanyl. *Anaesthesia* 1991; 46: 553–6.

45 Davies B, Tyers AG. Do patients like day case cataract surgery? *Br J Ophthalmol* 1992; 76: 262–3.

46 Barker JP, Vafidis GC *et al.* Plasma catecholamine response to caract surgery: a comparison between general and local anaesthesia. *Anaesthesia* 1991; 46: 642–5.

47 Campbell DNC, Lim M *et al.* A prospective randomised study of local versus general anaesthesia for caract surgery. *Anaesthesia* 1993; 48: 422–8.

48 Cook L, Lockwood J, Whitwam JG. True patient controlled sedation. *Anaesthesia* 1993; in press.

Chapter 14
General Anaesthesia for Outpatient Dentistry

A. Padfield

Without doubt the first routine form of outpatient, day-case, or ambulatory anaesthesia was that used for dental extractions and the original idiosyncratic method has persisted to the present day. As the 150th anniversary of Horace Wells' application of nitrous oxide for dental extractions approaches, the use of general anaesthesia for outpatient exodontia is declining in the UK.

In the 1860s Gardner Quincy Colton reputedly gave 24000 nitrous oxide anaesthetics for dental extractions over a period of 6 years. It is well-known that nitrous oxide is a very weak anaesthetic agent; to a greater or lesser extent unconsciousness has been produced with the 'help' of hypoxia. In the early 1990s the McKesson intermittent flow anaesthetic machine was introduced and, such was its popularity, that other manufacturers produced similar equipment. Nitrous oxide ('gas') became the preferred method with both dentists and patients, but has remained so only in the British Isles. By the end of World War II this type of outpatient general anaesthesia (GA) for dental extractions was becoming a peculiarly British speciality. In 1967 according to a report of a joint subcommittee of the Central Health Services Council, the majority (75%) of anaesthetics were administered in dental surgeries by general dental practitioners (GDPs) and family doctors with no postgraduate training [1].

Accurate figures are difficult to obtain but from the late 1950s onwards, the Dental Practice Board (DPB) (formerly Dental Estimates Board) has figures for the number of National Health Service (NHS) GAs paid for in England and Wales. These offer a crude guide to the frequency of GA in NHS general dental practice. Nearly 2 million GAs were paid for in 1958; but this figure had dropped to under 270000 in the most recent DPB report (1989/90). In the 1950s dental undergraduates in Sheffield would expect to anaesthetize 100 patients during their attachment to the General Anaesthetic Department. The subsequent decline in such experience in Sheffield is shown in Fig. 14.1 and this is also true in other dental schools throughout the UK. Though older dentists wish to retain the right to administer GA it is only a matter of time before all GAs will be carried out by trained medical anaesthetists. General dental practitioners prefer to work in their own offices or surgeries on a fee for service basis, whether government reimbursed or private. Younger GDPs recognize their lack of training at undergraduate level, that full monitoring is needed and that there is the financial disincentive of purchasing costly equipment both for anaesthesia and monitoring

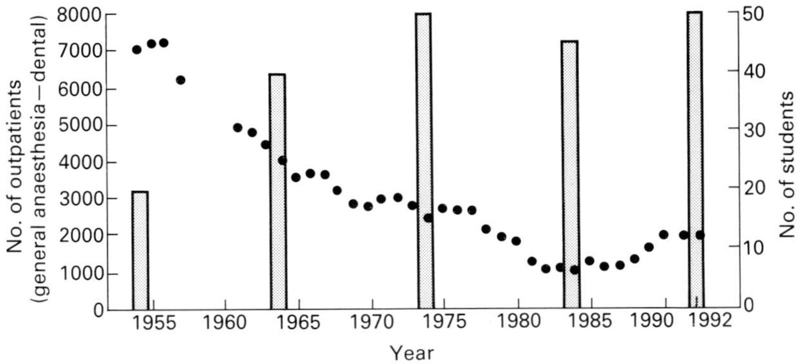

Fig. 14.1 Trend in number of dental extractions using general anaesthesia (dots) and examples of the number of dental students in the relevant year (bars) at Sheffield University Hospital.

coupled with low fee income. The graph shows a fall in the number of GAs during recent years which is a manifestation of the effect of Government action.

In October 1990 a new contract for dentists introduced a capitation payment for patient treatment. This was to stimulate preventive dentistry but it did away with many item-of-service payments, including fees for tooth extraction. In November 1990 a Department of Health Expert Working Party (the Poswillo Report) made many recommendations about improving staffing and facilities (especially monitoring) required if GA is to be administered in the dental surgery. Most of these were accepted by the Government in 1991. Hence more patients are now referred to hospitals and Community Dental Clinics for extractions under general anaesthesia which during the last 2 years has become a national trend (Fig. 14.1).

Moreover, the numbers of extractions and GAs have been declining over the past 40 years as general dental health has improved. This is due to many factors [2], the most influential being the reduced incidence of dental caries due to fluoride in toothpaste and also in those fortunate areas where the drinking water is fluoridated. There is also a distinct relationship with social class and affluence. There are proportionately fewer dental GAs administered in the richer south-east of England than in the industrial north (Dental Data Update 1988/89 DPB 1990) [3, 4] or in Scotland. Other factors include the increasing use of intravenous sedation, coupled with improved technical facilities in dental surgeries, wider acceptance of local analgesia, early use of antibiotics and the improved general health of the population as a whole.

Methods

In no other form of anaesthesia is the need for co-operation between surgeon and anaesthetist so vital. Outpatient dental anaesthesia as practised in the British Isles, breaks one of the fundamental golden rules of GA, i.e. the airway is not secured by endotracheal intubation despite the fact that it is compromised by the surgeon. The anaesthetist has to oxygenate and anaesthetize via the nasopharyngeal route and the surgeon must help by careful oral packing and by supporting the jaw.

GA for dentistry is now largely confined to children under 12 years of age. This is because adults will receive local analgesia with or without sedation for most extractions. GA will only be used for adults with severe acute infection where local analgesia has proved to be ineffective. In the author's institution 95·7% of patients anaesthetized in 1991 were under 16 years; with a mode age of 5 years and an average of 6.5 years. Nearly all children are fit for GA because any child with obvious pathology would not have been referred by the Childrens' Department. About 18–20% of children sent by GDPs to the Charles Clifford Dental Hospital (CCDH) for extractions under GA, are not referred for GA for various reasons. The most common medical problems that children present are:

1 Recent upper respiratory tract infection, which is not a contraindication if the nasal airway is clear.

2 Asthma which is rarely uncontrolled or severe enough to create problems with modern anaesthetic agents.

3 Heart murmurs which although thought to be functional still require antibiotic cover.

The presence of sickle cell trait is regarded by the author as a contraindication to outpatient dental GA for reasons which will be explained later. A further contra-indication is the extraction of more than 2–4 teeth in very small children (under 15 kg). Children of this size are usually under 3 years of age, and commonly have damaged their upper central incisors by falling. Alternatively, both upper and lower incisors are seriously carious because a sweetened dummy has been used for too long. If other, larger teeth are carious and need extraction then the pain, trauma and ensuing blood loss may indicate the need for inpatient management.

When seen in the GA department children are very often frightened or in pain or both. The accompanying parent may also be fearful, with unhappy personal memories of similar childhood experiences. It is difficult in the short time available to allay fear and anxiety. A sympathetic and caring attitude by all the staff together with the use of pictures and imagery to explain the process of anaesthesia, help to calm fears and make it an adventure. The use of a eutectic mixture of local anaesthetic (EMLA) cream on childrens' skin before venepuncture is well established, but the length of time needed before it works, about 1 h, makes its fully effective use difficult in a busy outpatient clinic. Parents are allowed to be with their child during the induction of anaesthesia but if they are frightened or unwilling they are not coerced. The bad psychological effect of a tearful terrified parent, in spite of previous, lengthy explanation and counselling during a child's anaesthetic induction, is probably greater than separation beforehand.

Volatile anaesthetic agents

The Jesuits hold that seven is the age of reason. Below this age the author uses inhalational induction of anaesthesia unless there is a request or other strong reason to the contrary while accepting that many anaesthetists use the intravenous route in relatively younger children. The volatile agent halothane transformed outpatient dental anaesthesia when introduced in the late 1950s, allowing the use of non-hypoxic mixtures of nitrous oxide and oxygen and being so much pleasanter than any previously used volatile anaesthetic agent. It is currently the agent of choice for the extremely short anaesthetics given in the UK for dental extractions. Halothane has a number of disadvantages which have caused a steady decline in its use in mainstream anaesthetic practice. These include liver damage which is very rare in small children [5] where the length of exposure to halothane is measured in minutes so that the production of significant amounts of metabolites is extremely small. The problem of arrhythmias is of greater importance and a number of studies have been carried out in the last few years comparing halothane with enflurane and isoflurane. Generally speaking there are more likely to be arrhythmias with halothane than with the other two agents [6]. However, there is no doubt that the quality of induction is smoother and easier using halothane, compared with isoflurane [7] and enflurane [8]. A study of paediatric outpatient anaesthesia in San Francisco was in agreement with both of these findings [9]. Speed of recovery to eye opening is faster with enflurane [10] but time to full recovery was found to be the same [11]. Another study found that recovery from isoflurane was significantly slower than from halothane and was more likely to be associated with coughing, salivation and laryngospasm [12]. From inpatient studies it is well known that arrhythmias are related to the extraction of teeth [13, 14]. The problem can be reduced by the administration of β-blockers orally as premedication

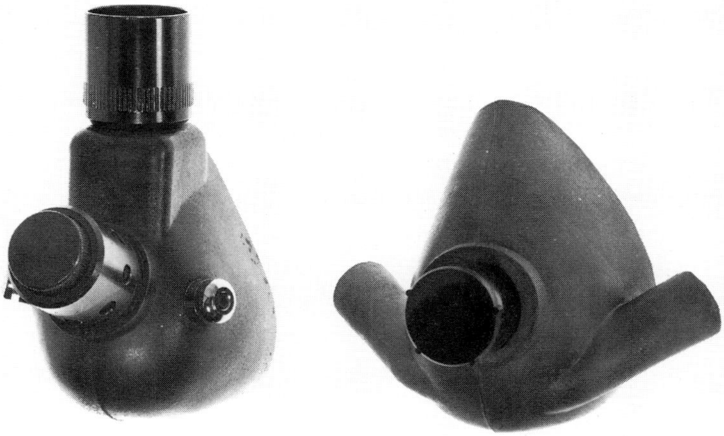

Fig. 14.2 Goldman dental mask (left) and McKesson dental mask (right).

[15] or intravenously during surgery [16]. However, it is very unlikely that there will be life-threatening arrhythmias during the very short GAs used in healthy children.

Inhalation induction and maintenance of anaesthesia is carried out using 70–75% nitrous oxide in oxygen with 0·5% halothane rising to 2% or more. Having introduced the child to the idea of a mask earlier ('flying' or 'diving') a Goldman or McKesson nasal mask (Fig. 14.2) is used from the outset, the child being encouraged to 'blow it away' if they object to the smell. (Alternatively, some practitioners may use a small amount of perfume sprayed in the mask to cover the smell which is particularly valuable with the ethers and could be useful with desflurane.) The advent of desflurane with the prospect of 'one breath' induction offers an alluring but expensive prospect to the paediatric dental anaesthetist [17], but it may not be a practical agent in the dental surgery or office if a standard vaporizer cannot be used or it becomes necessary to reduce costs.

Intravenous anaesthetic agents

Depending on the size and intelligence of the child, and usually in the 6–12 years old age group, a choice of inhalational or intravenous induction is offered. Except thiopentone, all the other commonly used intravenous induction agents are painful during injection. Thiopentone is quite unsuitable for nearly all forms of outpatient or day-case anaesthesia because of its prolonged metabolism after redistribution, giving a 'hangover' effect of at least 24 h. Etomidate is the most painful on injection, can cause thrombophlebitis and is associated with muscular activity which is more likely to occur in the unpremedicated patient. The pain and muscle movements associated with methohexitone are less severe than with etomidate and it is the cheapest intravenous agent at present. It is not as rapidly metabolized as propofol or etomidate but is significantly more rapid than thiopentone. Propofol is the most modern and expensive drug and although it causes pain on injection, abnormal muscle activity is not a problem. Propofol, however, does cause significantly more respiratory depression than methohexitone [18] and this may be a disadvantage when the anaesthetic is to be maintained inhalationally. A surprising finding in a recent study in dental practice was a more rapid recovery from methohexitone than propofol [19]. Pain during injection can be reduced by using larger veins than those on the dorsum of the hand, for instance the antecubital fossa. If some pain then occurs, exercising the hand will speed the blood flow and appears to alleviate the discomfort. The addition of a small quantity of 1–2% lignocaine to the intravenous agent is a common practice and may help to reduce pain. For the author methohexitone is the agent of choice, since it is less likely to cause bradycardia and severe hypotension. It is much cheaper and arguably a short sleep after the patient returns home, during the final metabolism of the drug, may well be beneficial.

Older children, from 10 years upwards, are often having extractions of adult-sized molar or premolar permanent teeth for orthodontic reasons, a not inconsiderable trauma in a child. It is exceptional for them not to receive an intravenous induction, after which, anaesthesia is maintained via a Goldman or McKesson nasal mask, using 70% nitrous oxide in oxygen and halothane 0·5–2%.

The problem of patients with sickle cell trait, referred to earlier, is that temporary loss of the airway may occur at any time during the procedure and cause hypoxia and hypercarbia. Although this may be rapidly and easily corrected when experienced personnel are working together, dental students and postgraduate trainees are less likely to overcome an airway problem as easily. Hypoxia and hypercarbia associated with sickle cell trait can cause serious sequelae. Sickle cell disease in the homozygous form is a much more serious pathophysiological problem. It should be managed in consultation with a haematologist or special clinic and may require preparation with exchange transfusion and inpatient treatment.

Outpatient dental GA is 'the last art form in anaesthesia' as it is presently practised in the UK.

Adult patients

Rarely, adult patients may need GA for simple dental extractions. There are only two groups where it is indicated: (a) those adults with child-like minds, i.e. the mentally challenged or handicapped who will not be able to co-operate in the use of local analgesia; and (b) patients with infected tooth sockets which require extraction to drain an absess. The first needs careful assessment as inpatient management may be required for many reasons, not least of which is the amount of co-operation which the patient can be expected to give. The second group only needs a short general anaesthetic if the surgeon is skilled and confident of removing the tooth intact. For example, the patient is made comfortable on the operating table, or in the dental chair, and asked to hold the dental prop between the teeth on the unaffected side. An intravenous injection of the preferred anaesthetic induction agent is given. As soon as the patient's eyes close, the dental pack is inserted and the tooth is extracted—a safe and efficient method, but not for the unskilled.

A more complicated type of oral surgery is the surgical removal of impacted wisdom teeth (third molars or eights). This is one of the commonest operations carried out in healthy young adults. It is the most frequently performed operation in UK private practice, according to one of the major health insurance groups (BUPA). The operation is now carried out as a day-case procedure in many dental and general hospitals.

Though the vast majority of such patients with third molar problems are medically healthy (ASA grade 1), careful surgical preoperative assessment is required to ensure that the duration and difficulty of the proposed surgery do not cause prolonged recovery or unexpected inpatient admission because of pain, tissue damage or haematoma, and loss of jaw movement with inability to take oral fluids or food, or a concern about tissue oedema and a potentially compromised airway. Preanaesthetic assessment carried out some days before surgery allows the anaesthetist to give psychological preparation and advice on postoperative problems as well as taking a medical history and examining the patient. Patients who are deemed to be unsuitable for day-case anaesthesia can be cancelled more amicably and under less pressure than when they are seen only an hour or minutes before surgery.

The most common reason for cancellation is obesity. Curiously, this is a condition frequently overlooked at the surgical consultation. Heavy smokers will be more likely to cough and develop laryngeal spasm and should be encouraged to give up for not less than a day or two preoperatively at least, to reduce their carboxyhaemoglobin levels.

Any medication other than simple analgesics or mild sedatives suggest that the patient may not be suitable for day-case surgery. Women in the first or third trimester of pregnancy should not be anaesthetized for any surgery except the most urgent or life-saving. Though the middle trimester is the safest time, removal of third molars is of no urgency and need not be contemplated. GA should only be used at this time if there is an acute abscess needing exodontia to allow drainage.

Nasal intubation is an essential part of any anaesthetic technique adopted and this may be facilitated in several different ways. The author continues to use the Magill method of blind nasal intubation: 5–10% carbon dioxide is added to the oxygen–nitrous oxide–volatile agent mixture after induction by a suitable intravenous induction agent. When the patient is hyperventilating, the nares and a plain nasal endotracheal tube are lubricated with KY jelly. The tube is passed gently down through the nose and into the nasopharynx. As it is advanced into the oropharynx beyond the base of the tongue, the anaesthetist listens for the noise of the patient's breathing and manipulates the tube towards the sound, usually by twisting the tube away from the side into which it was inserted. As inhalation occurs when the vocal cords are most widely separated the tube is pushed down firmly and should enter the larynx. At this point the anaesthetist must watch the neck in the region of the glottis to see where the tube goes. If it does not enter the larynx, correction of the location of the head from the usual 'sniffing the morning air' position and more or less twisting of the tube from one side to the other may be required. The use of suxamethonium causing severe muscle pain postoperatively as well as other more dangerous side effects is to be deplored, but paralysis with a non-depolarizing relaxant and subsequent intermittent positive pressure ventilation is often employed. Intubation may also be achieved in a spontaneously breathing patient by first deepening the level of anaesthesia using a volatile agent, and enflurane is the agent of choice because of its lesser respiratory depressant effect, and then spraying the vocal cords with 2% lignocaine before passing the tube. It is probable that blind nasal intubation causes less cardiovascular stimulation than the usual conventional laryngoscopic intubation.

Cardiac arrhythmias are well recognized in oral surgery and not infrequently occur during day-case wisdom tooth removal. They are usually associated with surgical manoeuvres such as drilling, chiselling and prising the roots from the jaw involving periodontal or root stimulation. The duration of arrhythmias is usually short, cardiac output is maintained, and they are normally of little consequence. However the intravenous administration of a β-blocker will prevent these arrhythmias but should be given in association with attention to any adverse physiological factors such as hypercarbia or hypoxia. Another simple way of avoiding arrythmias is to block the afferent pain impulses from the surgical site using local anaesthetic, i.e. a GA combined with local block introduced as soon as GA is induced.

Postoperative analgesia

Relief of postoperative pain is *the* growth area in anaesthesia at present. The cynic wonders when, enthusiasm having outweighed caution, the inevitable morbidity and mortality attendant on all medical intervention will cause a retrenchment. Most children hurt at play, pick themselves up literally and metaphorically and rapidly forget the pain they have suffered. Outpatient dental extractions if limited to a small number of teeth fall into a similar category, especially if relief of previous discomfort due to toothache is achieved. Oral analgesics are not well tolerated in a child immediately after GA and oral surgery, where nausea and vomiting are not uncommon.

Children having a large number of exodontia, regrettably still only too common, or older children having adult molars or premolars extracted solely for orthodontic reasons may suffer more lasting pain postoperatively. In these patients, paracetamol suppositories, inserted during the immediate recovery period, certainly provide analgesia. Local analgesic blockade before the extractions start are efficient for molar and premolar removal but may produce unwanted side effects. The non-steroidal anti-inflammatory drugs are probably superfluous in paediatric patients. They cause gastric irritation orally and are painful on intramuscular injection but can be given by suppository, e.g. diclenofac. In young adults following third molar surgery analgesia is nearly always essential. Intramuscular injection of non-steroidal anti-inflammatory agents, e.g. ketorolac (Toradal) at the end of surgery before the patient wakes or oral analgesics, which dissolve in water, later when the patient is able to swallow will alleviate the sometimes quite severe pain. The use of intravenous dexamethasone after induction of anaesthesia may help to control swelling and oedema postoperatively which aggravates the pain of surgery.

Sedation

Two forms of sedation are commonly used in outpatient dentistry. The first is known as relative analgesia (RA) and is induced by nitrous oxide at concentrations ranging from 5 to 70%. RA is actually the first (induction) stage of anaesthesia and is divided into three planes. In the first plane, often called inhalational sedation (5–25%) the patient becomes relaxed and co-operative with a mild degree of analgesia. Children are able to tolerate conservation treatment, and extractions with local analgesia, which they might not accept otherwise. Raising the concentration (20–55%) increases the analgesic property of nitrous oxide but the patient becomes less responsive. This plane is called dissociation sedation and the patient is sluggishly co-operative but still conscious and able to obey commands. The final plane (50–70% nitrous oxide) is that of total analgesia and is on the edge of the excitement stage and light GA. If the patient starts to close their mouth and fails to co-operate then the concentration must be reduced. A full description of this technique has been provided by Roberts [20, 21] and a study by Crawford [22] confirmed the efficacy of the method. It is essential that the dentist establishes rapport with the patient and the success of the technique relies very heavily on verbal encouragement and reassurance. It is not an area in which many, if any, medical anaesthetists have been involved.

Intravenous sedation using midazolam or diazepam is becoming more and more common in dental practice. It is particularly useful for patients with a high level of anxiety who have a phobia of local analgesia or dentistry in general. Details of the techniques used will be covered in Chapter 16. The most recent report of the DPB (1989/90) showed that the number of sedations of all types paid for, had risen to half the number of GAs (132 000:266 000).

Monitoring

The Poswillo Report [23], referred to above, has recommended that all patients having GA for dental surgery should be monitored at the levels recommended by the Association of Anaesthetists [24]. This means that pulse oximetry, electrocardiography (ECG) and non-invasive blood pressure measurement should be applied to all patients and intubated patients also require capnography. A pulse oximeter is easily attached, a blood pressure cuff may be put on fairly quickly without causing too much alarm but ECG electrodes, if correctly applied, necessitate a certain amount of undressing. Given the restlessness seen in the excitement stage with inhalational induction then the usefulness of ECG monitoring will be compromised by artefacts produced. The average duration of anaesthesia at CCDH in the author's hands was 6 min from the start of anaesthesia to the patient going into the recovery room (mode = 5 min). Compared to the time taken in general dental practice this is quite slow since anaesthesia is prolonged in a dental school by the inexperience of the student operators, but even this allows, at most, three blood pressure readings. Paradoxically, the Poswillo Report does not recommend that intravenous access should be mandatory for all outpatient dental GAs. Dentists are not well practised in obtaining venous access and would probably find it difficult in an emergency to treat any arrhythmias perceived. As far as sedation is concerned the Poswillo Report is equivocal; 'Pulse oximetry is desirable but not essential. Where it is used dentists should be aware of the significance of the readings'. A forthright recommendation that it is necessary would have been sensible, and it is interesting that the Poswillo guidelines are now being adopted widely as a necessary standard of practice, and have been accepted for eventual full implementation by the Department of Health.

Mortality

The mortality associated with GA for dental extractions in general dental practice is very low in comparison with any other branch of surgery. However, the death of a small child when it has been anaesthetized for what is perceived as a minor and trivial operation cannot fail to arouse strong emotions. Thirty-five years ago Bourne condemned the use of the upright dental chair when patients were anaesthetized for extractions [25]. He has returned to the theme over the years and suggested in 1986 that 80–90% of deaths were caused by fainting during induction or recovery, leading to cerebral hypoxia [26]. A number of authorities dispute Bourne's findings, notably Coplans and Curson [27–29]. They have made detailed studies of deaths related to dentistry and concluded that there was no relation to the posture of the patient. With the diminishing number of GAs given for outpatient exodontia it will be difficult to assess whether the implementation of the recommendations of the Poswillo Report will have an effect on mortality in this field.

Pollution

When gaseous induction and maintenance of anaesthesia is carried out by traditional methods, the prevention of pollution is virtually impossible. Expired anaesthetic gases escape from the open mouth, the nasal mask is not usually firmly applied initially and a high flow rate may be used. Various methods of reducing pollution have been suggested but none are very successful. Probably the best way to reduce the concentration of anaesthetic gases in the dental surgery is to provide 10 air changes per hour rather than the usual two [30]. Other methods used have included suction tubing attached to the front of the nasal mask, various forms of scavenging and the use of an intermittent flow machine with a lightweight Lack circuit [31]. It must not be forgotten that no clear evidence exists that anaesthetic pollution is harmful and that exposure times during dental outpatient GA are very short.

The future

As stated in the first paragraph, it is difficult to get accurate figures for the numbers of outpatient GAs for dentistry. At Guy's Hospital the numbers administered annually fell between 1914 and 1976 [32]. Until the emergence and acceptance of lignocaine as an efficient local anaesthetic, it was easier, and is still quicker, to use GA for exodontia particularly in children. Before the new contract, the more patients treated, the more the dentist earned and so GA was often used. Many patients fear intraoral needles and awareness of extraction and prefer to be 'asleep'. This preference has been encouraged and can now be satisfied by the use of sedation, although this is often overlooked as an option. As older dentists and medical practitioners who may give a thousand or more 'dental gases' a year retire, the expertise acquired over many years practice cannot be replaced. Dental undergraduates today cannot get useful practical experience of administering GA nor even become expert in extracting teeth from patients under GA. Anaesthetists trained in the last decade will seek to provide anaesthesia in a manner which they feel is the safest. This implies the use of endotracheal intubation. Intubation of the tens of thousands of children who will still require GA for exodontia will take longer, create iatrogenic complications and necessitate more hospital admissions. The use of the Brain laryngeal mask airway [33] may well be the answer but there are still some minor technical problems to be overcome.

References

1 Central Health Services Council. *Report of Joint Sub-committee on Dental Anaesthesia.* London: HMSO, 1967.

2 Padfield A. The future of general anaesthesia in the dental surgery. *J Roy Soc Med* 1989; 82: 30–2.

3 Dental Practice Board. *Annual Report 1989/90,* Appendix H, Table 1, p. 5.

4 Dental Practice Board. *FPC Series No. 7, General Anaesthetic and Sedation Techniques.* Dental Data Update 1988/89.

5 Stock JGL, Strunin L. Unexplained hepatitis following halothane. *Anesthesiology* 1985; 63: 424–39.

6 Casson WR, Jones RM. Cardiac rate and rhythm during anaesthesia for dental extraction. A comparison of halothane, enflurane and isoflurane. *Br J Anaesth* 1985; 57: 476–81.

7 Cattermole RW, Verghese C, Blair IJ, Jones CJH, Flynn PJ, Sebel PS. Isoflurane and halothane for outpatient dental anaesthesia in children. *Br J Anaesth* 1986; 58: 385–9.

8 Ryder W, Wright PA. Halothane and enflurane in dental anaesthesia. *Anaesthesia* 1981; 36: 492–7.

9 Fisher DM, Robinson S, Brett C, Gregory GA, Perin G. Comparison of enflurane, halothane and isoflurane for outpatient pediatric anesthesia. *Anesthesiology* 1984; 61: A427.

10 Strunin L, Strunin JM, Phipps JA, Corall IM. A comparison of halothane and enflurane (Ethrane) for outpatient dental anaesthesia *Br Dent J* 1979; 147: 299–301.

11 Hoyal RHA, Prys-Roberts C, Simpson PJ. Enflurane in outpatient paediatric dental anaesthesia. A comparison with halothane. *Br J Anaesth* 1980; 52: 219–22.

12 McAteer PM, Carter JA, Cooper GM, Prys-Roberts C. Comparison of isoflurane and halothane in outpatient paediatric dental anaesthesia. *Br J Anaesth* 1986; 58: 390–3.

13 Kaufman L. Cardiac arrhythmias in dentistry. *Lancet* 1965; ii: 287.

14 Rodrigo MRC, Moles TM, Lee PK. Comparison of the incidence and nature of cardiac arrhythmias occurring during isoflurane or halothane anaesthesia. Studies during dental surgery. *Br J Anaesth* 1986; 58: 394–400.

15 Hanna MH, Heap DG, Kimberley APS. Cardiac dysrhythmia associated with general anaesthesia for oral surgery. *Anaesthesia* 1983; 38: 1192–4.

16 Rollason WN, Bennetts FE, Clarke I. Cardiac dysrhythmias during outpatient dental anaesthesia with enflurane. The role of 'Beta blockade'. *Acta Anaesth Scand* 1984; 28: 497–502.

17 Jones RM. Desflurane and sevoflurane: inhalational anaesthetics for this decade? *Br J Anaesth* 1990; 65: 527–36.

18 Mackenzie N, Grant IS. Comparison of a new emulsion formulation of propofol with methohexitone and thiopentone for induction of anaesthesia in day cases. *Br J Anaesth* 1985; 57: 725–31.

19 Pollock JSS, Ferguson DM, Mackenzie NM. General anaesthesia in the dental surgery: a comparison of propofol and methohexitone. *Br Dent J* 1992; 173: 207–9.

20 Roberts GJ. Inhalation sedation (relative analgesia) with oxygen/nitrous oxide gas mixtures. 1. Principles. *Dental Update* 1990; 17: 139–46.
21 Roberts GJ. Inhalation sedation (relative analgesia) with oxygen/nitrous oxide gas mixtures. 2. Practical techniques. *Dental Update* 1990; 17: 190–6.
22 Crawford AN. The use of nitrous oxide–oxygen sedation with local anaesthesia as an alternative to general anaesthesia for dental extractions in children. *Br Dent J* 1990; 168: 395–8.
23 General anaesthesia, sedation and resuscitation in dentistry. *Report of an Expert Working Party, 1990.* London: Department of Health, 1990.
24 Association of Anaesthetists of Great Britain and Ireland. *Recommendations for Standards of Monitoring during Anaesthesia and Recovery*. London: Association of Anaesthetists of Great Britain and Ireland, 1988.
25 Bourne JG. Fainting and cerebral damage: a danger in patients kept upright during dental gas anaesthesia and after surgical operations. *Lancet* 1957; ii: 499–505.
26 Bourne JG. Deaths and posture in the dental chair: a 30 year perspective. *Today's Anaesth* 1986; 1: 29–33.
27 Coplans MP, Curson I. Deaths associated with general dental anaesthesia. *Br Med J* 1973; 1: 109–10.
28 Coplans MP, Curson I. Deaths associated with dentistry. *Br Dent J* 1982; 153: 357–62.
29 Coplans MP, Curson I. Deaths associated with dentistry and dental disease 1980–1989. *Anaesthesia* 1993; 48: 435–8.
30 Parbrook GD, Dale PD. Anaesthetic pollution in the outpatient dental surgery. *Anaesthesia* 1979; 34: 47–52.
31 Padfield A, Asbury JA. Economy and antipollution: the Lack circuit in outpatient dental anaesthesia. *Proc Ass Dent Anaesth* 1983; 1: 10–11.
32 Hutton AM, Wedley JR, Seed RF. Teaching of anaesthesia to dentists. *Br Dent J* 1978; 144: 35–9.
33 Bailie R, Barnett MB, Fraser JF. The Brain laryngeal mask. A comparative study with the nasal mask in paediatric dental outpatient anaesthesia. *Anaesthesia* 1991; 46: 358–60.

Chapter 15
Local Anaesthesia in Day-Case Surgery

W. W. A. Zuurmond and J. J. de Gange

Patients, scheduled for day-case surgery may be candidates for local, regional (locoregional) or general anaesthesia. Comparing locoregional to general anaesthesia, with special reference to day-case surgery, the main differences are:

1 Theoretically, locoregional anaesthesia offers for outpatients selective local action.

2 When applying locoregional anaesthetic techniques, many of the common side effects associated with general anaesthesia, such as postoperative nausea, vomiting, dizziness, sore throat and pain are avoided.

3 The risks of aspiration during locoregional anaesthesia are lessened [1]. Moreover, the incidence of problems and complications concerning the airway (e.g. difficult intubation, laryngospasm) and ventilation is lower. Nevertheless, locoregional anaesthesia may show other specific side effects and complications.

4 The experience of the patient concerning the incidence of minor discomfort during the perioperative period is greater during locoregional anaesthesia.

5 Locoregional anaesthesia requires a more prolonged induction time.

6 Locoregional anaesthesia is associated with failure: the possibility of inadequate analgesia, the unsuccessful block. A 100% success rate will never be achieved in performing locoregional anaesthesia for several reasons: anatomical variations, a procedure of unexpectedly long duration, inadvertent injection of the local anaesthetics, insufficient penetration of the local anaesthetic into the nerves, or other unknown reasons.

7 Locoregional anaesthesia for day-case surgery is not universally appropriate and proper selection of patients, procedures, anaesthetists and surgeons is essential for success [1].

Preassessment and preparation of the patient

Patients scheduled for day-case surgery, have to be selected preoperatively for locoregional anaesthesia. The preoperative assessment should not differ from the procedure concerning evaluation of patients for day-case surgery under general anaesthesia. The type of operation, the extent and site of the operation field, the patient's complete medical history and physical examination has to be reviewed.

Special attention should be paid to:

1 The patient's previous experience with locoregional anaesthetic techniques, including former treatments in the dental chair.
2 Bleeding disorders. The following questions are of special interest: Do you currently take anticoagulants, blood thinning medicine or non-steroidal anti-inflammatory drugs (NSAIDs)? Do you show bruises of more than 8 cm after minor trauma? Have you ever had prolonged or unusual bleeding from cuts, nosebleeds, minor bruises, tooth extractions or surgery? Before applying an invasive technique any bleeding disorders should be investigated.
3 Allergic reactions due to local anaesthetics, sun tan creams or cosmetics. Para-aminobenzoic acid or derivates, the main metabolites of the 'amino esters–local anaesthetics' may have the greatest potency to cause allergic reactions. These substances may be present in cosmetic and sun tan creams. Potentially all local anaesthetics may provoke an allergic reaction. Preservatives are added to unstable solutions and may also cause allergic reactions. The local anaesthetics, especially the amide type are stable but preservatives are added to stabilize vasoconstrictor agents. Multidose vials require the adding of antimicrobial agents, such as methylparaben or chlorocresol, to the local anaesthetic. The administration of chlorocresol, a neurotoxic agent, is not recommended.
4 Hyperventilation, fainting, seizures or convulsions. During sudden loss of consciousness or other emergencies preoperatively, the anaesthetist has to make a rapid and proper diagnosis before acting promptly. A knowledge of the medical history of the patient is mandatory to avoid therapeutic blunders.
5 Infection at the intended site of injection is an absolute contraindication for locoregional anaesthesia. Examination should be routine.
6 Drug therapy for chronic and acute medical conditions with special reference to antihypertensive, anti-epileptic and mood-altering drugs e.g. monoamine oxidase (MAO) inhibitors and tricyclic antidepressants.
7 Drugs interacting with local anaesthetics or vasoconstrictors have to be known to the anaesthetist.

Patients should be prepared for minor discomfort during the procedure. They have to know the consequences of the procedure under locoregional anaesthesia: the site of insertion of the needle(s), the existence and extent of the motor and sensory blockade, the possible sensations of numbness, paralysis and the potential complications. By being well-informed, patients are better prepared for the procedure.

Classification of the patient according to the ASA categories

After the evaluation of the medical history and physical examination patients require classification according to the ASA categories.

Patients falling into the ASA I and II categories are possible candidates for locoregional anaesthesia. ASA class III patients may be suitable if the medical condition is stable and the surgical procedure and the locoregional technique do not change the medical problems that the patient was managing at home before surgery [2].

The elderly patient scheduled for day-case surgery requires meticulous pre-assessment before being admitted. The acceptance of minor discomfort may be greater in the elderly patient and after spinal anaesthesia the incidence of postspinal puncture headache may be lower. However, conversely anatomical, systemic and pharmacological anomalies may frequently occur.

Psychological contraindications for locoregional anaesthesia are patients with:

1 Extreme anxiety and low tolerance for minor pain or discomfort.

2 Extreme anxiety concerning general anaesthesia. After being well informed patients have to choose a technique; making a choice out of negativism or mistrust should be avoided.

3 Extreme anxiety, refusal or an unco-operative attitude concerning locoregional anaesthesia.

Premedication

In day-case surgery rapid recovery from psychomotor disturbances is important to permit early discharge of patients. The best 'premedication' for the patient is to be well informed and reassured. Premedication may abolish one of the advantages of locoregional anaesthetic techniques, i.e. rapid recovery concerning psychomotor functioning.

Measuring only clinical parameters Jacobson *et al.* [3] found that oral diazepam decreased significantly preoperative discomfort and apprehension, without influencing the discharge time. Of course, the duration of the effect of oral premedicants or psychomotor functioning is dose-dependent. Nevertheless, measuring psychomotor functioning, premedicants such as diazepam or midazolam may show a longer duration of action than is desirable [4–6].

For day-case procedures the general rule has to be 'minimal or no premedication is advisable' [1, 7].

Sedation

If the patient experiences minor discomfort caused by insufficient analgesia, the anaesthetist or surgeon may complete regional blockade by local infiltration of the operation field. However, as a general rule, anaesthetists should administer general anaesthesia if a blockade is unsuccessful. Sedation of patients suffering from pain is contraindicated: the combination of sedatives and hypnotics often causes a state of uncontrolled unconscious sedation and delirious behaviour. The patients are then better off with general anaesthesia administered according to the standards of day case anaesthesia.

Sedation techniques have to be planned during the preoperative assessment and not improvised during the procedure. The incidence of complications increases, when local anaesthesia with sedation is administered [8, 9]. Careful titration of intravenous sedation shortly before or during the regional anaesthesia is only recommended if the patient can be supervised and controlled by an experienced second person (Chapter 16).

For locoregional anaesthesia verbal reassurance and communication is the best sedation technique, provided analgesia is adequate. The personal stereo has now been introduced into the operating theatre. The patient is requested to bring tapes of preferred music to listen to during the procedure.

Locoregional anaesthetic procedures for outpatients

General guidelines

1 The anaesthetist has to be skilled in performing locoregional anaesthetic techniques. Everyone who performs local anaesthetic techniques has to know: (a) the anatomy; (b) the permissable dose of the local anaesthetic in milligrams (Table 15.1); (c) the symptoms and therapy of toxic systemic reactions caused by local anaesthetics (Table 15.2); (d) the symptoms and therapy of allergic reactions (Table 15.3); and (e) the symptoms and therapy of vasovagal reactions (Table 15.4).

2 The surgeon has to be supportive of locoregional techniques. Preoperatively, in his or her contact with the patient and during intraoperative management, a positive attitude by the surgeon is mandatory. The surgery has to be performed gently, because the patient may perceive pressure as pain. Moreover, the locoregional anaesthesia is not always successful and sometimes additional infiltration of local anaesthetics is required. Everybody in the operating theatre should know that the procedure of administering locoregional anaesthesia may involve extra time. Co-operation between anaesthetist, surgeon and patient is of special importance.

3 Patient, anaesthetist and surgeon should all agree with the decision to perform a locoregional technique.

Table 15.1 The maximum dose in milligrams of local anaesthetics used in day-case surgery

Lidocaine plain	200
Lidocaine with adrenaline	500
Prilocaine plain	400
Prilocaine with adrenaline	600
Mepivacaine plain	350
Mepivacaine with adrenaline	350
Bupivacaine plain	150
Bupivacaine with adrenaline	150

Table 15.2 Symptoms and therapy of systemic toxic reactions of local anaesthetics

Signs	Therapy
Drowsiness Dizziness Tinnitus Numbness of the tongue Anxiety Confusion Emotional lability Difficulty with speech Blurred vision	Observation Oxygen by face mask Diazepam 10 mg i.v.
Muscle 'twitching'	—
Convulsions	Assisted ventilation with 100% oxygen Diazepam
Loss of consciousness Coma	Endotracheal intubation Assisted ventilation Controlled ventilation
Hypotension Bradycardia	Infusion of fluid. Vasoconstrictor Anticholinergic (atropine, glycopyrrolate)
Respiratory arrest Cardiac arrest	Basic life support

Table 15.3 Symptoms of an allergic reaction to local anaesthesia. For therapy see Chapter 4

Signs
Exanthema Stomach cramps Itching Urticaria Quincke's oedema Sweating Red-coloured face
Respiratory insufficiency Bronchospasm
Hypotension
Convulsions
Cardiac arrest

Table 15.4 Symptoms and therapy of vasovagal reaction

Signs	Therapy
Pale colour	Atropine 0·5 mg i.v.
Sweating	Infusion of fluid
Bradycardia	Oxygen by mask
Hypotension	
Nausea and vomiting	
Loss of consciousness	

4 The administration of local anaesthesia and the operation should be performed separately; the time between locoregional procedures and the start of the operation has to be at least 5–10 min for infiltration, 10–15 min for peripheral nerve blocks and 15–30 min for central neural blockades.

5 An indwelling intravenous needle or catheter should be inserted into a peripheral vein in all cases other than possibly small procedures using infiltration anaesthesia. The patient has to be monitored adequately during the perioperative period: electrocardiogram (ECG), heart rate, systolic and diastolic arterial blood pressure and oxygen saturation by pulse oximetry. Oxygen and resuscitation equipment should always be available.

6 Avoid intravascular injection by aspirating before injection.

7 Only the smallest amount of the local anaesthetic in a solution of the lowest possible concentration, that will give the desired effect, should be used [1].

8 Emergency patients may receive locoregional anaesthesia. However, such patients cannot be treated on a day-case basis as described in this chapter since their preparation, preoperative evaluation, physical and mental condition may differ to a great extent.

9 In choosing the appropriate local anaesthetic for outpatient surgery, the anaesthetist has to make a profile of the desired effects. Procaine and chloroprocaine (not available in Europe) have the shortest duration of action. However, being ester-type local anaesthetics, these drugs are associated with potential allergic sensitivity. Generally, there is no indication for using the ester-type of local anaesthetics. The intermediate-acting amide local anaesthetics, lidocaine, prilocaine and mepivacaine are the drugs of choice for outpatient anaesthesia. Adding a vasoconstrictor to the local anaesthetic prolongs the duration of action. The long-acting local anaesthetics of the amide-type, bupivacaine and etidocaine, may be useful if prolonged blockade is needed. Discharge from the outpatient ward may be delayed, otherwise the patient has to be instructed to protect the numb extremity or area from external injury. A prolonged stay in the recovery area is to be preferred to the potential risk of sending the patient home with a motor and/or sensory block.

Locoregional anaesthetic techniques for day-case surgery may be divided into four categories:

1 Topical anaesthesia
2 Infiltration techniques: (a) extravascular; (b) intravascular; and (c) intra-articular.
3 Conduction anaesthesia: (a) peripheral nerve blockade; and (b) plexus blockade.
4 Central neural blockade: (a) intrathecal anaesthesia; and (b) epidural anaesthesia.

Also, locoregional and general anaesthesia or sedation can be combined.

Topical anaesthesia

For topical anaesthesia liquids, sprays, creams, ointments or gels can be applied to the skin or mucous membrane to block the nerve terminals near the surface of the skin or mucosa.

The most effective of these topical preparations contain the base form of the local anaesthetic agent. Despite the proximity of the nerve terminals to the surface of the skin, the onset of effect is at least 60 min after administration of the topical agent. Concerning the administration of topical anaesthesia to mucosae, the onset time is 2–3 min and absorption of the local anaesthetic is rapid. Local anaesthetic sprays tend to have a bad taste and may induce salivation especially if the spray contacts the tongue. The normal duration of mucosal analgesia is 15–30 min.

Recommended drugs and dosage: (a) for the skin, the eutectic mixture of local anaesthetic (EMLA), a 50:50 mixture of 25 mg lidocaine and 25 mg prilocaine per millilitre as an oil–water formulation; and (b) for the mucosa, lidocaine 2, 4 or 10% either as spray or ointment is the most appropriate topical anaesthetic.

Indications include superficial but painful skin procedures. A thick layer of EMLA cream on the dorsum of the hand covered with a plastic dressing before venipuncture to prevent pain is especially suitable for children, and also for adults if venipuncture is expected to be painful. Absorption of EMLA produces pallor, oedema and vasoconstriction. Applying glyceryl trinitrate ointment just distal to the EMLA cream patch promotes vasodilatation and prevents blanching of the skin [10]. Sprays, gels and ointments are used for topical anaesthesia of the airways, in urology and eye surgery for small procedures of short duration.

Contraindications include a known allergy for local anaesthetics, and skin destined for keratinocyte culture [11].

The rapid absorption of the highly concentrated local anaesthetic in sprays may cause systemic reactions if the permissable dose is exceeded: count the sprays one by one!

Extravascular infiltration techniques

The majority of minor surgical procedures may usually be performed with infiltration anaesthesia administered by the surgeon. Innervation of subcutaneous areas of the

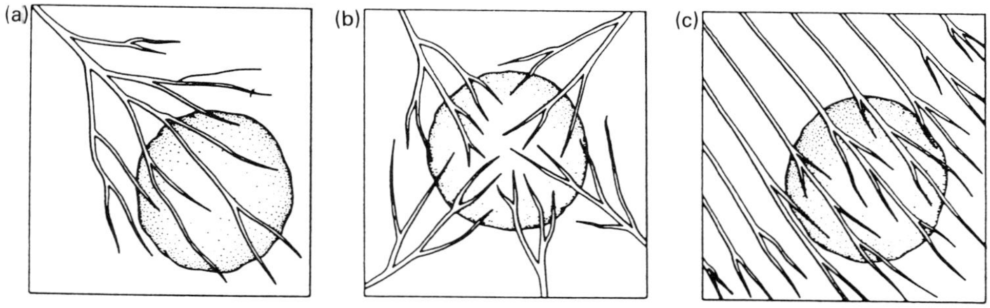

Fig. 15.1 The types of innervation of subcutaneous tissue: (a) convergent; (b) divergent; and (c) parallel.

body may be divided into three types (Fig. 15.1): (a) convergent; (b) divergent; and (c) parallel.

The subcutaneous injection of a local anaesthetic causes blockade of the branches of the sensory nerves of the cutis, subcutis and subfascial tissue. Local infiltration is simple and safe and may be subdivided into two methods: (a) direct infiltration of the operation site; and (b) field block. Direct infiltration is indicated only for small areas. Conduction analgesia is the method of choice for the convergent type of innervation; the field and infiltration blocks are the proper methods for the divergent or parallel type of innervation.

Direct infiltration

Fanwise infiltration from the centre of the area to be anaesthetized is the technique of choice, avoiding intravascular injection by aspirating before injection. A solution of 0·5 or 1% lidocaine or prilocaine with or without adrenaline or noradrenaline 1:200 000 should be used.

Indications include removal of superficial scars, lesions or small tumours. Postoperative pain relief can be obtained by infiltration of the wound with the longer acting local anaesthetic bupivacaine [12]; or infiltration of the mesosalpinx after tubal sterilization with yoon rings [13].

Contraindications include a known allergy to local anaesthetics. Complications are rare.

A disadvantage of this technique is the distortion of the anatomy of the operation site.

Field block

Fanwise infiltration of the local anaesthetic from two points at both sides of the operation site (Fig. 15.2) is the technique of choice. A solution of 0·25–0·5% lidocaine or prilocaine should be used with or without adrenaline. The concentration of

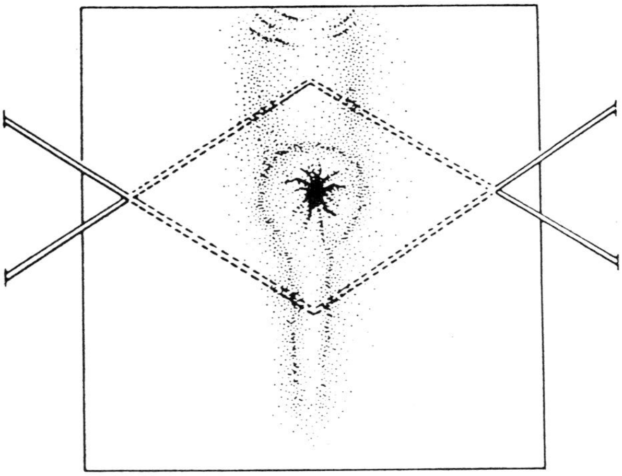

Fig. 15.2 Field block for haemorrhoidal operation.

adrenaline has to be lower than 1:200000. By injecting bupivacaine, the duration of the analgesic period may be prolonged. In tissues supplied with endarteries, only local anaesthetic solutions without adrenaline should be administered. The maximum dosage of the local anaesthetic should not be exceeded. An amount of 7–10 ml of local anaesthetic solution is required for each 10 cm^2.

Indications include operations on the skin and subcutaneous tissue (Figs 15.3 & 15.4), and haemorrhoidal operations (Fig. 15.2). Contraindications include a known allergy for local anaesthetics. Complications include overdose by exceeding the maximum dosage of local anaesthetic or vasoconstrictor. Detailed knowledge of the type of innervation of the operation field is mandatory.

Intravascular regional anaesthesia

Intravenous regional anaesthesia is an effective and reliable method of producing analgesia of an extremity with a rapid onset and recovery. The intravascular administration of a local anaesthetic into a tourniquet occluded limb causes analgesia distally to the inflated cuff.

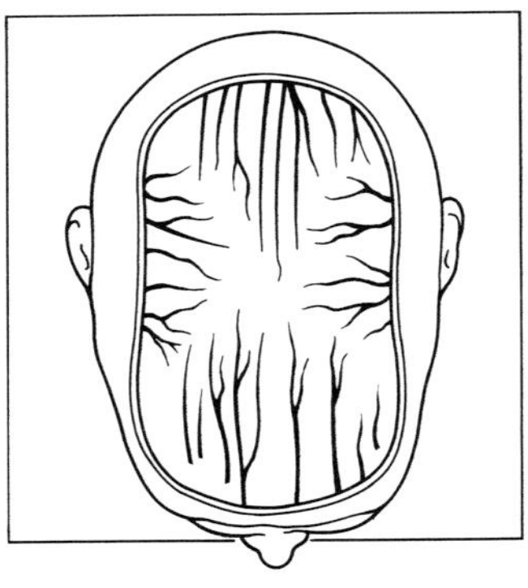

Fig. 15.3 Innervation of the subcutaneous tissue of the skull.

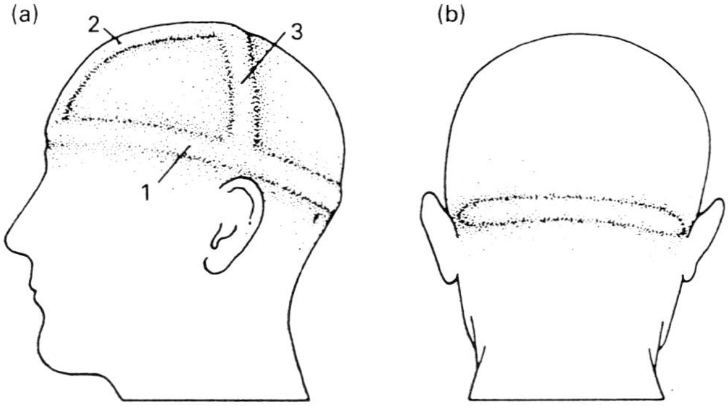

Fig. 15.4 Field block subcutaneous tissue of the skull: (a1) temporal; (a2) sagittal; (a3) parietal; and (b) occipital.

An indwelling plastic intravenous catheter is inserted into a peripheral vein of the involved extremity. It is mandatory to insert a second intravenous catheter in the opposite extremity for use in case of emergency. Exsanguination of the extremity prior to injection is required for achieving a better operation field and probably for better local action of the anaesthetic. This may be obtained by elevation of the extremity for a few minutes and by the use of an Esmarch bandage. The patient has to be warned to expect minor discomfort and must be willing to accept the tourniquet pressure before the onset of the blockade.

Before the procedure the pneumatic cuffs and the equipment, especially the tubing system and the dials have to be tested for proper functioning. Using a double pneumatic cuff system, first the proximal pneumatic cuff is inflated. After the block is established, the distal cuff is inflated, and thereafter the proximal one can be deflated.

After release of the tourniquet at the end of the procedure mild systemic toxic reactions may occur. Intermittent deflations of the tourniquet with a cycling regimen of a 10 s deflation interval followed by a 1 min period of reinflation, is recommended to minimize possible toxic reactions [14].

The patient has to be monitored adequately during the perioperative period: ECG, heart rate, arterial blood pressure and SaO_2.

Lidocaine and prilocaine are the local anaesthetic drugs of choice for this block; with bupivacaine, cardiotoxicity may occur and this agent is *not* recommended for intravenous regional anaesthesia. Comparing lidocaine and prilocaine, no differences were found in terms of onset, duration and quality of anaesthesia. However, the blood concentrations of prilocaine were lower and this may indicate a greater margin of safety in terms of potential systemic concentrations after release of the tourniquet [15].

Methaemoglobin formation observed with prilocaine only occurs at a dose greater than 600 mg [16]. The dosages of either lidocaine or prilocaine for the upper and lower extremity are 40 ml 0·5% and 75–100 ml 0·25% respectively. The onset time of intravenous regional anaesthesia is 3–7 min. After cuff release, post-tourniquet analgesia varies between 5 and 8 min. By increasing the concentration of prilocaine, without exceeding the maximum dose of 4–5 mg kg^{-1}, analgesia after release of the tourniquet can be extended to more than 15 min [17].

This technique is suited for soft tissue operations, that take less than 90 min to perform. It is the tourniquet time which is the limiting factor. Analgesia is inadequate for operations with major involvement of bone or nerve tissue.

Absolute contraindications include: (a) a known allergy for local anaesthetics; (b) patients with sickle cell disease; and (c) infections. Intravenous regional anaesthesia is relatively contraindicated in patients with neurological or vascular disease of the involved extremity and in patients showing a low tolerance for pain or psychological instability.

Inadvertent accidental or premature release of the pneumatic cuff during the first 20–40 min may lead to excessive local anaesthetic blood levels in the systemic circulation and hence to severe toxic reactions.

Leakage of the local anaesthetic agent beneath the cuff, due to unsatisfactory pneumotourniquet placement or technique, may also lead to systemic toxicity during the procedure. The hypothetical leakage of local anaesthetics via the interosseous vessels is of minor importance.

The postoperative pain relief is of short duration. Patients require a recovery time of at least 2 h after the procedure. Adequate pain relief has to be established and premature discharge of the patient may lead to vasovagal reactions.

Intra-articular techniques

Periarticular infiltration and intra-articular instillation of local anaesthetics for arthroscopic knee surgery may be an alternative to regional or general anaesthesia.

Technique according to Erikson [18]: after local infiltration of the skin and underlying tissues over the anterior side of the knee, being the place of insertion of the arthroscope, and also lateral to the upper lateral corner of the patella, being the place of insertion of the local anaesthetic, lidocaine or prilocaine, combined with adrenaline, is injected into the knee joint. The patient is then asked to move the joint for 2–5 min. Supplementary doses of diluted lidocaine and adrenaline 1:200000 may be administered during the procedure if necessary. During surgery the knee joint can be irrigated.

Based on patient comfort and the absence of systemic toxicity, lidocaine concentrations of 1 or 1·5% with adrenaline may be preferred over 0·5% solutions; 20 ml is instilled intra-articularly for knee arthroscopy. The mean duration of analgesia is 6 h [19].

Indications include both arthroscopy of the knee and therapeutic procedures by arthroscope (menisectomy, removal of loose bodies). This technique is also useful in combination with general anaesthesia, to provide postoperative analgesia.

Contraindications include a known allergy for local anaesthetics, patients who show a low tolerance for pain or psychological instability, and the use of a tourniquet.

The technique is controversial; Milligan *et al.* [20] could not find any postoperative pain relief after the postoperative intra-articular insertion of bupivacaine. Smith *et al.* [21] found a more rapid recovery and mobilization and less opioid requirement after intra-articular bupivacaine administration, compared with placebo, after completion of the arthroscopy under general anaesthesia.

Moreover, this anaesthetic technique has to be supplemented with sedation techniques, for example inhalation of nitrous oxide and oxygen (50:50 mixture) by mask in about one-third of patients [19].

Probably its success is based upon the skills and cooperation of the members of the team.

Conduction analgesia

Peripheral nerve blockade

Digital nerve block

The two dorsal and two ventral branches of the nerves innervating the digit or toe, can be blocked by an injection of a total of 2 ml lidocaine or prilocaine, without vasoconstrictors, from a dorsolateral point at the base of the phalanx. Digital nerve block can also be produced by injection of the common volar digital nerves near their bifurcation between the metacarpal heads.

Lidocaine or prilocaine 1% is the concentration of choice. Digital blocks have to be performed without vasoconstrictors. Compression of the nerves has to be prevented by injection of a volume of less than 2 ml.

Indications include small operations on the finger or toe.

Contraindications include a known allergy for local anaesthetics and patients with small vessel diseases.

Gangrene or necrosis of the finger may occur when using vasoconstrictors, applying a small tourniquet at the base of the finger longer than 15 min; or when administering too much volume at the base of the phalanx.

The digital nerve block is usually administered by the surgeon. Other peripheral nerve blocks are relatively infrequently performed in most surgical cases when compared to the number of plexus or intravenous regional blocks which produce more complete analgesia.

Plexus blockade

The upper extremity; brachial plexus block (Fig. 15.5)

The axillary approach. The arm must be abducted to an angle of 90°, externally rotated and resting comfortably. The landmark of the axillary brachial plexus is the brachial

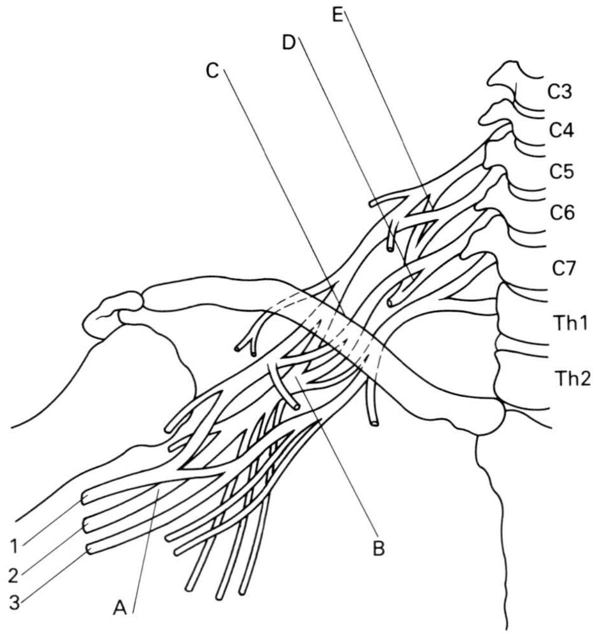

Fig. 15.5 Approaches for plexus blockade of the upper extremity: A, axillary; B, infraclavicular; C, supraclavicular; D, subclavian perivascular; and E, interscalene—(1) median nerve, (2) radial nerve, and (3) ulnar nerve.

artery, as high in the axilla as possible. The main three methods of localizing the axillary brachial plexus are:

1 Insertion of the catheter in the plexus sheath.

2 Eliciting paraesthesia.

3 Using a nerve stimulator.

Baranowski and Pither [22] advocate after their study of 100 patients, the nerve stimulator technique, in view of the possible risk of neurological damage associated with eliciting paraesthesia and the technical difficulties with the catheter technique. Using a nerve stimulator, the upper extremity has to be controlled by a second person to prevent inadvertent movements.

The disadvantage of the axillary approach is the difficulty in blocking the musculocutaneous nerve, innervating the dorsal area of the forearm and the axillary nerves. Spread of the anaesthetic agent in the sheath to the musculocutaneous nerve may be encouraged by closing it off distal to the point of injection during administration of the local anaesthetic solution. The axillary nerves innervating the lateral arm region can be blocked by supplementary infiltration of the upper arm with lidocaine 1% if a tourniquet is required during the operation.

To obtain satisfactory anaesthesia 20–40 ml lidocaine, mepivacaine or prilocaine 1% with or without adrenaline 1:200000 should be administered.

Indications include operations on the hand and forearm, provided that the musculocutaneous nerve and the lateral distal part of the upper arm are also blocked.

Contraindications include: (a) a known allergy for local anaesthetics; (b) infected glands in the axilla; (c) if abduction of the arm to 90° is not possible; and (d) bleeding disorders.

Complications include inadvertent intra-arterial injection, or systemic toxic reactions.

Interscalene 'one needle' technique [23]. The head is turned to the opposite side and the shoulder is depressed to lower the clavicle. Finding the interscalene groove is essential for the success of this technique. A horizontal line is drawn laterally from the cricoid cartilage to indicate the level of the C6 transverse process.

The patient is asked to lift the head to detect the lateral border of the sternomastoid muscle. Fingers must then be placed behind the lateral border of the sternomastoid muscle which is rolled backwards over the scalenus anterior muscle until the groove between scalenus anterior and medius is reached.

At the level of C6 a 4–6 cm short bevel needle is inserted, through a skin weal of 1% lidocaine, medially and directed about 15° dorsally and 45° caudally.

Before making contact with the transverse process paraesthesias are felt by the patient. Paraesthesias to the shoulder may be due to contact with the suprascapular nerve which lies outside the plexus. The use of a nerve stimulator is recommended. Aspiration prior to injection of the local anaesthetic solution prevents inadvertent vascular or cerebrospinal fluid spread. The recommended dosage is 20–40 ml lidocaine or prilocaine 1% or 1·5%.

Indications include procedures on the shoulder and upper arm. Often the median and ulnar nerve are inadequately blocked.

Contraindications include bleeding disorders and impaired pulmonary function.

Phrenic nerve paresis was reported in 100% of patients during interscalene block [24] and a reduction in pulmonary function of approximately 25% may be expected [25].

This technique should be avoided in patients with impaired pulmonary function. Bilateral blocks should not be performed. Discharging the patient after the block has worn off and using lidocaine or prilocaine as local anaesthetic agents is the safest regimen. The patient has to be prepared for the consequences of an eventual blockade of the recurrent laryngeal nerve or stellate ganglion causing hoarseness, difficulty in swallowing, dyspnoea and Horner's syndrome respectively.

Pneumothorax, inadvertent epidural or intrathecal administration of the local anaesthetic is possible but should not occur if the correct needle and technique are used [26].

With brachial plexus block, venous access must be assured in the opposite limb and the patient has to be monitored adequately (see General guidelines, above; and Chapter 22).

The axillary approach to the brachial plexus is the safest method. However, for operations on the shoulder and upper arm, the interscalene technique has to be preferred; the discomfort for the patient may be expected to be high.

The use of bupivacaine for interscalene block is not appropriate for outpatients: discharging patients with an impairment of pulmonary function of about 25% has to be prevented. The anatomy of the brachial plexus allows several more approaches for blockade, applying a 'one needle' technique. Three other approaches are frequently used in clinical practice: (a) perivascular subclavian [27]; (b) supraclavicular [28]; and (c) infraclavicular [29].

The blocks around the clavicle, the supraclavicular area, perivascular subclavian and infraclavicular areas, may be associated with pneumothorax, thus creating a major complication. Symptoms of pneumothorax may arise insidiously after discharge of the patient. The incidence of pneumothorax after supraclavicular blockade may be relatively high compared to the other blocks, but even if the incidence of pneumothorax after the perivascular subclavian or infraclavicular approach is relatively low, refraining from performance of all these blocks, increases safety in day-case patients.

The lower extremity, lumbosacral plexus block

The plexus lumbosacralis can be approached by two main pathways: the dorsal or the ventral inguinal route.

Psoas block. The blockade involves the ventral branches of the lumbosacral plexus between L1 and S3, including the genitofemoral, lateral cutaneous femoral, femoral and obturator nerves. The sciatic nerve is often only partially anaesthetized and a supplementary block of this nerve is sometimes necessary, provided the maximum dose of local anaesthetic is not exceeded.

The patient is positioned with the affected side uppermost. The use of a neurotracer is recommended. The needle is inserted following the landmarks described by Chayen [30]: processus spinosus L4, 3 cm caudal and 5 cm lateral (Fig. 15.6).

When contraction of the lower limb is observed, injection of the local anaesthetic

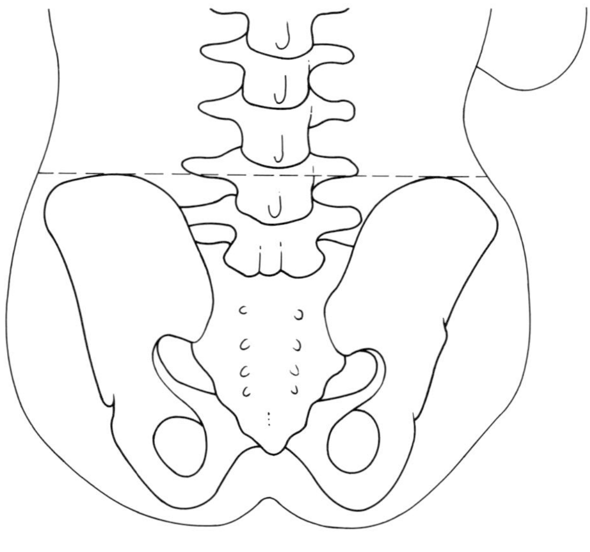

Fig. 15.6 Psoas blockade. Surface measurements for the point of injection: 3 cm caudal and 5 cm lateral below the upper level of the iliac crests.

can be performed after an aspiration test to exclude the presence of blood or cerebrospinal fluid.

The 'three in one block', inguinal approach to the lumbosacral plexus. In 1973 Winnie *et al.* [31] described a method which allows the blockade of the obturator, femoral and lateral femoral cutaneous nerves applying a 'one needle technique' in the paravascular inguinal region. These three nerves emerge from the lumbar plexus and are located between the psoas major muscle ventrally and the quadratus lumborum dorsally.

If an anaesthetic solution is injected around the femoral nerve, 2 cm caudal from the ilioinguinal ligament and 1–1·5 cm lateral from the femoral artery, the solution will rise in the sheath between the two muscles and all three nerves are blocked. The cephalad spread of the solution is encouraged by compression of the tissues caudal to the point of injection during the administration of the local anaesthetic agent. When locating the femoral nerve, the use of a neurostimulator is recommended to prevent inadvertent damage to the nerve by the 'seeking for paraesthesias method'.

To ensure complete surgical anaesthesia of the lower limb, the obturator, femoral, lateral femoral cutaneous and the sciatic nerves have to be blocked.

Sciatic nerve block [32]. The patient is placed on the side opposite to the one which is to be blocked. The main landmarks are the greater trochanter and the posterior superior iliac spine. From the midpoint of a line between these two points, a second line is drawn at a 90° angle in a caudal direction.

The point of insertion of the needle is located at a distance of 3 cm from the base line, perpendicularly to the skin. A nerve stimulator should be used. After localizing the sciatic nerve, 10–15 ml of the local anaesthetic solution is sufficient to provide blockade.

Recommended drugs and dosage for the psoas and sciatic nerve block or 'three in one' plus sciatic nerve block are lumbosacral plexus block 30 ml lidocaine or prilocaine 0·5–1% with adrenaline 1:200000. Supplementary sciatic nerve block: 10 ml lidocaine or prilocaine 1% with adrenaline 1:200000.

Indications for this technique include operations on the lower extremity and arthroscopic procedures of the knee or ankle. Contraindications include a known allergy for local anaesthetics and bleeding disorders.

Complications for psoas block include particularly the following: (a) mild hypotension due to unilateral involvement of the sympathetic chain; and (b) inadvertent epidural injection of local anaesthetics by improper needle technique.

For both psoas block and 'three in one block' toxic systemic reactions by overdose may occur especially when the lumbosacral plexus block and sciatic nerve block are combined without controlling the maximum dose.

The advantages of plexus blockades of the lower extremities over spinal or epidural anaesthesia are a lower incidence of:

1 Hypotension.

2 Nausea and/or vomiting.
3 Bladder or bowel dysfunction.
4 Total block.
5 Back or headaches.

The disadvantages are:

1 More complicated and often multiple needle techniques.
2 Higher incidence of systemic toxicity by the greater amount of local anaesthetic agent.

The permissible dose of local anaesthetic must not be exceeded. Using plain solutions the local anaesthetic concentrations in plasma may be higher than when administering solutions with adrenaline. Using bupivacaine, the duration of the blockade may be too prolonged for discharging patients after day-case surgery [33].

Central nerve blockades

Epidural anaesthesia

The epidural space (extradural space, peridural space) is the space between two layers of the dura mater. The outer layer is formed by the ligaments and periosteum lining the vertebral canal, extending from the foramen magnum to the sacrococcygeal membrane; the inner layer is the actual, so called, dura mater spinalis.

The contents of the epidural space are adipose areolar tissue, connective tissue, veins, lymphatics and the segmental mixed spinal nerves, crossing the epidural space before exiting from the spinal canal through the intervertebral foramina. Epidural anaesthesia is produced by injection of a local anaesthetic agent after inserting a needle into the epidural space. The possible sites of action of the local anaesthetic drugs administered into the epidural space include the nerve trunks in the paravertebral space, the dorsal root ganglia, the vertebral spinal roots and the spinal cord itself [34].

An epidural block can be performed in either a lateral or sitting position. The lateral position may be preferred because of the lower incidence of fainting.

Recommended drugs and dosage for epidural anaesthesia are 20 ml lidocaine 2%, 20 ml prilocaine 2% or 20 ml mepivacaine 2%.

The blockade may be prolonged if adrenaline 1:200000 is added to the local anaesthetic solution. The usual duration of the blockade with and without adrenaline is 60–180 and 60–90 min respectively. Placement of a catheter in the epidural space and the administration of incremental doses is recommended, if there is uncertainty concerning the length of the procedure. The long-acting local anaesthetics bupivacaine and etidocaine are not recommended for this blockade in day-case surgery.

Indications for epidural anaesthesia in day-case surgery include hernia repairs, minor urological operations and gynaecological operations. Discomfort and shoulder pain during the procedure may occur if laparoscopies are performed with epidural anaesthesia. Operations on the lower limbs may also occur under epidural anaesthesia.

Contraindications for epidural anaesthesia include patient refusal, bleeding disorders, infection near the site of injection, chronic backache or headache and a known allergy for local anaesthetics.

Other contraindications are diseases of the cardiovascular system and neurological disorders. Septicaemia or shock are not normally present in patients scheduled for day-case surgery.

Immediate complications include:

1 Inadequate block or patchy analgesia.

2 Total spinal anaesthesia by inadvertent injection of the local anaesthetic into the subarachnoid space.

3 High blockade.

4 Systemic toxic reactions due to either inadvertent intravenous injection or inappropriate dosage.

5 Vasovagal reactions.

6 Nausea and vomiting.

7 Hypotension and cardiovascular depression.

8 Inadvertent puncture of the theca.

Entering the subarachnoid with an epidural needle is a serious complication. The incidence of postspinal headache is significant. If the patient is not hospitalized, communication with the patient at home is important to ensure correct treatment.

Late complications include backache, urinary retention, and postural hypotension.

Caudal anaesthesia

The needle is inserted into the epidural space via the sacral hiatus. The epidural space in the sacrum is an extension of the epidural space of the lumbar region. The anaesthetist must be aware of this, particularly concerning sterility measures. After positioning of the patient, in the lateral or prone position, the anaesthetist can palpate the sacral spines in a caudal direction and will recognize a distinct depression just below the last sacral spine. If the finger is then moved in a cephalad direction, the outlines of the space are defined. A needle is inserted at a right angle to the skin until a bony resistance is met.

It is then angled at 30° to the plane of the sacrum and advanced in a cephalad direction until a distinct 'plop' is felt. After aspiration and if no blood or spinal fluid is obtained, the local anaesthetic can be injected. During injection the tissue over the sacrum should be palpated to detect subcutaneous infiltration.

Recommended drugs and dosage are 20 ml lidocaine or prilocaine 2% with or without adrenaline 1:200000.

Indications include perineal surgery and painful urological and gynaecological examinations.

Contraindications are essentially the same as for lumbar epidural anaesthesia.

The failure rate of this blockade is relatively high. Anatomical variations may occur in 10% of the patients [35]. Moreover, leakage of the local anaesthetic solution via the sacral foramen may result in insufficient analgesia. At the level L5–S1 the epidural space is anatomically narrowed from an average width of 6–2 mm [36] and this may prevent cephalad spread of the local anaesthetic. Analgesia up to a level of T10–T12 is required for haemorrhoidectomy. Further complications are similar to the lumbar epidural approach.

Spinal anaesthesia

The intrathecal space surrounds the spinal cord between pia and arachnoid mater. Its lower limit is the termination of the dural sac at the second sacral vertebral level and cranially it communicates with the cerebrospinal fluid in the cranium [37].

The injection of a local anaesthetic solution in the cerebrospinal fluid results in spinal anaesthesia: a temporary autonomic, sensory and motor block of the nerve roots which come in contact with the anaesthetic solution. It may be better to call spinal anaesthesia, subarachnoid or intrathecal anaesthesia (or analgesia).

Although it is possible to introduce local anaesthetic agents at any level, insertion of the needle below the termination of the spinal cord, i.e. below the second lumbar vertebra is preferable to prevent inadvertent trauma of the spinal cord.

Spinal anaesthesia can be performed in a lateral or in a sitting position. The lateral position has a lower incidence of fainting.

Recommended drugs and dosage are 2–3 ml lidocaine 5% in glucose with or without adrenaline.

Indications and contraindications are similar to the epidural technique.

Acute complications include the following:

1 Hypotension and cardiovascular depression.
2 Vasovagal reactions.
3 Nausea and vomiting.
4 High blockade.

Late complications include:

1 Postspinal puncture headache.
2 Backache.
3 Urinary retention.
4 Postural hypotension.

When comparing the lumbar and caudal epidural approach in day-case surgery, the lumbar approach is more elegant, precise, reliable and the local anaesthetic is injected in a much cleaner area.

Comparing the spinal and epidural techniques there are various essential differences. The epidural space has to be detected by the loss-of-resistance or hanging-drop method, while the intrathecal space is more simply detected by the free flow of cerebrospinal fluid from the needle. The higher success rate of spinal intrathecal anaesthesia is probably due partly to this factor, because the anatomical end-goal of spinal anaesthesia is more easily obtained. Moreover, leakage via the intervertebral foramina may occur whilst administering the local anaesthetic into the epidural space and may result in insufficient blockade.

In spinal anaesthesia, the local anaesthetic is administered into a closed fluid system and therefore it is a more reliable technique, with less tendency to cause incomplete blocks or missed segments.

The amount of local anaesthetic used for spinal anaesthesia is lower and the anaesthetic agents are mixed with the cerebrospinal fluid. In epidural anaesthesia the epidural space has to be filled with the local anaesthetic. Consequently, systemic toxic reactions due to high plasma concentrations are more likely to occur during epidural anaesthesia.

The speed of onset is faster in spinal anaesthesia, and the motor blockade is more pronounced.

Spinal anaesthesia, using an intermediate-acting local anaesthetic should theoretically be ideal for outpatients. However, spinal anaesthesia may be associated with the late complication of postspinal puncture headache.

The spinal block is not a contraindication to early ambulation and discharge of patients. It has been shown that the incidence of headaches is the same whether the patient is placed in the flat position for 24 h or allowed to sit up or be ambulatory [32, 38].

After intrathecal anaesthesia patients will be discharged from the outpatient ward. However, 1 or even 3 days later, postspinal puncture headache may occur. One of the purposes of day-case surgery for the patients, 'feeling themselves again' as soon as possible, has not been achieved when this complication occurs. It requires treatment listed in Table 15.5. Home follow-up and communication (for example by telephone) with the patient after discharge is mandatory after day-case surgery and especially after spinal anaesthesia. When a patient suffers from postspinal puncture headache, and communication, for what ever reason, is poor, hospitalization is indicated. Proper technique, appropriate choice of a 25 or 26 G spinal needle without cutting bevels and correct placement of the needle may decrease the incidence of postpuncture headache.

Young people are more prone to develop postspinal puncture headache, being the major group of patients in day-case surgery.

The incidence of postspinal puncture headache after day-case surgery varies from 37 to 5·2% [39–41]. The use of spinal anaesthesia for day-case surgery is controversial

Table 15.5 Therapy for postspinal puncture headache

Bedrest
Non-steroidal anti-inflammatory drugs
Abdominal binder
Measured oral intake of at least 3 l day^{-1}
Epidural blood patch after 3 days of headache

[42–44]. However, patients older than 50 years may be good candidates for this technique.

The alternatives are the plexus blockades (lower extremity) or epidural anaesthesia.

Discharge criteria and hospitalization

Minimal general criteria for discharge of patients from hospital are:

1 Stable vital signs for 1 h.
2 Orientation in person, time and place.
3 No surgical complications (bleeding).
4 Ability to walk without support.
5 Ability to tolerate fluids.
6 No or minimal emesis.
7 Ability to urinate.
8 Pain controllable with oral NSAIDs or paracetamol.

The postoperative residual analgesia after locoregional anaesthesia is one of the benefits of this technique. However, disadvantages of discharging a patient with a still existing motor or sensory blockade are:

1 The numbness of the extremity or operated area may lead to accidental damage of the affected part of the body.

2 The block wears off at home and additional pain therapy often becomes mandatory. The patient has to be instructed and supplied with analgesics for adequate pain relief at home: oral NSAIDs or paracetamol should be prescribed to be taken orally at fixed intervals.

Before discharging patients lumbosacral plexus blocks, spinal and epidural blockade should have completely worn off.

Extra attention should be paid to the following discharge criteria for spinal and epidural blocks [45]:

1 Possibility of plantar flexion of the big toe and ability to walk.

2 Return of sensation in perianal area (S4–S5) and ability to urinate. Using the intermediate-acting local anaesthetics the problem of urinary retention is only temporary. Before leaving the day-case ward patients must have urinated.

3 Absence of postural hypotension; patients can dress themselves and can sit for at least 1 h without feeling dizzy.

Psychomotor disturbances after locoregional anaesthesia may be expected for 1–1·5 h after 200 mg plain lidocaine whereas 500 mg lidocaine with adrenaline, 3 mg kg^{-1} of plain mepivacaine or prilocaine did not impair psychomotor skills [46].

After the administration of psychotropic drugs psychomotor functions may be disturbed dependent on the type of drug and the dosage. A wide variety of tests have been applied for creating criteria for discharge of patients, from the patients ability to walk to the use of advanced computerized test methods. Recovery tests should be complete, reliable and valid to permit conclusions to be drawn from their results [47] (Chapter 6).

Table 15.6 Minimum and maximum time of the usual duration of locoregional techniques [50] in minutes using the dosage described in the text

	L	L+	M	M+	P	P+
Local infiltration	30 60	120 360	45 90	120 360	30 90	
Conduction	50 200	120 180	50 200	120 180	50 200	120 180
Plexus	60 90	120 140	60 120	120 140	60 120	
Epidural	60 90	60 180	60 120	60 180	60 120	
Spinal	60 90	90 135				

L, lidocaine plain; L+, lidocaine with adrenaline; M, mepivacaine plain; M+, mepivacaine with adrenaline; P, prilocaine; P+, prilocaine with adrenaline.

To avoid inappropriate discharge, the physician has to assess the patient for home readiness. The patient must be accompanied by a responsible person.

For hospital admission, criteria should also be established: surgical complications, severe pain, persistent nausea and vomiting are the most common reasons for hospital admission. Meridy [48] stated that the number of patients transferred from a day-care unit to an inpatient setting can serve as an index of outcome, the hospital admission index (HAI). The HAI in his study was 2·4%; patients who had received local anaesthesia showed a lower HAI. However, comparing local and general anaesthesia, Grimes *et al.* [49] established that after suction curettage abortions, similar degrees of overall safety were found, although each technique was associated with a different spectrum of complications. After oral surgery in young patients Muir *et al.* [51] could find no difference in postoperative sequelae. In the Federated Ambulatory Surgery Association study [8, 9], the incidence of complications after local anaesthesia and general anaesthesia was not different if local anaesthesia was combined with sedation. Recovery times after locoregional and general anaesthesia have been compared by several authors [1, 48]. However, a proper comparison between the techniques demands a review of the total procedure, including induction times and the duration of the blockade (Table 15.6) [50].

References

1 Bridenbaugh LD. Regional anaesthesia for outpatient surgery. A summary of 12 years' experience. *Canad Anaesth Soc J* 1983; 30: 548–52.

2 Carlton JE. Local anaesthesia for day stay surgery. *Baillière's Clin Anaesth* 1990; 4: 691–712.

3 Jacobsen H, Hertz JB, Johansen K, Hansen A, Kolliker K. Premedication before day surgery. *Br J Anaesth* 1985; 57: 300–5.

4 Short TG, Galletly DC. Double-blind comparison of midazolam and temazepam as oral premedicants for outpatient anaesthesia. *Anaesth Intens Care* 1989; 17: 151–6.
5 Korttilla K. Postanaesthetic cognitive and psychomotor impairment. *Int Anesth Clin* 1986; 24: 59–74.
6 Rettig HC, Haan P de, Zuurmond WWA, Leeuwen L van. Effects of hypnotics on sleep and psychomotor performance. A double-blind randomised study of lormetazepam, midazolam and zoplicone. *Anaesthesia* 1990; 45: 1079–82.
7 Aken H van. General versus locoregional anaesthesia for outpatient surgery. In: Kallar SK, Whitwam JG, eds. *Outpatient Anaesthesia, Proceedings of an International Symposium*. Antwerp, Belgium, 9 June 1988. Bussum: Medicom Europe 1988: 67–76.
8 Federated Ambulatory Surgery Association. *Special Study I*. Federated Ambulatory Surgery Association, Alexandria, VA 1986.
9 White PF. Outpatient anesthesia. In: RD Miller, ed. *Anaesthesia*, 3rd edn. New York: Churchill Livingstone, 1990.
10 Teillol-Foo WLM, Kassab JY. Topical glyceryl trinitrate and eutectic mixture of local anaesthetics in children. A randomized controlled trial on choice of site and ease of venous cannulation. *Anaesthesia* 1991; 46: 881–4.
11 Mountford EM, Blight A, Chesire IM, Levick PM. Adverse effects of lignocaine (lidocaine) on skin destinated for keratinocyte culture. *J Invest Dermatol* 1991; 97: 746.
12 Reid MF, Harris R, Phillips PD, Barker I, Pereira NH, Bennett NR. Day-case herniotomy in children. A comparison of ilioinguinal nerve block and wound infiltration for postoperative analgesia. *Anaesthesia* 1987; 42: 658–61.
13 Thomson RE, Wetchler BV, Alexander CD. Infiltration of the mesosalpinx for pain relief after tubal sterilization with yoon rings. *J Reprod Med* 1987; 32: 537–9.
14 Sukhani R, Garcia CJ, Munhall RJ, Winnie AP, Rodvold KA. Lidocaine disposition following intravenous regional anesthesia with different tourniquet deflation technics. *Anesth Analg* 1989; 68: 633–7.
15 Bader AM, Concepcion M, Hurley RJ, Arthur GR. Comparison of lidocaine and prilocaine for intravenous regional anaesthesia. *Anesthesiology* 1988; 69: 409–12.
16 Harris WH, Cole DW. Methaemoglobin formation and oxygen transport following intravenous regional anaesthesia using prilocaine. *Anesthesiology* 1968; 29: 65–9.
17 Tryba M, Zenz M, Hausman E. Prolonged analgesia after tourniquet cuff release following i.v. regional analgesia with prilocaine. *Br J Anaesth* 1983; 55: 631–4.
18 Eriksson E. Local anaesthesia for athroscopy. In: Eriksson E, ed. *Illustrated Handbook in Local Anaesthesia*, 2nd edn. Copenhagen: Schultz Forlag 1979: 149–50.
19 Dahl MR, Dasta JF, Zuelzer W, McSweeney TD. Lidocaine local anesthesia for arthroscopic knee surgery. *Anesth Analg* 1990; 71: 670–4.
20 Milligan KA, Mowbray MJ, Mulrooney L, Standen PJ. Intra-articular bupivacaine for pain relief after arthroscopic surgery of the knee joint in daycase patients. *Anaesthesia* 1988; 43: 563–4.
21 Smith J, Hemelrijck J van, White PF. Effects of local anaesthesia on recovery after outpatient arthroscopy. *Anesth Analg* 1991; 73: 536–9.
22 Baranowski AP, Pither CE. A comparison of three methods of axillary brachial plexus anaesthesia. *Anaesthesia* 1990; 45: 362–5.
23 Winnie AP. Interscalene brachial plexus block. *Anesth Analg* 1970; 49: 455–66.
24 Urmey WF, Talts KH, Sharcock NE. One hundred percent incidence of hemidiaphragmatic paresis associated interscalene brachial plexus anesthesia as diagnosed by ultrasonography. *Anesth Analg* 1991; 72: 498–503.
25 Urmey WF, McDonald M. Hemidiaphragmatic paresis during interscalene brachial plexus block: effects on pulmonary function and chest wall mechanics. *Anesth Analg* 1992; 74: 352–7.

26 Urmey WF. Brachial plexus block. *Curr Opinion Anaesth* 1992; 5: 666–7.
27 Winnie AP, Collins VJ. The subclavian perivascular technique of brachial plexus anesthesia. *Anesthesiology* 1964; 25: 353–63.
28 Kulenkampf D. Die Anaesthesierung des Plexus brachialis. *Zentralbl F Chir* 1911; 38: 1337–50.
29 Raj PP, Montgomery SJ, Nettles D, Jenkins MT. Infraclavicular brachial plexus block. A new approach. *Anesth Analg* 1973; 52: 897–903.
30 Chayen D, Nathan H, Chayen M. The psoas compartment block. *Anesthesiology* 1976; 45: 95–9.
31 Winnie AP, Ramamurthy S, Durrani Z. The inguinal paravascular technic of lumbar plexus anaesthesia. The '3-in-1 block'. *Anesth Analg* 1973; 52: 989–96.
32 Moore DC. Regional block. *A Handbook for Use in the Clinical Practice of Medicine and Surgery*, 4th edn. Springfield Illinois: Charles C Thomas, 1965.
33 Odoom JA, Zuurmond WWA, Sih IL, Bovill J, Osterlof G, Ooosting HV. Plasma bupivacaine concentrations following psoas compartment block. *Anaesthesia* 1986; 41: 155–8.
34 Cousins MJ, Bromage PR. Epidural blockade. In Cousins MJ, Bridenbaugh PO, eds. *Neural Blockade in Clinical Anesthesia and Management of Pain*, 2nd edn. Philadelphia: JB Lippincott, 1988: 306–10.
35 Collins VJ. *Principles of Anesthesiology*, 2nd edn. London: Lea & Febiger, 1976: 725.
36 Cheng P. Epidural space. Anatomical and clinical aspects. *Anesth Analg* 1963; 42: 398–411.
37 Bridenbaugh PO, Greene NM. Spinal (subarachnoid) neural blockade. In: Cousins MJ, Bridenbaugh PO, eds. *Neural Blockade in Clinical Anesthesia and Management of Pain*, 2nd edn. Philadelphia: JB Lippincott, 1988: 215–42.
38 Carbaat P, Crevel van H. Lumbar puncture headache: Controlled study on the preventive effect of 24 hours' bedrest. *Lancet* 1981; ii: 1131–5.
39 Flaaten H, Raeder J. Spinal anaesthesia for outpatient surgery. *Anaesthesia* 1985; 40: 1108–11.
40 Clarke GA, Power KJ. Spinal anaesthesia for day case surgery. *Ann Roy Coll Surg Engl* 1988; 70: 144–6.
41 Mulroy MF, Neal JM, Bridenbaugh LD, Palmen B. Is post-spinal headache more frequent in outpatients? *Regional Anaesth* 1989; 14 (suppl): S2.
42 Lee JA, Atkinson RS. Spinal anaesthesia and day care surgery? (Editorial). *Anaesthesia* 1985; 40: 1059–60.
43 Lee JA, Atkinson RS. Spinal anaesthesia and day care surgery? (Correspondence, 1979). *Anaesthesia* 1986; 41: 650–1.
44 Flaaten H. Spinal anaesthesia and day care surgery? (Correspondence). *Anaesthesia* 1986; 41: 650–1.
45 Plug AE, Aasheim GM, Foster C. Sequence of return of neurological function and criteria for safe ambulation following subarachnoid block (spinal anaesthetic). *Canad Anaesth Soc J* 1978; 25: 133–9.
46 Korttila K. Recovery and driving after brief anaesthesia. *Anaesthetist* 1981; 30: 377–82.
47 Zuurmond WWA, Balk VA, Dis H van, Leeuwen L van, Paul EAA. Multidimensionality of recovery from anaesthesia. Analysing six recovery tests. *Anaesthesia* 1989; 44: 889–92.
48 Meridy HW. Criteria for selection of ambulatory surgical patients and guidelines for anesthetic management: A retrospective study of 1553 cases. *Anesth Analg* 1982; 61: 921–6.
49 Grimes DA, Schulz KF, Cates W, Tyler CW. Local versus general anesthesia: Which is safer for performing suction curettage abortions? *Am J Obstet Gynecol* 1979; 135: 1030–5.
50 Philip BK, Covino BG. Local and regional anesthesia. In: Wetchler BV, ed. *Anesthesia for Ambulatory Surgery*, 2nd edn. Philadelphia: JB Lippincott, 1991: 309–65.
51 Muir VMJ, Leonard M, Haddaway E. Morbidity following dental extraction. *Anaesthesia* 1976; 31: 171–80.

Chapter 16
Sedation and Sedoanalgesia

J. G. Whitwam and Chen Wang

Endoscopic and other procedures which come under the general heading of minimally invasive therapy are being practised by a progressively wider spectrum of specialists for a greater range of both diagnostic and increasingly complex therapeutic procedures, particularly in the fields of gastroenterology, interventional radiology and endoscopic surgery [1].

Many such procedures can cause anxiety amounting to fear and feelings of panic, particularly when the airway is compromised as may occur during endoscopy. Fear more than pain is a major stimulus to increased sympathetic activity, causing problems such as hypertension, arrhythmias, an increase in the myocardial oxygen demand to supply ratio with the risk of myocardial infarction which will be compounded by hypoxaemia. Alternatively some patients, for example those with arthritis, may find the need for immobility on hard surfaces for long periods causes discomfort and restlessness.

Apart from anxiolysis, amnesia is also a desirable state in such patients ensuring that they have no fear of returning for further procedures.

Sedoanalgesia

Whenever possible, pain at the site of intervention, and hence nociceptive reflexes, should be obtunded using local anaesthesia. However, even under these circumstances, complete management of the patient includes sedation, not only to allay anxiety but also if the procedure is prolonged or uncomfortable. A combination of local analgesia and sedation is termed sedoanalgesia [1].

When local analgesia is not feasible, for example in colonoscopy, some gynaecological procedures, such as oöcyte retrieval and various interventional procedures, it may become necessary to administer a centrally acting analgesic drug, which may have the potential to act synergistically with the sedative drug causing deep sedation or the induction of anaesthesia with loss of verbal communication. In addition airway obstruction and severe respiratory and cardiovascular depression can occur. At any subsequent enquiry such an event would require the practitioner and assistant to be competent in the conduct of anaesthesia and resuscitation to standards required by specialists in anaesthesia and whenever possible polypharmacy should be avoided except by suitably trained practitioners [2]. Many procedures require general

Table 16.1 Definition of sedation and anaesthesia

Sedation
Verbal communication maintained
Appropriate, albeit sluggish, response to command
Simple classification of grades of sedation
1 Unsedated or aroused—anxious
2 Anxiolysis—awake, not anxious
3 Sedation—sedated, speech slurred
4 Deep sedation—eyes closed, may fall asleep if unstimulated, rousable, appropriate responses to command
Anaesthesia
5 Eyes closed, loss of verbal communication, may respond to physical stimulation, but unrousable
6 Unresponsive

anaesthesia, e.g. laparoscopic and thoracoscopic surgery and should not be attempted using sedation.

Objectives of sedation

1 Behavioural. Anxiolysis, reduction of attention, amnesia, maintenance of verbal communication and co-operation by the patient.
2 Physiological. Retention of a brisk glabellar tap eye blink response, reduction of sympathetic activity and possibly also muscle tone.
3 Monitoring. Arterial oxygen saturation (SaO_2) near presedation values and greater than 90%.

A simple classification of levels of sedation and the definition of anaesthesia and sedoanalgesia is shown in Table 16.1.

Drugs available for sedation

Some of the more commonly used ones are summarized in Table 16.2. All drugs used for the induction of anaesthesia by the intravenous route can be administered in smaller doses to provide sedation. Inhalational anaesthetic agents with analgesic properties, e.g. nitrous oxide, have been used widely in obstetrics and dentistry, but their use is limited and in decline. Anaesthesia is induced intravenously by four principal drug types and a variety of combinations of these.
1 Classical intravenous induction agents, effective within one arm–brain circulation time, e.g. (a) barbiturates—thiopentone, methohexitone; (b) imidazole derivative—etomidate; and (c) phenol derivative—propofol.
2 Opioids—pethidine, morphine, fentanyl, alfentanil, sulfentanil, nalbuphine, pentazocine.

Table 16.2 Drugs used for sedation and analgesia

BZD	**α_2 adrenoreceptor agonists**
Midazolam (Versed, Hypnovel)	Clonidine
Diazepam (as diazemuls)	Dexmetomidine
Flunitrazepam (Rohypnol)	**Combinations**
Lorazepam (Ativan)	BZD i.v. + opioid
Opioids	e.g. midazolam
Morphine	+
Meperidine (Pethidine)	Pethidine i.m., i.v.
Fentanyl	Morphine i.m.
Alfentanil	Fentanyl i.v.
Sufentanil	Alfentanil i.v. bolus or infusion
Nalbuphine	Sufentanil i.v.
Pentazocine	Nalbuphine
Butorphanol	Pentazocine
NSAIDs	NSAIDS
Ketorolac (Toradol)	e.g. Ketorolac, Diclofenac
Diclofenac (Voltarol)	Ketamine + BZD
Intravenous anaesthetic agents	e.g. Midazolam i.m. + ketamine i.m.
Propofol	lorazepam p.o. + ketamine i.m.
Methohexitone	Propofol
Inhalational anaesthetic agents	Propofol }
Nitrous oxide	+ } Propal
Other	Alfentanil }
Barbiturates	Alfentanil [107]
e.g. pentobarbitone	Infusion (1–5 μg kg^{-1} min^{-1})
Butyrophenones	+
e.g. droperidol	Midazolam i.m.
Arylcyclohexylamine	
e.g. ketamine	

BZD, benzodiazepine; NSAID, non-steroidal anti-inflammatory drug.

3 Phencyclidine derivative—ketamine.
4 Benzodiazepines (BZD)—midazolam, diazepam.

Other drugs such as droperidol or α_2 adrenoreceptor agonists (e.g. clonidine) are sometimes used as adjuncts to the other groups of drugs.

With the exception of the BZDs and the opioids, the therapeutic window available for sedation, before the induction of anaesthesia, can be extremely narrow. For example, propofol is a highly potent and extremely short-acting anaesthetic drug which is playing a rapidly increasing role in anaesthetic practice, particularly day-case and intensive care, particularly when administered by infusion [3–5]. Sedation, light and deep anaesthesia occur at plasma levels of 2, 3 and 6 μg ml^{-1} respectively. Thus it is easy to achieve and maintain anaesthesia but, in view of the individual variation in response of patients to the drug, it is much more difficult to quickly establish and maintain a constant level of adequate sedation, e.g. within 5 min, with no risk of trespassing into anaesthesia either at the start or at a later stage. Propofol can cause apnoea and severe cardiorespiratory depression in anaesthetized patients although intraoperative patient controlled sedation with propofol by infusion has been described [6]. However it remains an anaesthetist's or intensivist's drug and at present its use requires at the very least monitored anaesthetic care (MAC), i.e. the presence of an anaesthesiologist. These remarks are particularly apposite, for example to gastro-intestinal endoscopy, with the need for a rapid turnover of patients and where the presence of anaesthetists on the one hand and personnel trained, practised and certified in anaesthesia and resuscitation on the other, is unusual.

Opioids may be used alone to cause analgesia and sedation, but they can cause severe respiratory depression, bradycardia and muscle rigidity. They always introduce an incidence of nausea and vomiting. However their current safe application in patient controlled analgesia (PCA) implies that they can be used providing the doses and conditions of administration are carefully controlled.

Ketamine produces a state called 'dissociative anaesthesia' and has a relatively long duration of action. Its side effects include hypertension, tachycardia, a rise in intracranial pressure and severe, unacceptable, dysphoric effects [7]. Although these can be ameliorated by BZDs they preclude its use in routine clinical practice. It is an invaluable drug for the induction of anaesthesia with only minimal cardiovascular and respiratory depression in difficult or emergency situations, e.g. in radiodiagnostic and therapy departments and in the trauma services. It is also widely used by many anaesthetists, often in combination with midazolam, for the induction of anaesthesia for major procedures, particularly in critically ill patients [8, 9].

Benzodiazepines, because of their wide margin of safety and ease of administration, are used not only by anaesthetists but also by a wide spectrum of practitioners, both medical and dental, with little or no formal training in anaesthesia. The reason is that given good patient selection, an appreciation of the sensitivity of the elderly to sedative drugs, knowledge of the recommended doses in normal subjects, and an element of good sense, it is possible to practise safe sedation with little risk of inducing anaesthesia.

The development and introduction of midazolam provided for the first time a short-acting water soluble BZD which, by also providing a high level of amnesia and virtually no enterohepatic circulation in normal subjects, represents a major advance in sedation therapy. The subsequent development and introduction of flumazenil now allows the termination of BZD-induced sedation at will, which has major implications not only for safety but also potentially for health economics.

Thus many drugs can be adapted for sedation given adequate resources, i.e. time, anaesthetists, infusion pumps and recovery facilities. As a result, at present any practical discussion of sedation for endoscopic procedures has at its central theme the pharmacology and application of the BZDs, specifically midazolam, its interactions with other drugs, principally the opioids, and the combined use of midazolam and flumazenil [10]. The most recent report by a working party commissioned by the Royal College of Surgeons of England on guidelines for sedation by non-anaesthetists stresses the central role of midazolam for intravenous sedation, and its interaction with opioids, and nitrous oxide, for sedoanalgesia [11]. 'The anaesthetic agents ketamine and propofol cannot be recommended as sedatives at present.' The volatile anaesthetic agents cannot be relied upon to provide sedation as defined, and the specific antagonists flumazenil and naloxone should be immediately available.

Practical considerations

Conduct of sedation and sedoanalgesia

External stimuli can reduce the effectiveness of sedative drugs. The environment should be orderly and quiet with carefully planned illumination such that the total candela in the patients' view are reduced to only a necessary minimum. After initial work-up and stabilization of sedation, repeated cuff blood pressure measurements are best avoided since the cuff causes discomfort and may arouse the patient. Monitoring equipment should be muted apart from alarms. Some surgeons prefer to work with music in the background which also helps many patients to relax.

In view of the current mortality rates and critical incidents there should be prerequisites before any sedation procedure is commenced.

1 Continuous venous access via an intravenous cannula.

2 Availability of continuous monitoring with both a pulse oximeter and electrocardiogram (ECG).

3 Both the practitioner and assistant should have recently certified evidence of training in cardiopulmonary resuscitation.

4 Resuscitation equipment, i.e. oxygen delivery and ventilation systems, suction, defibrillator and drugs required for resuscitation should be immediately to hand.

5 There should be the possibility of rapid transfer for full critical care facilities (e.g. intensive care, operating theatres, transfusion).

The issues to consider during work-up and management of patients undergoing sedoanalgesia are summarized in Table 16.3.

If a patient becomes excessively restless there are three potential events to consider:

1 Is the patient hypoxic? Inspect SaO_2, blood pressure, ECG, heart rate.

2 Is the patient oversedated and entering light anaesthesia? Check verbal communication and response to command.

3 Is the patient undergoing a genuine paradoxical reaction to the BZD sedation [12]?

The patient's 'minder' should encourage the patient to take a few deep breaths from time to time, providing this does not induce coughing, and this may be all that may be required to improve the SaO_2. Alternatively oxygen therapy should be introduced. Arguably, whenever possible, oxygen administration should be routine throughout any sedation procedure, preferably using a face mask, or if inappropriate, e.g. during gastroscopy, nasal prongs or catheters. Flumazenil in a dose of 0·5–2 mg i.v. should be sufficient to lighten sedation or reverse paradoxical reactions.

Table 16.3 Sedoanalgesia—considerations for good practice

Work up to consent	
Sources of information	Referring physician Patient Relatives
Problem patients (probably 3–5% of all patients are unsuitable and better managed using anaesthesia)	Young anxious females Large males Drug/alcohol abusers Psychologically disturbed Language difficulty
Pain management	Pre-, peri- and postoperative
Procedural safety	Staff Training Attitudes Working environment Monitoring (heart rate, blood pressure, electrocardiogram, SaO_2) 'Minder'—anaesthetist or member of staff with adequate training Recovery facilities Discharge procedures

Techniques of sedation

In terms of sedating the nervous system the barbiturates and opioids have served practitioners of medicine well. In more recent times BZDs, because of their inherent safety, have assumed a major role in sedation, particularly by practitioners without formal anaesthetic training. In the last 4 years both midazolam and propofol have been used to provide patient controlled sedation (PCS).

BZDs are active by all routes of administration, sublingual, nasal, anal, rectal, subcutaneous, intramuscular and intravenous and have been used for clinical sedation by all these routes. However, because of the immediacy and predictability of the intravenous route discussion of the use of BZDs will largely be restricted to this route of administration.

The best form of analgesia is infiltration of local anaesthetic, Bier block or nerve block. When combined with sedation it constitutes sedoanalgesia and local anaesthesia combined with sedation, using a single drug, is now the recommended method in dentistry following the Poswillo Report [2]. The use of centrally acting analgesic drugs may be necessary, e.g. gastrointestinal endoscopy and some radiological procedures when there should be a major reduction in the dose of one or both drugs, i.e. either the analgesic or the sedative, to avoid the inadvertent induction of anaesthesia. When propofol is combined with opioids severe bradycardia can occur and cardiac asystole has been reported (Chapter 2).

Table 16.4 Intravenous techniques for sedation

Methods	Drug	Patient selection	Duration of procedure	Flumazenil
Titration	Midazolam	All patients	Any	In critically ill or elderly to terminate residual effects of sedation
Bolus	Midazolam	ASA I/II Controlled III < 65 years of age	Short	In UK, except as emergency drug
Patient controlled	Midazolam Propofol	All patients who can co-operate: at present restricted to patients < 65 years old	Extended	$\pm$

Sedation may be induced by the intravenous route by titration, bolus or patient controlled techniques (Table 16.4).

Midazolam is the drug of choice for general sedation practice by practitioners without any training in anaesthesia. However, both propofol and midazolam have been used for demand sedation. Whenever propofol is in use it is always prudent that an anaesthetist should be present.

Titration

In reality this rarely occurs. For BZDS it implies the use of up to two to three doses i.v. at 3 min intervals, i.e. the time to maximum effect, which is impractical when the procedure may last only a few minutes. The aim would be to work towards a satisfactory end point and in adult patients whose general condition is good, this usually requires a total dose in the range of 0·04–0·07 mg kg^{-1} of midazolam which is normally given as a rapid or slow bolus. For most practitioners the slow bolus is regarded as titration.

However in the elderly or adult patients with poor physical status a total dose of 0·25–0·5 mg of midazolam i.v. should be administered in a well diluted solution, e.g. 1 mg ml^{-1} and 7 min allowed to observe the effect. On the basis of this 'test' dose, which may be all that is required, further incremental doses up to a total of 2–3 mg may be appropriate. It is very important in the elderly to take time to settle them and such patients should receive oxygen therapy, e.g. via a Hudson or MC mask or an anaesthetic circuit. In old or ill patients the use of flumazenil should be considered to terminate sedation immediately the procedure is complete and hence minimize the peak duration of effect of the sedative drug.

Bolus dosing

Because of the slow onset times of BZDs it is usual for even the most patient clinician to use an unnecessarily large dose for sedation, i.e. to overdose. Bolus dosing implies that a preset dose is injected, well diluted, e.g. 1 or 2 mg ml^{-1} during a period of 30–60 s and the i.v. cannula should then be flushed with saline. It is recommended that the sedative dose should be reduced by one-third from the data sheet recommendation (0·07 mg kg^{-1}) for both midazolam [13] and diazepam [13, 14] and many clinicians work in a dose range of 3–5 mg of midazolam i.v. depending on the size and perceived anxiety of the patients, with rapid introduction, for example, of a gastroscope when the drug shows an effect. Clearly in view of the variability of response of patients to midazolam, and depending on the speed of the procedure further incremental doses of 1–2 mg may be required.

Sedation using bolus doses of propofol has been compared with midazolam [15] and bolus doses of midazolam have been compared with propofol infusions for sedation for outpatient bronchoscopy [16]. Bolus doses of propofol should not be administered by practitioners without training and experience in anaesthesia.

Patient controlled sedation (PCS)

For any but the shortest procedures the future safe practice of sedation probably lies in allowing the patients to control their own sedation. Patient controlled intravenous therapy, initially introduced for analgesia (PCA), was first adapted for controlled anxiolysis using diazepam by Galletly *et al.* [17] and more recently for perioperative sedation (PCS) using either midazolam or propofol [18–20].

PCA systems are designed for use with analgesic drugs, usually opioids, for many hours or days, when there is ample time to modify the protocol of use to meet the needs of individual patients. The requirements for sedation practice in relation to interventional therapy are more demanding, since a satisfactory result has to be achieved within a few minutes and the duration of the procedure will usually be a matter of minutes or only a few hours. It seems unlikely that an unmodified PCA system would be suitable for sedation for interventional procedures with the rapidly varying levels of discomfort and anxiety seen intraoperatively.

In practice, attempts to use PCA systems for PCS have necessitated an initial anaesthetist-administered bolus of sedative [18] or fentanyl [19]; the demand system is then used to maintain the sedation.

For example Osborne *et al.* [18] used an initial bolus dose of 0·7 mg kg^{-1} i.v. of propofol with further doses of 0·7 mg kg^{-1} i.v. on demand with a dose infusion time of 3 min and a subsequent lock out time of 1 min. In a more recent paper this group compared propofol with midazolam. All patients initially received 0·7 μg kg^{-1} fentanyl followed by a bolus dose of either propofol 20 mg or midazolam 0·5 mg and then further doses during 6 s, at an infusion rate of 1200 ml l^{-1}, with a lock out time of

1 min. This technique was used to support the use of local analgesia for extraction of third molar teeth [19]. Patient controlled sedation for day-case surgery has also been described by Grattridge [20].

True PCS

True PCS would allow patients to establish their own level of sedation, which they could subsequently either maintain or vary as required. Such a system, combined with psychomotor tests, would also provide an objective method for comparing the relative potencies and efficacy of anxiolytic and sedative drugs.

For this purpose a PCA pump (PCA, Graseby Medical) with a maximal infusion rate of 200 ml h^{-1} (i.e. $\approx$ 3·3 ml min^{-1}) is modified by removal of the lock out interval. The pump is loaded with either midazolam 10 mg in 30 ml saline or propofol 300 mg, i.e. 30 ml, and narrow bore infusion tubing is also primed with the solution of drug before connection to the patient via an intravenous cannula. Each successful patient demand delivers either 3 mg propofol or 0·1 mg midazolam, i.e. 0·3 ml of drug solution. The time for the injection of each 0·3 ml dose is 5·4 s and this is in effect a lock out time, since the administration of another dose cannot be triggered, even though the patient may make an unsuccessful demand by pressing the button, until the previous one is delivered. Thus the maximum dose of 1·1 mg of midazolam or 33 mg of propofol per minute is a consequence of the maximum infusion rate of the pump which can be modified.

So far this technique has been used comparing midazolam and propofol for sedation on patients undergoing ultrasound guided oöcyte retrieval for *in vitro* fertilization [21]. The sedation is combined with 20 ml lignocaine (1%) injected into the vault of the vagina and the administration of three doses of alfentanil (200 μg i.v.) in relation to insertion of the vaginal speculum and needle entry into each ovary. The patients receive oxygen therapy throughout (4 l min^{-1} via a Hudson mask).

The procedure was successfully completed in all patients so far studied. At no point did the oxygen saturation fall below 96% and cardiovascular stability was maintained throughout.

All patients drank and ate within 20 min of the end of the procedure, and all had dressed, and were ready to leave within 1 h. Flumazenil was neither required nor used in this study.

Pain at the infusion site was a problem in the propofol group, despite the use of intravenous lignocaine, and 19 of 25 patients studied required a second dose of intravenous lignocaine despite which some patients complained that the sedation was more painful than the procedure.

The patients were assessed clinically and with a battery of psychomotor tests. Although they self-administered a wide range of doses of the drugs, they all achieved similar sedation levels.

This technique offers one of the best possibilities for providing safe extended sedation for example during interventional radiology or endoscopic procedures.

Sedation end-point

It is difficult to assess the end-point of sedation during the intravenous administration of BZDs or other drugs. Suffice it to say that the recommended classical sign of drooping of the eyelid, causing partial closure of the eyes so that the lid covers half the eye, represents unnecessarily deep sedation. The best end-point depends on the 'body language' of the patient combined with their subjective feeling of relaxation and loss of anxiety. For example, the shoulders and facial muscles relax, and the feet rotate outwards slightly as the muscle tension associated with anxiety is removed.

Other sedation techniques

In global terms, ketamine is probably the most widely used drug with anaesthetic properties, which is the ultimate practical expression of its versatility and safety. It is therefore widely used for analgesia, sedation and anaesthesia, either intramuscularly or intravenously. Oral BZDs are also effective sedative drugs, none better than lorazepam, while midazolam, being water soluble can be used intramuscularly [22].

Because of the shortage of anaesthetically trained personnel, most departments of gastroenterology and radiology have had to evolve 'safe' systems for their own use which suit their purposes.

Lorazepam 2 mg orally followed after about 30–40 min by ketamine 0·5 mg kg^{-1} or 0·25 mg kg^{-1} i.v. provides up to 2 h sedation time for minimally invasive procedures. However this may not 'fit' day-case requirements, but midazolam 0·1 mg kg^{-1} i.m. combined with either oral ketorolac 10 mg administered 1 h previously or an infusion of alfentanil i.v. for example in a dose of 1–5 $\mu g\ kg^{-1}\ min^{-1}$ [23] may provide an adequate technique in some situations, e.g. as an adjunct to local analgesia. Alternatively, midazolam 0·1 mg kg^{-1} i.m. and ketamine 0·25 mg kg^{-1} i.m. can be combined to provide an extended period of sedation. Another technique combines local analgesia with midazolam i.m. or i.v. and a diclenofac suppository, e.g. for prostatectomy [1].

Complications of sedation

The most serious complication of sedation is the inadvertent induction of anaesthesia, loss of the airway and severe cardiovascular or respiratory depression causing hypoxaemia [24, 25]. Another problem is the depression of laryngeal and airway reflexes, which would facilitate aspiration of materials in the oropharynx such as secretions, debris or gastric content and the latter is most likely to occur during the withdrawal of a gastroscope or if the patient regurgitates or vomits. Drummond [26] has recently reviewed existing information on anaesthesia, sedation and airway reflexes.

Essential safety measures, i.e. in addition to the prerequisites for sedation outlined above are:

1 The patient should be on an 'operating' table which allows easy movement of the patient into a lateral position with head down tilt.
2 Powerful suction with a variety of attachments, both rigid and flexible, should be immediately available.
3 Oxygen therapy with a system for manual inflation of the patient with someone competent in its use.
4 Drugs. In addition to required drugs for resuscitation, i.e. normally adrenaline and atropine, flumazenil should always be available when BZDs are in use, and also naloxone if opioids are being administered.
5 In addition to the endoscopist or radiologist a competent trained assistant should be continuously present.

Conclusions

Sedation is practised widely with remarkably few critical incidents. However, each year there are a number of clinical disasters usually due to drug overdose, general mismanagement of the patient, failure in early recognition of the start of the onset of a serious problem and inability to deal with it once recognized. A recent survey, about to be published, suggests that the mortality rate following upper gastrointestinal endoscopy may be as high as 1 in 2000 [27].

For example, a pulse oximeter alarm is a late event since by the time it is triggered the patient is already entering a critical state. In the hospital setting reliance on the general 'crash call' team is unacceptable and each unit where sedation is practised, e.g. endoscopy, cardiology and arthroscopy clinics, radiology departments and scanning units, should be self-sufficient in staff, equipment and drugs for the immediate first phase management of critical situations, while more experienced and trained personnel are summoned, e.g. from the department of anaesthesia.

The best approach to the problem is prevention. This involves better training schedules than exist at present and good patient selection and preparation.

The development of techniques for PCS on the one hand and safer analgesic drugs on the other are becoming increasingly important because of the rapid increase in minimally invasive therapy. The need for research and development in this field to improve patient care is urgent. Chapter 17 on demand sedation reviews some of the theoretical considerations involved in the design of safe demand sedation systems.

Acknowledgements

Parts of this chapter have been rewritten, with permission, from Whitwam JG. Drugs for sedation. In McCloy R, ed. *Quality Control in Endoscopy. Report of an International Forum*. Berlin: Springer-Verlag, 1991: 3–21. © Springer-Verlag.

References

1 Birch BRP, Anson KM, Miller RA. Sedoanalgesia in urology: a safe, cost-effective alternative to general analgesia. A review of 1020 cases. *Br J Urol* 1990; 66: 342–50.

2 Department of Health Standing Dental Advisory Committee. *Report of an expert working party. General Anaesthesia, Sedation and Resuscitation in Dentistry.* London: HMSO, 1991.

3 Cockshott ID. Propofol (Diprivan). Pharmacokinetics and metabolism—an overview. *Postgrad Med J* 1985; 61 (suppl 3): 45–50.

4 Mackenzie N, Grant IS. Propofol for intravenous sedation. *Anaesthesia* 1987; 42: 3–6.

5 Roberts FL, Dixon J, Lewis GTR, Tackley RM, Prys-Roberts C. Induction and maintenance of propofol anaesthesia. A manual infusion scheme. *Anaesthesia* 1988; 43 (suppl): 14–17.

6 Rudkin GE, Osborne GA, Curtis NJ. Intra-operative patient-controlled sedation. *Anaesthesia* 1991; 46: 90–2.

7 Thompson GE, Moore DC. Ketamine, Diazepam and Innovar. A computerised comparative study. *Anesth Analg.* 50: 458–63.

8 Podlesch I, Dähn H, Engel M. Anaesthetic and side effects of midazolam and ketamine in surgical patients. *Anesthesiology* 1985; 62: 68.

9 Seitz W, Lübbe N, Hamkens A, Bornscheuer A. Midazolam–Ketamin Kombinationsanaesthesie bei traumatologischen Eingriffen. *Anaesthetist* 1987; 37: 231–7.

10 Thomson D (ed.). Midazolam and flumazenil—the agonist–antagonist concept for sedation and anaesthesia. Proceedings of an international symposium, April 1989. *Acta Anaesth Scand* 1990; 34 (suppl 92): 1–109.

11 Royal College of Surgeons of England. *Report of Working Party. Guidelines for Sedation by Non-Anaesthetists.* London: Royal College of Surgeons of England, 1993.

12 Ricou R, Forster A, Bruckner A, Chastonay P, Gemberle M. Clinical evaluation of a specific benzodiazepine antagonist (Ro15-1788). Studies in elderly patients after regional anaesthesia under benzodiazepine sedation. *Br J Anaesth* 1986; 58: 1005–11.

13 Bell GD, Antrobus JHL, Lee J, Coady T, Morden A. Bolus or slow titrated injection of midazolam prior to upper gastrointestinal endoscopy? Relative effect on oxygen saturation and prophylactic value of supplemental oxygen. *Alim Pharmacol Ther* 1990; 4: 393–401.

14 Swain DG, Ellis DJ, Bradby H. Rapid intravenous low-dose diazepam as sedation for upper gastrointestinal endoscopy. *Alim Pharmacol Ther* 1990; 4: 43–8.

15 Patterson KW, Casey PB, Murray JP, O'Boyle CA, Cunningham AJ. Propofol sedation for outpatient upper gastrointestinal endoscopy: comparison with midazolam. *Br J Anaesth* 1991; 67: 108–11.

16 Crawford M, Pollock J, Anderson K, Glavin RJ, MacIntyre D, Vernon D. Comparison of midazolam with propofol for sedation in outpatient bronchoscopy. *Br J Anaesth* 1993; 70: 419–22.

17 Galletly DC, Short TG, Forrest P. Patient administered anxiolysis—a pilot study. *Anaesth Intens Care* 1989; 17: 144–50.

18 Osborne GA, Rudkin GE, Curtis NJ, Vickers D, Craker AJ. Intraoperative patient controlled sedation. *Anaesthesia* 1991; 46: 553–6.

19 Rudkin GE, Osborne GA, Finn BP, Jarvis DA, Vickers D. Intraoperative patient controlled sedation. Comparison of patient-controlled propofol with patient-controlled midazolam. *Anaesthesia* 1992; 47: 376–81.

20 Grattridge P. Patient controlled sedation using propofol in day surgery. *Anaesthesia* 1992; 47: 683–5.

21 Cook LB, Lockwood GG, Moore CM, Whitwam JG. True patient-controlled sedation: a new concept. *Anaesthesia* 1993; 48: 1039–44.

22 McAteer EJ, Dixon J, Whitwam JG. Intramuscular midazolam. A comparison of midazolam with

papaveretum and hyoscine for intramuscular premedication. *Anaesthesia* 1984; 39: 1177–82.
23 Alfentanil infusion. In: Dollery CT, ed. *Therapeutic Drugs*. Edinburgh: Churchill Livingstone, 1991: A43–6.
24 Whitwam JG. The use of midazolam and flumazenil in diagnostic and short surgical procedures. *Acta Anaesth Scand* 1990; 34 (suppl 92): 16–20.
25 Whitwam JG. Resedation. *Acta Anaesth Scand* 1990; 34 (suppl 92): 70–4.
26 Drummond GB. Upper airway reflexes (Editorial). *Anaesthesia* 1993; 70: 121–3.
27 Quine MA, Ball GD, McCloy RF, Charlton JE, Devlin HB, Hopkin A. Complications of upper gastrointestinal endoscopy; in preparation.

Chapter 17
Patient Controlled Sedation

L. B. Cook and J. G. Whitwam

Many procedures do not require general anaesthesia, but are sufficiently unpleasant or uncomfortable to merit a degree of sedation. The aim is to produce a relaxed comfortable patient, able to maintain their own airway. The depth of sedation required varies with the procedure, the patient's personality, and other intangibles such as the reassurance of the medical and nursing staff.

The doses of a sedative agent required to achieve and maintain a given depth of sedation vary widely among patients. Should a previously well-sedated patient become anxious, or uncomfortable, prompt administration of further drug may be necessary.

Titration of sedative drugs to an individual patient's needs, while universally advocated, is far from universally practised. It carries costs in terms of time, and expensively acquired skills (often in demand elsewhere). The alternative approach, which usually works well, is simply to give a relatively large dose of sedative, likely to sedate the majority of patients adequately. The variability of response to sedative agents means that such an approach will lead to a degree of oversedation in some patients, which seldom causes overt problems, and is arguably less troublesome than coping with undersedated patients.

However, intraoperative oversedation is not entirely innocuous. Patients require longer to recover, increasing the demand on recovery beds and nursing time. Not infrequently oversedation leads to morbidity or death.

An increasing number of minimally invasive (e.g. radiological) procedures can last a considerable time. These patients cannot be sedated throughout to a required, but varying, level with a single dose of any drug. These procedures demand considerable skill and concentration from the practitioner, who cannot at the same time be expected to continuously supervise the patient's sedation level.

It is impracticable to demand a trained anaesthetist at every site and at all times when sedation is administered. The advent of patient controlled sedation (PCS) may, however, offer an effective alternative. Patients can choose, within limits, how sedated they wish to be. Patient controlled analgesia (PCA) is now widely used postoperatively; it gained acceptance when the medical and nursing professions recognized that the one person uniquely well qualified to assess the patient's pain was the patient. If the principle holds true for postoperative use, then why not during a procedure? And who is the person most competent to judge the extent of a patient's anxiety or discomfort? Again, surely the patient.

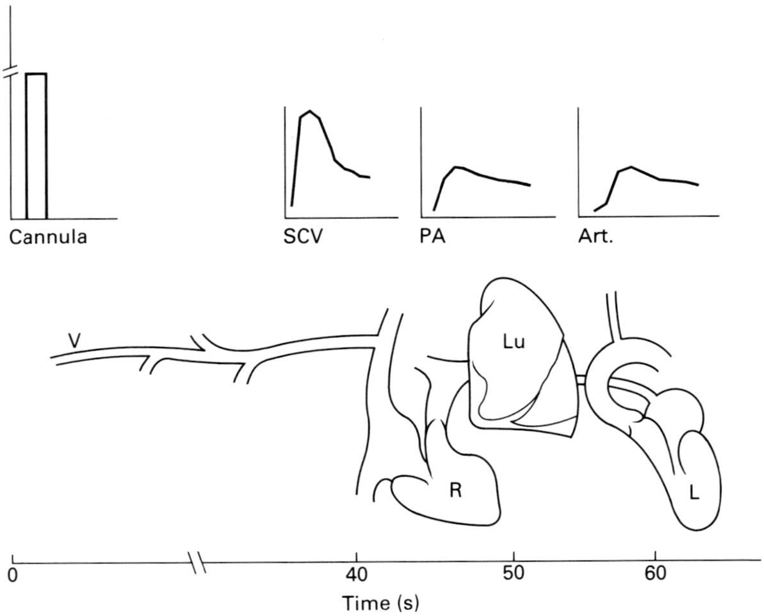

Fig. 17.1 The fate of a rapid bolus injection made into a vein on the dorsum of the right hand. The fate of the drug as it passes from the hand vein (V) through the right heart (R), lungs (Lu) and left heart (L) to the systemic circulation is shown against the time scale at the bottom of the figure. Plots of concentration against time are shown for the subclavian vein (SCV), pulmonary artery (PA) and radial artery (art.). The delay in the appearance of the drug and the reduction in its peak concentration are clearly seen. (L. B. Cook, unpublished observations.)

Pharmacokinetic principles

PCS utilizes the principle of the feedback loop to achieve and maintain sedation. To request sedation the patient presses a button on a hand-held device. This sends a signal to the microprocessor controlling a syringe driver, which delivers a predetermined dose of sedative drug via an intravenous cannula.

The fate of an intravenous bolus is outlined in Fig. 17.1. Even if the bolus is given rapidly, there is always a delay before its peak effects are seen: the drug spreads into the network of veins, whence it is washed out by the blood perfusing the arm. It is diluted in the central and pulmonary circulations, before reaching the brain.

This process takes a variable time. In young, healthy individuals, the peak effects of commonly used anaesthetic agents are seen after 30–90 s. In the elderly, and others with slow circulation the peak effects may not be seen for 2–5 min.

This delay, commonly called the arm–brain time, is considered further in the section on safety. Its importance stems from the fact that the drug which has been delivered, but not yet taken effect constitutes a reservoir, which may lead to overdose.

Figure 17.2 shows the effect of a succession of equal boluses. Also shown is the effect of the same boluses given slowly (in effect a continuous infusion). In both cases

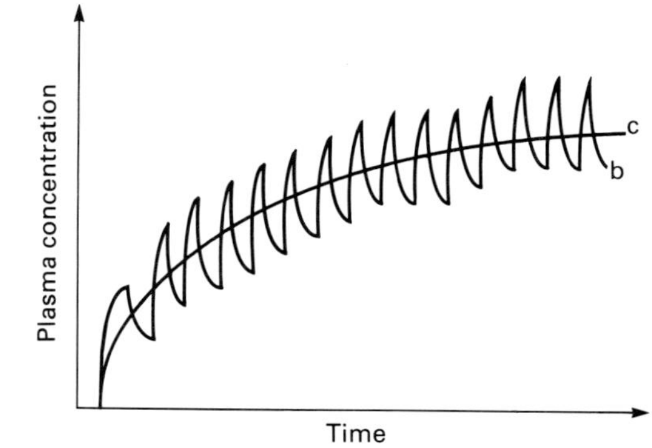

Fig. 17.2 Whether the drug is given as a series of boluses (b), or a continuous infusion (c), the plasma concentration reaches a plateau when the rate of clearance from the central circulation equals the mean infusion rate.

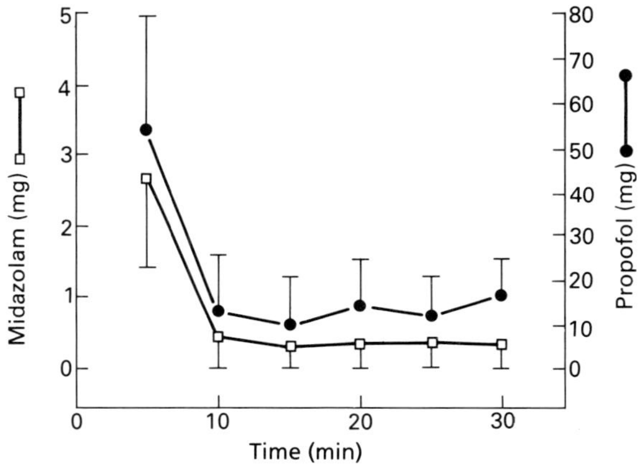

Fig. 17.3 The mean doses of midazolam (□) and propofol (●) administered by a patient controlled system during each 5 min period. The error bars show the standard deviation. Redrawn from [6] with permission.

the plasma concentration eventually reaches a plateau, where the amount of drug cleared from the central circulation equals the rate of administration. To achieve adequate plasma levels of a sedative agent quickly, an initial bolus or fast infusion is necessary. Thereafter smaller doses or reduced infusion rates suffice to maintain the desired plasma concentration.

Figure 17.3, for example, shows the doses of midazolam and propofol taken by a group of patients using a PCS system. Note that the mean infusion rate during the first 5 min is around five times the rates subsequently required. Note also that, although these were all similar patients undergoing the same procedure, there is great variation in the doses actually required.

The equipment

Although it is theoretically possible to design a PCS system around any means of drug administration (e.g. a drip counter), in practice all work to date has been done with microprocessor-controlled syringe drivers. Most syringe drivers are mains-powered, usually incorporating a rechargeable battery. Many incorporate the ability to

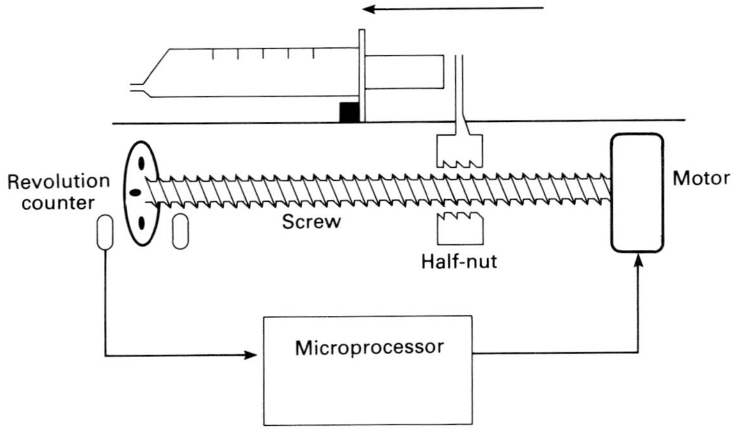

Fig. 17.4 The plunger of the syringe is gripped securely by the assembly which includes the half-nut. The latter engages, locking into position on the screw. Since the diameter of the syringe is known, the microprocessor is able to determine how far the plunger must move to administer the desired dose. In order to administer a dose, the microprocessor switches on the motor, rotating the screw a precalculated number of revolutions. The accuracy of this process is enhanced by the revolution counter, which allows feedback to the microprocessor. Each rotation of the screw moves the half-nut, and hence the plunger, a known distance. Occlusion or high pressure sensing is now standard. The sensors may be incorporated into the narrow-gauge infusion tubing ('wet-side'), or be within the pump ('dry-side'). In the former, pressure may be measured directly, and increasing sophistication means that other potential hazards such as disconnection or air bubbles may also be detected. In the latter, the maximum force which the half-nut is allowed to exert is preset. In the event of occlusion this force is exceeded, and the motor is disengaged from the screw by a clutch mechanism. The discrepancy between the rotation of the motor and the feedback from the revolution counter is indicated to the microprocessor and an occlusion alarm is triggered.

'recognize' the type of syringe used, helping ensure accuracy in the dose delivered. The mechanical principle is shown in Fig. 17.4.

The pump should be electrically safe, and pose no hazard if used, for example, during diathermy. The number of demands for sedation, and doses given may be displayed or printed. Recently, provision has been made to link such pumps to an oximeter [1]; if the oxygen saturation falls below the limits set on the monitor, the infusion pump is automatically switched off.

The microprocessor at the heart of such pumps receives instructions from two sources. Control algorithms governing its main functions are supplied in 'read only memory' (ROM), written by the manufacturer and incorporated in permanent form on the chip. These routines enable the microprocessor to determine the diameter of the syringe, calculate how far the plunger must move to infuse a given dose, and how many rotations of the screw are required to achieve this. They turn the motor on, measure the number of revolutions, and check that the pressure generated is not too high. They also process the interception of signals from the patient-control device.

Certain instructions must be set by the physician responsible for the sedation. These include the dose to be infused, and the lock-out period (see below). A range of other

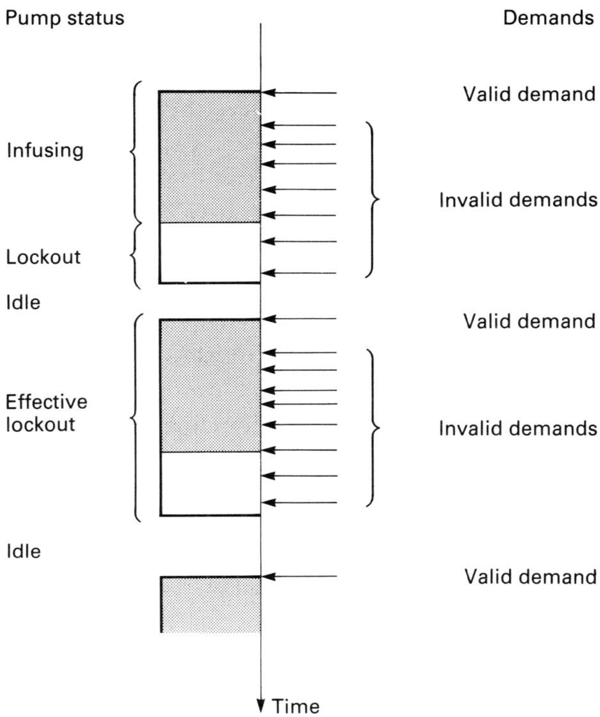

Fig. 17.5 The principle of patient-controlled infusion devices. Following a valid demand the preset dose is infused. Demands made during the infusion, or during the lock-out period which follows are invalid and have no effect. After the end of the lock-out period the pump remains idle until the next demand.

options such as recording the number of demands and doses via a remote printer may be available. A *valid* demand causes the pump to infuse the preset dose. The rate at which the dose is infused is usually fixed for any given pump; it is termed the *nominal infusion rate*. Additional demands received while the pump is infusing are *invalid* and ignored. After the dose has been delivered, the lock-out period set by the physician begins. Demands during the lock-out are also invalid. After the end of the lock-out period, the next demand will be valid, causing the delivery of a further dose. The principle is illustrated in Fig. 17.5.

Principles of PCS

The maximum mean infusion rate (MMIR)

Because lock-out time begins *after* a dose has been infused, the *minimum* interval between doses is the *sum* of the lock-out and the time taken to infuse the dose. This interval is the *effective lock-out* time.

If a patient always presses the button the moment the lock-out period expires, drugs will be delivered at the fastest rate of which the system is capable. This is the MMIR. Because the pump is idle during the lock-out, this will be less than the nominal infusion

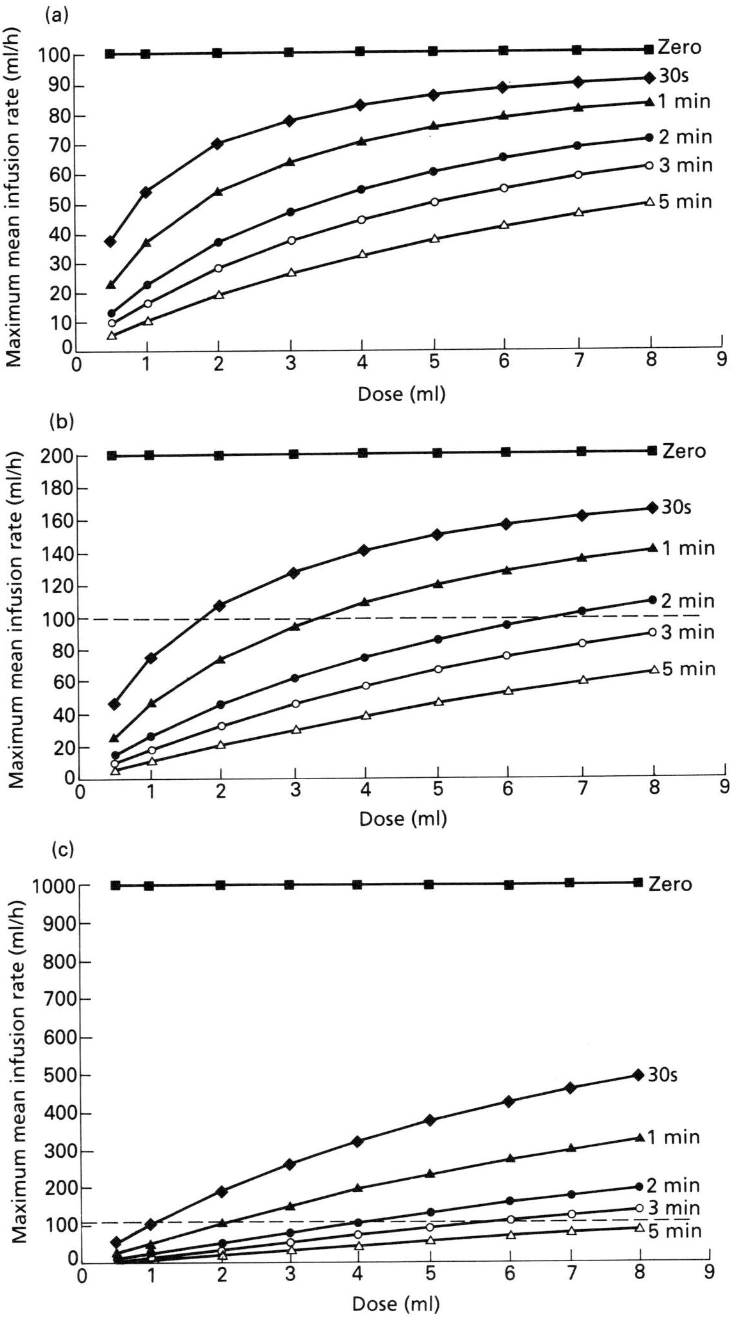

Fig. 17.6 The maximum mean infusion rate (MMIR), plotted against the dose set for various lock-out intervals. The nominal infusion rate is (a) 100 ml h^{-1}, (b) 200 ml h^{-1}, and (c) 1000 ml h^{-1}. The dotted line shows MMIR of 100 ml h^{-1}. Each line represents the relationship between the dose set and the MMIR for a given lock-out time.

rate (the infusion rate during delivery of a dose). The MMIR is central to consideration of both the efficacy and safety of the system.

Given the nominal infusion rate, lock-out and dose, the MMIR can be calculated as follows:

$$\text{MMIR} = \frac{\text{time to infuse dose}}{(\text{time to infuse dose} + \text{lock-out})} \times \text{nominal infusion rate} \tag{1}$$

this may be simplified to

$$\text{MMIR} = \frac{\text{dose}}{\text{effective lock-out}}. \tag{2}$$

Suppose that the pump settings are as follows:

nominal infusion rate	100 (ml h^{-1})
dose	2 ml
lock-out period	3 min

since the nominal infusion rate of 100 ml h^{-1} is 1·67 ml min^{-1}, and

$$\text{time to infuse dose} = \frac{\text{dose}}{\text{nominal infusion rate}},$$

in this case each dose will take $2/1.67 = 1{\cdot}2$ min to infuse. The effective lock-out will therefore be 1·2 min longer than the 3 min set, i.e. 4.2 min. Hence, using equation (1) above:

$$\text{MMIR} = \frac{1{\cdot}2\ \text{min}}{4{\cdot}2\ \text{min}} \times 100\ \text{ml h}^{-1} = 28{\cdot}6\ \text{ml h}^{-1}.$$

Alternatively, from equation (2):

$$\text{MMIR} = \frac{2\ \text{ml}}{4{\cdot}2\ \text{min}} = 0{\cdot}48\ \text{ml min}^{-1} = 28{\cdot}6\ \text{ml h}^{-1}.$$

In the example, although the nominal infusion rate is 100 ml h^{-1}, the maximum rate at which the system can deliver sedation is less than 30 ml h^{-1}. The graphs in Fig. 17.6 illustrate the variation of MMIR for various nominal infusion rates. Note that a given MMIR can be achieved in many different ways. For instance, an MMIR of 100 ml h^{-1} can be achieved with a nominal infusion rate of 100 ml h^{-1}, and no lock-out. It could also be produced by a nominal infusion rate of 600 ml h^{-1}, a dose of 2 ml, and a 1 min lock-out, or by a nominal infusion rate of 200 ml min^{-1}, a dose of 5 ml, and a 90 s lock-out.

Efficacy and safety

All PCS regimens require a balance between efficacy and safety. This is especially so because the requirements for, and susceptibility to sedative drugs vary widely: a dose just sufficient to sedate one patient may anaesthetize another. The challenge is to design a system capable of offering sedation to all, and still make self-administration of a dangerous overdose impossible.

Efficacy

As discussed in the section on pharmacokinetic principles, an initial bolus or fast infusion is required to establish sedation. Thereafter, the requirement will be for smaller or less frequent doses. Should the patient experience discomfort or anxiety, sufficient drug should be available to rapidly deepen or re-establish the sedation.

In the case of propofol, for instance, a dose of 30–50 mg (3–5 ml) is usually required to establish sedation, although some patients may need twice this. Thereafter an infusion of 100–600 mg h^{-1} will usually maintain sedation. Inadequate sedation may be treated with a bolus of, say, 10–30 mg.

Rapid infusion is necessary to produce sedation reasonably quickly. Similarly, requests for more sedation should result in rapid infusion of an adequate dose. This reassures the patient, who gains confidence in the method, and feels in control. A sluggish response, or inadequate doses, drain the patient's confidence since the cause of the discomfort persists, pressing the button appears to have no effect and this may in itself increase the anxiety.

In many cases patients who initially require relatively deep sedation are happy to reduce it during the procedure secure in the knowledge that they can rapidly increase their level of sedation at will.

Safety

Let us consider two patients. One is extremely anxious, clears sedative drugs rapidly, and is naturally resistant to their effects. The other is determined to anaesthetize himself. How can the same system provide the high doses of drugs required by the first patient, without permitting the second to achieve anaesthesia?

Provided that patients are capable of pressing a button to request additional sedation, arguably they are not oversedated, and, if they lose consciousness, they will no longer press the button. However, ensuring safety is not that simple.

The danger, impelling the patient from heavy sedation towards anaesthesia, consists of all the drug which takes effect after the patient becomes incapable of pressing the button.

The safety of a given system may be quantified by asking this question: if the patient loses consciousness immediately after pressing the button, how much additional drug will then take effect? The less this is, the safer the system. This amount will be referred to as the maximum possible overdose (MPO) expressed as a volume (ml of solution).

This amount will, of course include the dose delivered as a result of the last demand. It may also include a variable amount which was delivered as a result of previous demands, but which has not yet reached the brain or taken full effect. Here the concept of the arm–brain circulation time representing a potential reservoir of drug is crucial.

For the purposes of this discussion, the arm–brain time includes all the factors which delay the onset of peak sedative effect following intravenous drug administration: transit time to the brain, time to cross the blood–brain barrier, and time to take effect on neurones.

In the remainder of this section, the influence of various factors is explored, and a strategy suggested by which safety may be maximized.

Suppose, for example, it is decided that to sedate most patients adequately, and allow rapid augmentation of sedation at will, an MMIR of 100 ml h^{-1}, or 1·67 ml min^{-1}, is required. As discussed above, this might be achieved in many different ways (see Fig. 17.6). Which is safest?

Safety may be quantified in terms of the maximum possible overdose and this may be calculated for any given arm–brain time, and any infusion system. For the simplest system (100 ml h^{-1}, no lock-out, Fig. 17.6a), this becomes:

$$\text{MPO} = \text{arm–brain time} \times \text{MMIR} + \text{dose} = \left(\frac{\text{arm–brain time}}{\text{time to infuse dose}}\right) \times \text{dose} + \text{dose}.$$

Where the dose is expressed in volume (ml of solution). At the other end of the spectrum lies rapid drug delivery, plus a lock-out interval (Fig. 17.6c). Here the calculation is more complex. If the lock-out interval is greater than the arm–brain time, then the maximum possible overdose is simply the dose set. If not, then it is equal to the dose set, plus the number of such doses which could be delivered during the arm–brain time:

$$\text{MPO} = \left[\text{integer}\left(\frac{\text{arm–brain time}}{\text{effective lock-out}}\right)\right] \times \text{dose} + \text{dose}.$$

Figure 17.7 shows the influence of dose and lock out on the MPO for two systems. As the arm–brain time increases, so does the maximum possible overdose. In the simple system (no lock-out and MMIR equal to the nominal infusion rate) for a given arm–brain time the MPO increases linearly with dose.

In the more complex system (virtually instantaneous drug delivery, MMIR maintained at 100 ml h^{-1} with lock-outs) the result is less obvious. The minimum MPO is always produced by a lock-out slightly in excess of the arm–brain time. However, this turns out to be critical, because a lock-out slightly less than this dramatically increases the MPO. Note that this is true for all arm–brain times. Use of a much smaller dose, sufficient to ensure a lock-out much less than the arm–brain time, reliably produces MPOs close to the minimum. Used in this way, the performance of the system is indistinguishable from that of the simple zero-lock-out system.

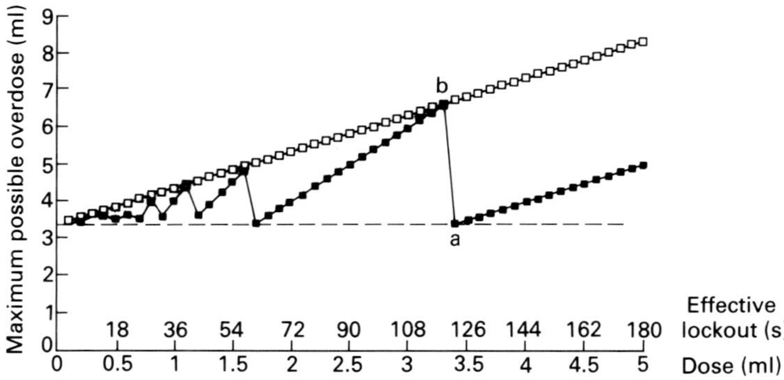

Fig. 17.7 The arm–brain time is 120 s. MMIR is 100 ml h^{-1}. Slow infusion with zero lock-out compared with very rapid infusion with lock-out. The following points should be noted:

1 The maximum possible overdose (MPO) is never less than the mean infusion rate multiplied by the arm–brain time. For example, if the MMIR is 100 ml h^{-1} (1·67 ml min^{-1}), and the arm–brain time is 2 min, then no combination of dose or lock-out can reduce the MPO below 3·33 ml. This is represented on the graph by the dashed line.

2 Increases in the arm–brain time, or the mean infusion rate, inevitably increase the MPO.

3 For the simplest system (no lock-out, where MMIR is the nominal infusion rate), the MPO increases linearly with the dose.

4 For more complex systems, incorporating lock-out intervals, the MPO is minimized by a lock-out slightly greater than the arm–brain time (point a). If the arm–brain time lengthens, however, to slightly exceed the lock-out, then the MPO increases sharply (point b).

5 In both systems, use of small doses will minimize the MPO.

It should thus be clear that the main effect of a lock-out is to reduce the MMIR. This reduces both the MPO and the efficacy. It is legitimate to use a lock-out in this way, but systems incorporating lock-outs are not inherently safer than those without. It bears repeating that no combination of dose and lock-out can reduce the MPO to less than the product of the arm–brain time and the MMIR. Attention should therefore rather be focused on matching the MMIR to the anticipated requirements of the population to be sedated.

Practical points

Syringe drivers

Currently, there are no commercially available syringe drivers designed for PCS. Most investigators have used a PCA syringe-driver intended for use with opioids. These are less than optimal in several respects.

The commonly used opioids have an onset of action within 5–15 min, and a duration of action of 1–2 h. The requirement is thus for a dose of 1–3 ml, with an effective lock-out of 5–10 min. A nominal infusion rate of 100 ml h^{-1} is common, and adequate for this purpose. Most PCA devices will not accept a lock-out time of less than

3 min. Suppose that a dose of 3 ml is chosen; reference to equations (1) and (2), pp. 279–80, and Fig. 17.6 will show that the MMIR of such a pump will be 37·5 ml h^{-1}.

It will be apparent that, if the volume of drug required to achieve sedation is of the order of 5 ml, as it is in the case of propofol, then this initial dose would require 7 min to infuse. This is unacceptably long.

Currently the options are:

1 If the physician administers the first dose, then the patient can use the system to maintain sedation from then on. Although the MMIR is too slow for the induction of sedation, it should suffice to maintain it.

2 If a more concentrated solution of drug is used, then the MMIR required will be lower. This is not possible with propofol, since around 5 ml of (10 mg ml^{-1}) solution is required to initiate sedation, but other drugs, such as midazolam, are presented as more potent solutions.

In the future as manufacturers of syringe drivers appreciate the potential of the technique, it is to be hoped that a new generation of pumps optimized for sedation rather than analgesia will become available. Already one manufacturer produces a pump with a nominal infusion rate of 100 ml h^{-1} which will accept a lock-out as low as 1 min. A dose of 3 ml produces a MMIR of 64 ml h^{-1}, which is more practical for purposes of sedation. If a longer lock-out is used, the pump may be used as intended for PCA but the option of use for sedation has at least been provided.

Monitoring

This has been considered elsewhere in this book. The same standard of monitoring should obtain, whatever the method used to administer sedative drugs. In our opinion, this should include oximetry, and possibly electrocardiogram (ECG). Communication with the patient provides the best monitoring available.

Choice of drug

All published work has used either propofol or midazolam. This is not surprising, as the kinetics of propofol are more suited to non-cumulative infusions than other intravenous anaesthetic agents, and midazolam is the shortest acting sedative benzodiazepine.

There appears to be little to choose between midazolam and propofol. The slightly faster onset time of propofol will reduce the MPO, compared with midazolam; this effect may, however, be more than offset by the greater margin of safety of the latter drug.

Recovery after equisedative doses of either drug is rapid. Early recovery is faster with propofol, but the difference is not great [2]. Against this may be set the problem of pain at the cannula site, which is a feature of propofol, and the availability of flumazenil to reverse the effects of midazolam, should this become necessary.

Patient selection

Psychology

Almost all young healthy patients may use PCS. It might be anticipated that very anxious patients would make poor subjects, but this does not appear to be the case provided the system has the capacity to produce adequate sedation, i.e. has a sufficiently high MMIR.

Some patients state that they would prefer to be asleep and that, if allowed to use the device, they will simply press the button until they put themselves to sleep. This is not a contraindication to PCS. Usually, once these patients convince themselves that pressing the button does produce sedation, they relax and use it sparingly. If the system is correctly set, then if they do try to anaesthetize themselves, they will not succeed.

The exception may be the highly intelligent, articulate, extremely anxious patient, who denies any need for sedation, but reacts violently at any attempt to carry out the procedure. Such patients often will not sedate themselves adequately, and have a miserable time. Should this happen, and they do not respond to a direct request to press the button more often, administration of supplementary drug will be necessary.

Physiology

As has been discussed above, the safety and the efficacy of the system are dependent on the MMIR, and the arm–brain time. The MMIR can be reduced to suit the population to be sedated, either by means of lock-outs, or by reducing the concentration of drug in the infusion.

Nothing can be done, however, to offset the effect of a long arm–brain time. This applies particularly to the elderly, where the potential for overdose is most worrying. A combination of a basal infusion of sedative, supplemented on patient demand, might be preferable to the simple PCS systems described so far. No results of work in this patient group are yet available, and caution is indicated.

Choice of procedure

Use of PCS has so far been largely confined to procedures performed under local or regional anaesthesia, e.g. dentistry. In these areas it is remarkably successful. It remains to be seen whether it can be successfully used for more stressful procedures such as gastroscopy or bronchoscopy.

Use of analgesics

There is considerable synergy between sedative drugs and opioid analgesics. A previously adequately sedated patient may become comatose remarkably quickly, if opioids are administered with sedative drugs, and a person capable of managing general anaesthesia should be available.

It may be that prior administration of a non-steroidal anti-inflammatory drug (NSAID) reduces the requirement for opioids thereby ameliorating the problem. For some procedures, however, opioids cannot reasonably be avoided and the best technique for combining PCS with opioid administration is unknown. Among the options are:

1 Prior administration of the opioid [2]. If the opioid has already exerted its effects, then patients should require and take less sedative, and compensation for the synergy will be automatic. The MMIR needed will be lower, and the system should be adjusted with this in mind, to reduce the potential for overdose. A beneficial effect is that a standard PCA pump may then suffice.

2 Using the opioid as the sedative [3]. If a short-acting opioid is used, it may be that other sedative agents will not be required in some patients.

3 Mixing the sedative and opioid drugs. The PCS system could be filled with, for example, a mixture of propofol and alfentanil. Theoretical objections include the fact that the relative requirement for analgesics and sedatives varies among patients. However, the mixture produces good results in anaesthetist controlled sedation [4], and initial experience with its use in PCS systems, has been encouraging.

Setting up and using the device

Once set up for a given patient population, the syringe driver should require minimal adjustment. It is impossible to predict the doses required in any individual patient which is one of the main reasons for using PCS. There is, for example, little correlation between patient weight or age and the doses required [5, 6]. Individually adjusting the pump settings for each patient is thus not only unnecessary, but also impossible.

Consider the requirements of a group of young, fit, adult women. Mean doses to establish sedation will be of the order of propofol 50 mg, or midazolam 3 mg. If the pump is to be used to establish sedation, then to be practical these doses must be delivered over not more than, say 2–3 min.

For undiluted propofol, then, the pump must be capable of infusing at least 5 ml over 3 min. Hence the MMIR must be at least 1·67 ml min^{-1}, or 100 ml h^{-1}. In practice, the MMIR should be higher, as some patients will require larger doses. There are many ways to achieve a given MMIR, but settings may be chosen to minimize the potential for overdose. In practice this entails using a small dose (Fig. 17.7).

The MMIRs of PCA pumps do not approach these rates. If an unmodified PCA device is to be used, the operator must first establish sedation, then allow the patient to use the device to maintain sedation. For propofol, the mean infusion rate to achieve this is around 180 mg h^{-1} (18 ml h^{-1}), but individual patients at times require twice this rate, or more. Here the potential for overdose is almost nil, but the problem is to achieve an adequate MMIR. If, for example, the minimum lock-out which can be set is 3 min, and the nominal infusion rate is 100 ml h^{-1}, then reference to Fig. 17.6a shows that the dose must be set to at least 3–5 ml, to reach these rates of administration.

We have used a modified PCA pump which can be used without a lock-out period, allowing a MMIR of 200 ml h^{-1} [6]. This gives an effective lock-out of 5·4 s when used with a 0·3 ml dose. Under these conditions we have found that both propofol 10 mg ml^{-1} and midazolam 0·3 mg ml^{-1} allow satisfactory PCS in a young, healthy population.

Summary

PCS is in an early stage of development, with many problems still to be addressed. Nonetheless it already offers good quality, safe and cost-effective sedation. Work in progress should shed light on the problem of incorporating potent analgesics into the technique, possibly as an admixture of propofol and alfentanil. The range of drugs used with the technique is also expected to be extended.

Although standard PCA pumps can be used for this technique, its full promise may only be fulfilled when purpose-designed syringe drivers become available.

References

1 Juhl G. Der Infucommand. Ein PCA-Gerat mit pulsoximetrischer Boluskontrolle (The Infucommand. A PCA (patient-controlled analgesia) device using pulsoximetric bolus control). *Anaesthetist*, 1990; 39: 236–9.

2 Rudkin GE, Osborne GA, Finn BP, Jarvis DA, Vickers D. Intra-operative patient-controlled sedation. Comparison of patient-controlled propofol with patient-controlled midazolam. *Anaesthesia* 1992; 47: 376–81.

3 Ghouri AF, Taylor E, White PF. Patient-controlled drug administration during local anesthesia: a comparison of midazolam, propofol, and alfentanil. *J Clin Anesth* 1992; 4: 476–9.

4 Sherry E. Admixture of propofol and alfentanil. Use for intravenous sedation and analgesia during transvaginal oocyte retrieval. *Anaesthesia* 1992; 47: 477–9.

5 Grattidge P. Patient-controlled sedation using propofol in day surgery. *Anaesthesia* 1992; 47: 683–5.

6 Cook LB, Lockwood GG, Moore CM, Whitwam JG. True patient controlled sedation. *Anaesthesia* 1993; 48: 1039–44.

Chapter 18
Anaesthetic Circuits and Ventilation Systems

M. K. Chakrabarti, P. Ravussin and J. G. Whitwam

Anaesthetic breathing systems

Anaesthetic breathing systems consist primarily of breathing tubes or ducts, reservoir bags, one-way valves, carbon dioxide absorbers and appropriate connectors for delivering anaesthetic gases, agents and oxygen from delivery systems, e.g. anaesthetic machines, to the patients.

There are two main types of system for general anaesthesia: (a) semi-open; and (b) semi-closed or closed. The semi-open breathing systems have been classified as Mapleson A, B, C, D and E [1, 2] (Fig. 18.1). However, in practice the commonly used breathing systems are Mapleson A (Magill circuit) and Mapleson D and E (T-piece circuits). All other systems are modifications or combinations of these two systems.

The efficiency of a breathing system is normally measured by the anaesthetic fresh gas flow requirements to eliminate carbon dioxide. The lower the requirement of anaesthetic gas or loss of anaesthetic gas from the breathing system, the higher will be the efficiency with major cost savings and also less potential pollution of the atmosphere. However, one of the problems in assessing published data and statements about breathing circuits is that 100 ml kg^{-1} min^{-1} is considered to be the normal ventilation requirement which is not the actual ventilation requirement for every patient. During anaesthesia it is normally decreased, so that the efficiency of these circuits is sometimes overstated.

The semi-closed or closed breathing systems incorporate a carbon dioxide absorbing chamber containing a chemical compound, e.g. soda–lime, so that the expired gas can be reused, i.e. rebreathed, wholly or partially after the absorption of carbon dioxide from the exhaled gas.

Semi-open breathing systems

Mapleson 'A' (the Magill attachment). In this breathing system the overflow 'blow off' way valve is placed near the patient connection, i.e. upstream in the breathing duct or tube, and the reservoir bag is placed distally from the valve, close to the source of fresh gas, i.e. downstream in the wide bore breathing tube [1, 3] (Fig. 18.2). Anaesthetic fresh gas flows from the anaesthetic machine into the reservoir bag during expiration and also into the patient during inspiration. This system is very efficient during

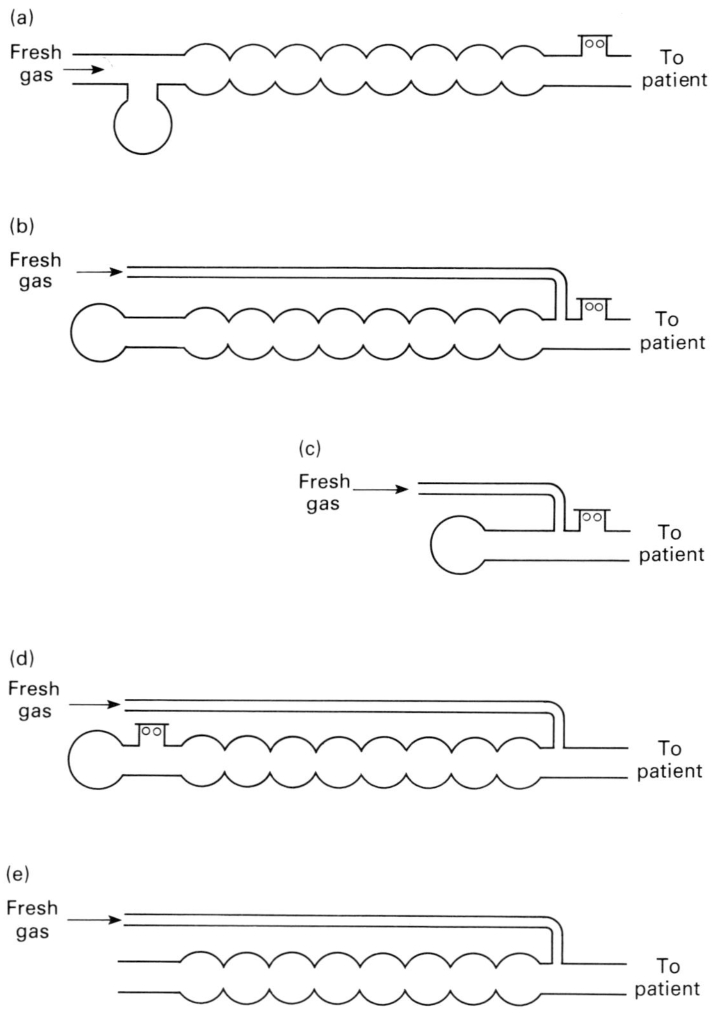

Fig. 18.1 Semi-open breathing systems (Mapleson A, B, C, D and E): A, also referred to as Magill attachment; E, Ayre's T-piece.

spontaneous breathing but becomes less efficient during assisted or controlled ventilation of the patient as the overflow valve requires to be restricted to allow positive pressure ventilation of the lungs. Under such conditions gas escapes during forced inspiration rather than expiration, leading to rebreathing unless a high fresh gas flow is used. Therefore the Mapleson 'A' breathing system is mainly used during spontaneous breathing when only about 70% of the minute ventilation ($\dot{V}$) of fresh gas flow, i.e. equivalent to alveolar ventilation volume, $\dot{V}_A$, is required since the dead space gas, not exposed to the pulmonary circulation is recycled.

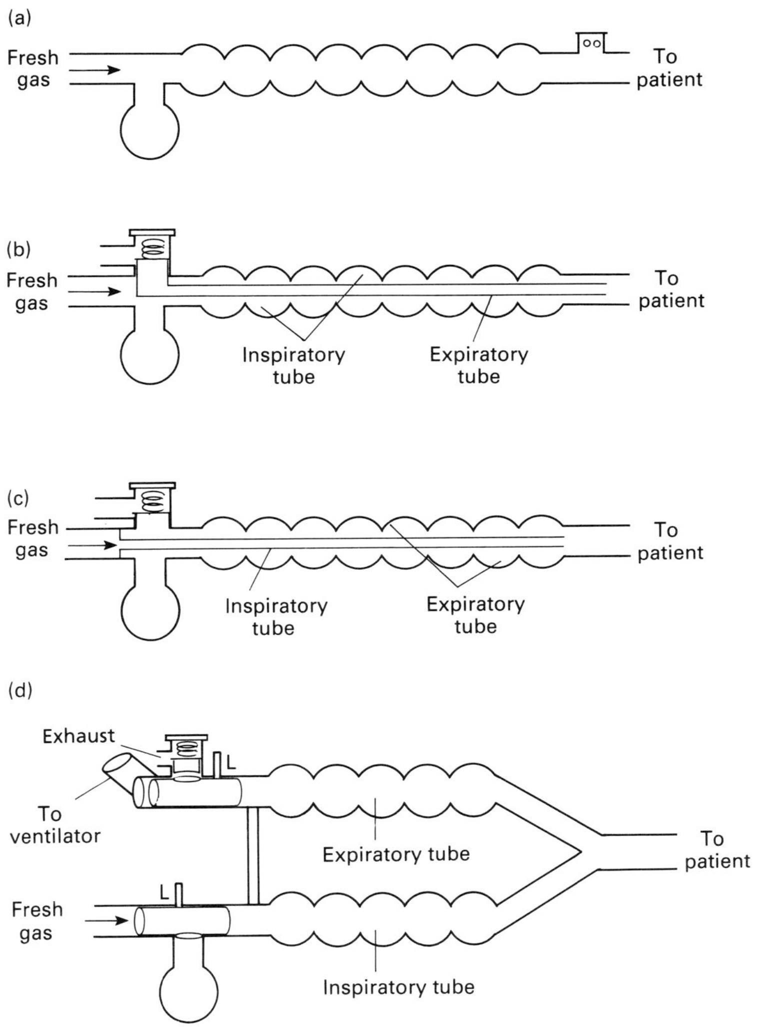

Fig. 18.2 Commonly used semi-open breathing systems. (a) Mapleson 'A' (Magill) type; (b) Lack system; (c) Bain system; and (d) Humphrey combined A, D and E system. With the levers (L) in the vertical position it functions as a Mapleson 'A' system for spontaneous breathing. With the levers in the horizontal position it functions as Mapleson 'D' and 'E' systems for mechanical ventilation.

*Lack-Mapleson 'A' breathing system.** This breathing system utilizes the principle of the Mapleson 'A' system but consists of two breathing tubes, one for the inspiratory and

* The normal reference point is the connection with the ventilating tubes near the patient's mouth. Proximal or upstream in the breathing circuit refers to this point. Distal or downstream refers to the point of the circuit away from the patient close to the delivery system. However, for jet ventilation proximal is still the patient's mouth, whereas distal refers to the jet orifice in the patient's airway which is further upstream towards the alveoli.

the other for the expiratory breathing phase. The 'blow off' valve is placed distally at the end of the expiratory tube and the reservoir bag is placed at the proximal end of the inspiratory tube, i.e. near the gas outlet from the anaesthetic machine [1, 3] (Fig. 18.2b). As a result the fresh gas flow requirement is very similar to the Mapleson 'A' system. However, it is claimed to be slightly more efficient as rebreathing of expired gas may be totally prevented. It is also easy to scavenge the expired gas from the overflow valve which is near the machine and not the patient. Disadvantages include necessity for two breathing tubes, making it more cumbersome and expensive, and also difficulty in adjusting the overflow valve during manual ventilation.

Bain system. In this system, the fresh gas flow is supplied through a coaxially placed narrow tube inside a wide bore breathing tube but in principle it is functionally similar to the Mapleson 'D' breathing system [4] (Fig. 18.2c). Some of the advantages claimed are warming of the inspired gas and ease of use. However, unless the expiratory outer tube is of wider bore, the resistance to breathing can be relatively high. Fresh anaesthetic gas flow requirement is similar to the Mapleson 'D' system during spontaneous breathing, and varies from one to three times the normal minute ventilation depending on the breathing pattern and expiratory time, but can be decreased below 1 min volume by allowing some rebreathing with increased tidal volumes during controlled mechanical ventilation.

Humphrey breathing system. This breathing circuit can be used as either a Lack–Mapleson 'A' or Mapleson 'E' (T-piece) by the use of two levers for spontaneous breathing or mechanical ventilation respectively without changing the system (Chapter 11). One lever is used to open or close the inlet of the reservoir bag and the other is used to bypass the overflow 'blow off' valve [5] (Fig. 18.2). When both the levers are vertical, i.e. opening the inlet of the reservoir bag for the fresh gas to flow in and connecting the overflow 'blow off' valve at the expiratory tube outlet, it is most suitable for spontaneous breathing with the efficiency of Lack–Mapleson 'A' systems. When the levers are placed in the horizontal position the breathing system becomes a Mapleson 'E' system and a ventilator can be connected at the expiratory end. In this configuration the inlet of the reservoir bag is closed and the overflow valve is bypassed (Fig. 18.2). This breathing system is also available in coaxial form and has similar advantages to the Bain system, i.e. a single duct. The main advantage claimed for the Humphrey breathing system is that it is suitable for both spontaneous breathing and mechanical ventilation without the need for a change of breathing system. However, it has the disadvantage of two breathing tubes and in coaxial form the resistance to breathing may be increased unless a wide bore external tube is used.

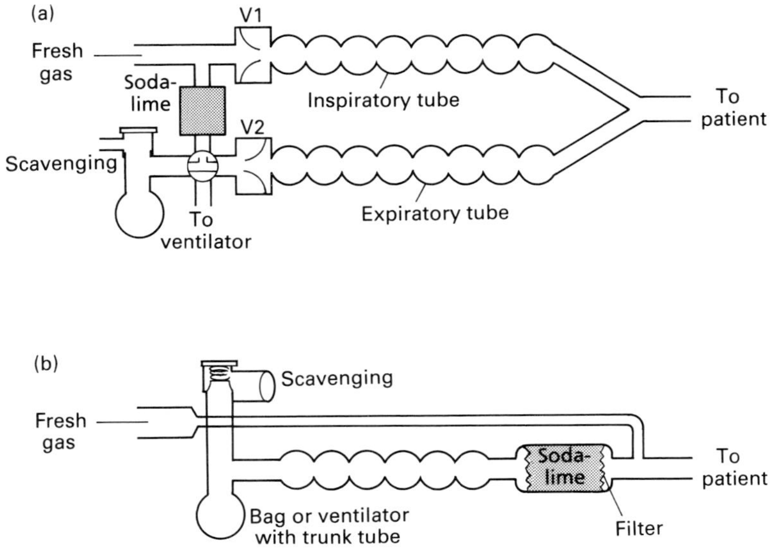

Fig. 18.3 Low flow breathing systems, i.e. with CO_2 absorption. (a) Circle system for semi-closed or closed breathing arrangement; and (b) to-and-fro breathing system.

Semi-closed and closed breathing systems

Circle system. Semi-closed and closed breathing systems are the most efficient with regard to utilization of anaesthetic gas and vapours since the elimination of carbon dioxide does not depend on the fresh gas flow. The most common system is called the circle system and is composed of two one-way valves in the breathing tubes and one overflow 'blow off' valve (Fig. 18.3). A reservoir bag collects the expired gas which is partially or fully rebreathed after absorption of carbon dioxide by a soda–lime canister (Fig. 18.3). Fresh anaesthetic gas is supplied to the circuit and if it exceeds the patient's consumption the excess gas is blown out through the outflow 'blow off' valve. Under such conditions the system is called a low-flow semi-closed breathing system and the fresh anaesthetic gas supply will be much less than the normal minute volume. However, if the anaesthetic fresh gas supply equals the patient's consumption and no excess gas escapes, it becomes a closed system. In a low flow or semi-closed system anaesthetic fresh gas flow in excess of $1\ l\ min^{-1}$ and up to $4\ l\ min^{-1}$ is widely used. However, initially a high fresh gas flow of at least 1 min normal volume is necessary for a few minutes to flush the circle system and wash out the patient's lung nitrogen. In a normal adult approximately 1 litre of nitrogen still remains in the tissues and will be eliminated slowly during several hours of anaesthesia.

Advantages of the circle system include minimum anaesthetic gas and agent requirement, making the system cost-effective and less liable to pollute the atmosphere. Also the inspiratory gas is well humidified and comparatively warm due to preservation of expired moisture and heat, and also to the water and heat generated by the chemical reaction of soda–lime and carbon dioxide. However, there are also a few disadvantages apart from it being cumbersome and difficult to sterilize quickly.

With totally closed systems, when only basal anaesthetic gas flow is supplied to meet the patient's oxygen consumption and anaesthetic requirement, the concentration of anaesthetic agent in the inspired gas will not be the same as that delivered at the outlet of the vaporizer and there may not be any relationship between the inspired concentration and vaporizer settings. The inspired concentration will always be lower in the breathing circuit because the anaesthetic vapour delivery will be inadequate at the very low gas flow and a normal setting of a conventional vaporizer. Therefore a much higher setting of the vaporizer concentration is required to meet the required inspired concentration. Under these conditions it is essential to have an anaesthetic agent monitor in the breathing system to provide an accurate measurement of its concentration in the inspired gas, i.e. delivered to the mask or tracheal tube.

However in a semi-closed circle system, using anaesthetic gas flows over 2 l min^{-1} a reasonable relationship between the inspired concentration of the anaesthetic agent and the vaporizer setting is normally achieved.

A circle system as a semi-closed or closed breathing system is suitable for both spontaneous breathing and mechanical ventilation. However, for a totally closed breathing system a dedicated mechanical ventilator is normally required, whereas with a semi-closed system any ventilator can be used with a single trunk connection. In low flow semi-closed systems cost-effectiveness is relatively less compared to the totally closed system but they are safer to use. Simple disposable circle systems with prepacked soda–lime are now available (e.g. Intersurgical, Wokingham).

Low flow to-and-fro breathing system (Waters). An example of a to-and-fro breathing system is the classical 'Waters' canister. It consists of a soda–lime chamber and a wide bore breathing tube. A low flow of anaesthetic fresh gas is supplied by a narrow tube near the tracheal tube connection. There are no valves [6] (Fig. 18.3). This breathing system is suitable for both spontaneous breathing and mechanical ventilation.

Use of this low flow to-and-fro breathing system can reduce the cost of anaesthetic gases and also pollution. However, as in the circle system, an anaesthetic agent monitor will be essential when the fresh gas flow is much less than 2 l min^{-1}. Disadvantages include the soda–lime canister which needs to be near the patient, which cannot be large and has to be changed during long procedures lasting over 2–3 h unless higher fresh gas flows are used. It also requires good filtering to prevent soda–lime dust reaching the patient's airways. However, for short day-case surgery the simplicity of the system, without any valves and its suitability for both spontaneous breathing and mechanical ventilation has major advantages. This system also provides adequate heat and humidity in the inspired gas. A disposable to-and-fro breathing system has been developed and is now commercially available (Intersurgical UK in collaboration with the Department of Anaesthesia at the Royal Postgraduate Medical School).

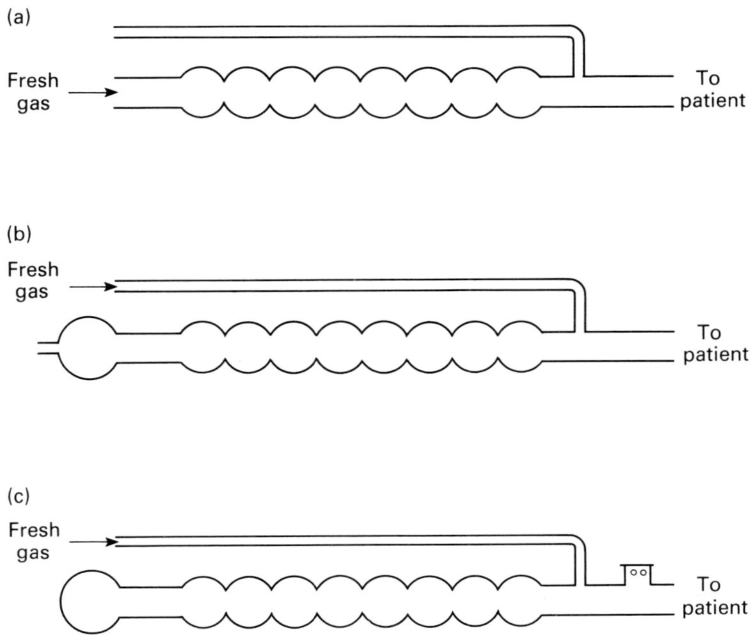

Fig. 18.4 Breathing systems used in paediatric (small children). (a) Mapleson 'E' (Ayre's T-piece) system; (b) Jackson Rees modification of T-piece system; and (c) Mapleson 'B' system.

Ventilation systems

For most purposes any suitable ventilator can be used and positive pressure ventilation can be applied using a laryngeal mask airway [7] in addition to the conventional tracheal tube. However, in endoscopic surgery (e.g. laser therapy or diagnostic procedures) of the airways, the recommended methods of ventilation are either jet ventilation in the airways [8] or external cuirass ventilation [9–11]. Total intravenous anaesthesia (TIVA) with or without the use of muscle relaxants is recommended [9, 12, 13].

Conventional paediatric circuits are illustrated in Fig. 18.4. Artificial ventilation is achieved in very small children with paediatric or perinatal ventilators, or with paediatric attachments to conventional adult ventilators. Alternatively the classical Jackson Rees system (Fig. 18.4b) can be used for prolonged manual ventilation.

Jet ventilation

Using the cricothyroid route a catheter can be introduced alongside the endoscope or a tracheal tube, as illustrated in Figs 18.5 and 18.6 may be used.

One of the major advantages of these techniques is that at ventilation frequencies above 100 breaths min^{-1} with an I:E ratio of 1:1 no debris will enter the lungs

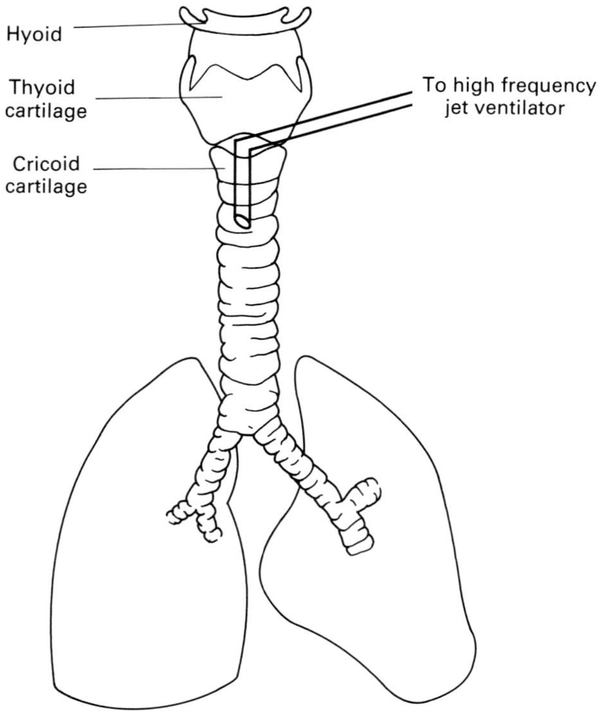

Fig. 18.5 Transtracheal high frequency jet ventilation for laryngoscopy, bronchoscopy and endoscopic surgery including laser surgery, or emergency ventilation for failed intubation.

providing the surgery is above the tip of the ventilating catheter. The main physiological events are summarized in Appendix 3.

Safety

The problem with higher frequencies of ventilation is the time constant of the lungs, i.e. compliance (C) × airways resistance (R). At higher frequencies gas trapping in the lungs occurs which at very high frequencies causes high intrapulmonary pressures and circulatory impairment with the possibility of secondary organ damage.

Routine minimal monitoring is required together with additional monitoring (Table 18.1). The principal danger is overinflation of the lungs with compromise of the circulation and a tape measure or stethograph around the thorax provides a simple monitoring device. The end expiratory pressure in the airways will indicate upper airway obstruction which must be corrected immediately. The ventilator should cut out in response to a rapid large rise in airway pressures to avoid continuing to drive gas into the lungs until the problem is remedied or a large aperture, relieving cricothyroidotomy can be performed. Alternatively, in a dire emergency several large (13 FG) i.v. cannulae can be introduced into the trachea via the cricothyroid membrane.

The end tidal carbon dioxide concentration is easily measured by slowing the respiratory rate to 30 breaths min^{-1}, i.e. within the response time of the sampling infra-

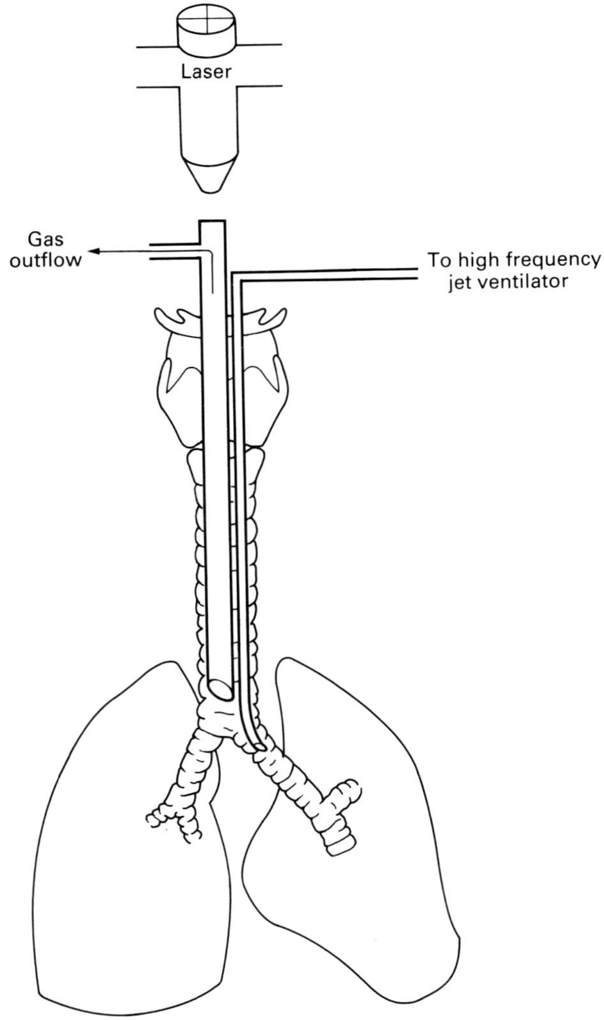

Fig. 18.6 One lung high frequency jet ventilation for laser surgery.

Table 18.1 Monitoring during high frequency jet ventilation

Routine blood pressure, SaO_2, electrocardiogram, heart rate
$F_{\acute{E}}CO_2$. This is easily measured by reducing the ventilation frequency to 30 breaths min^{-1}, sampling the expired alveolar gas for three to four breaths and then returning to the higher frequency. Interrupted high frequency ventilation (see text) [15] will do this automatically. It allows the measurement of $F_{\acute{E}}CO_2$ and the trapped gas volume above functional residual capacity as a V_E
The jet ventilator must have a means of measuring pressure in the airway linked to an alarm and a machine cut out
A tape measure or stethograph around the thorax will indicate over distension
Arterial blood gas and pH measurements represent the final comprehensive analysis of ventilation but while desirable should not be a mandatory requirement for day-case anaesthesia, no matter what the form of ventilation

red analyser for three to four breaths [14]. Alternatively interrupted high frequency ventilation can be used. In this system the ventilator automatically stops several times each minute (e.g. 6–8) which reduces mean airway and intrathoracic pressures, allows the lung to deflate, providing an additional V_T, assisting carbon dioxide removal, and also allows the measurement of the trapped gas volume and the alveolar carbon dioxide concentration [15].

Cuirass ventilation

Traditional cuirass ventilation is normally a negative pressure ventilation system mimicking spontaneous breathing. During the inspiratory phase a negative pressure is created by suction within a shell surrounding the thorax and abdomen which causes expansion of the thorax and an increase in the negative intrathoracic pressure. Gas is drawn into the lungs due to their expansion. Expiration is either passive or active. These are very efficient and in normal volunteers without anaesthesia and severe hyperventilation is possible [16]. Recently a more modern system has been introduced [17] in which higher frequencies of ventilation are possible and the expiratory residual capacity can be adjusted to any desired level.

The disadvantages of these systems include potential aspiration, particularly at normal frequencies of ventilation, it may be difficult to undertake surgery of the chest wall, they require almost airtight fitting of the shell and therefore a number of different sized shells are required, bruising may occur at the contact area and the pump is often large with a high noise level.

Padfield and Stamp [18] have reviewed the precautions required in the use of lasers in the airway.

References

1 Mapleson WW. The elimination of rebreathing in various semi-closed anaesthetic systems. *Br J Anaesth* 1954; 26: 323–32.

2 Willis BA, Pender JW, Mapleson WW. Rebreathing in a T-piece: volunteer and theoretical studies of the Jackson Rees modification of Ayre's T-piece during spontaneous respiration. *Br J Anaesth* 1975; 47: 1239–46.

3 Humphrey D. The Lack, Magill and Bain anaesthetic breathing systems: a direct comparison in spontaneously breathing anaesthetized adults. *J Roy Soc Med* 1982; 75: 513–24.

4 Bain JA, Spoerel WE. A streamlined anaesthetic system. *Canad Anaesth Soc J* 1972; 19: 426–35.

5 Humphrey D. A new anaesthetic breathing system combining Mapleson A, D and E principles. *Anaesthesia* 1983; 38: 361–75.

6 Waters DJ, Mapleson WW. Rebreathing during controlled respiration with various semi-closed anaesthetic breathing systems. *Br J Anaesth* 1961; 33: 374–81.

7 Wilson JG. The laryngeal mask in paediatric practice (Editorial). *Br J Anaesth* 1993; 70: 124–5.

8 Chollet-Rivier M, Ravussin P. Midazolam-flumazenil vs. propofol in ambulatory ENT endoscopic procedures. *Eur J Anaesth* 1992; 9: 377–85.

9 Morgan M, Lumley J, McCormick PW, Stradling P. Anaesthesia for bronchoscopic photography. *Anaesthesia* 1969; 24: 343–54.

10 Hill S. Clinical applications of body ventilators. *Chest* 1986; 90: 897–905.
11 Dilkes MB, Hayek Z. *The Hayek Oscillator—an Invaluable Aid to Anaesthesia in Endolaryngeal Surgery. Fifth Annual Trauma Anaesthesia and Critical Care Symposium*. Amsterdam, Mosby Yearbook Inc., 1992.
12 Paes ML. General anaesthesia for carbon dioxide laser surgery within the airway. *Br J Anaesth* 1987; 59: 1610–20.
13 Crawford M, Pollock J, Anderson K, Glavin RJ, MacIntyre D, Vernon D. Comparison of midazolam with propofol for sedation in outpatient bronchoscopy. *Br J Anaesth* 1993; 70: 419–22.
14 Whitwam JG, Chakrabarti MK, Konarzewski WH, Askitopoulou HA. A new valveless all-purpose ventilator. Clinical evaluation. *Br J Anaesth* 1983; 55: 1017–23.
15 Chakrabarti MK, Swenzen GO, Whitwam JG. Intermittent high frequency ventilation: a new mode to measure changes in lung volume and alveolar gas concentration, enhance CO_2 elimination and reduce intrapulmonary pressures. *Acta Anaesth Scand* 1988; 32: 295–303.
16 Whitwam JG, Boetner RB, Gilger AP, Littell AS. Hyperventilation brain damage and flicker. *Br J Anaesth* 1965; 38: 846–52.
17 Hayek Z, Sohar E. External high frequency oscillation—concept and practice. *Intens Care World* 1993; 10.
18 Padfield A, Stamp JM. Anaesthesia and laser surgery. *Eur J Anaesth* 1992; 9: 353–66.

Paediatric Anaesthesia

Chapter 19
General Principles of Paediatric Day-Case Anaesthesia

N. S. Morton and D. Lord

Selection of suitable procedures

A wide range of paediatric surgical and medical diagnostic and therapeutic procedures are suitable for day-case surgery (Table 19.1). Most will require general anaesthesia or supervised sedation although in older co-operative children, superficial operations can be carried out under local anaesthesia.

The procedure should take less than 1 h and should be performed by skilled senior staff or trainees under the closest supervison, it should *not* involve opening of a body cavity, should *not* carry a serious risk of bleeding or body fluid loss requiring replacement and should *not* require prolonged postoperative pain control.

Individual surgeons vary in their views concerning suitable procedures. For example, many feel that orchidopexy, hypospadias correction or bilateral procedures are too difficult to manage as day cases. Although adenoidectomy and adeno-tonsillectomy are often carried out as day cases in North America, the current consensus in the UK is that these procedures are not suitable because the risks of primary haemorrhage in the first 12 h postoperatively are 0·47% and 0·44% for adenoidectomy and for tonsillectomy respectively [1]. Some surgeons in the UK are prepared to undertake both these procedures on a 'short overnight stay' basis and some carry out adenoidectomy on a 'same day' basis, provided the patient can be observed afterwards for 6–12 h. Good follow-up and rapid access to help at home are vital for success. It is likely that day-case management will be more widely adopted when the results of clinical audit projects in this field are published showing an acceptable outcome.

Procedures requiring tracheal intubation are to be avoided where possible, particularly in children under 6 years of age. As modern tube materials are less irritant, the incidence of postextubation stridor [2] can be minimized by meticulous selection of the correct diameter of endotracheal tube. The laryngeal mask airway (LMA) has been a significant advance in allowing operations upon the head and neck without the need for tracheal intubation [3]. Most day-case ear, nose and throat (ENT), dental, ophthalmology and plastic surgical operations listed in Table 19.1 can be performed with the aid of the LMA.

Selection criteria for paediatric day care need to be rigorously adhered to if complications are to be minimized. Age, intercurrent and familial medical disorders

Table 19.1 Range of suitable procedures for paediatric day care

Surgical

Diagnostic

Endoscopy ± biopsies: upper GI, colonoscopy, sigmoidoscopy, proctoscopy, cystoscopy
Examinations under anaesthesia
Evoked response audiometry
Measurement of intraocular pressure
Biopsies: skin lesions, bone, muscle
Arthroscopy, arthrograms

Therapeutic

General surgery: herniotomy (inguinal, femoral, epigastric, umbilical); hydrocele; perianal procedures; skin lesions; preauricular sinus; external angular dermoid; removal of sutures; frenulectomy
Urology: STING; circumcision; glansplasty; meatotomy; urethral dilatation; hypospadias repair/revision; prepucial adhesions; penoscrotal web; orchidopexy; fixation of testis; vulval warts; labial adhesions
ENT: myringotomy ± grommets; nasal manipulation; removal of aural or nasal foreign body; antral lavage; nasal cautery; adenoidectomy; adenotonsillectomy
Dental: extractions; restorations; periodontal treatment; biopsies; minor oral surgery; fissure sealants
Ophthalmology: probing tear duct; chalazion; strabismus surgery; skin and eyelid lesions
Orthopaedics: plaster casts; removal of sutures, metalwork, leg-lengthening devices; injection of bone cysts; intra-articular injections; minor hand surgery, trigger thumb, excision of ganglion; minor toe surgery
Plastic surgery: change of dressings; removal of sutures; superficial lesions; scar revision; prominent ears

Medical

Diagnostic

Blood sampling; bone marrow sampling; lumbar puncture; lymph node biopsy; needle aspiration cytology; metabolic/endocrine tests; CT scan; MRI scan

Therapeutic

Venesection; intrathecal injection; radiotherapy; change of urinary catheter; interventional radiology/cardiology

CT, computerized tomography; GI, gastrointestinal; MRI, magnetic resonance imaging.

and psychosocial factors have to be considered in addition to the surgical and anaesthetic factors noted above.

Age

The healthy full-term neonate may be suitable for brief day-case surgery provided none of the other exclusions apply and a trained senior paediatric anaesthetist and surgeon perform the procedure. This type of work must be a regular feature of their practice so that skills are maintained and the facilities must be appropriate for such small patients with access to inpatient neonatal care if required [4].

The premature neonate cannot safely undergo surgery as a day case before reaching 60 weeks postconceptual age because of the risk of significant perioperative apnoea [5]. Even then, other complications of prematurity may rule out day-case management.

Intercurrent and familial medical disorders

The majority of children selected for day care should be normal healthy children with a specific problem requiring investigation or treatment. Children with mild systemic disease or well-controlled more severe disease can be managed on a day-case basis. Mentally handicapped children often receive superior care at home from dedicated parents who are more familiar with their individual needs. Children with stable treated asthma, epilepsy and corrected simple congenital heart defects are suitable, provided antibiotic prophylaxis against subacute bacterial endocarditis is given when required. Corrected patent ductus arteriosus, atrial and ventricular septal defects and coarctation of the aorta are examples. Only those with larger repaired defects or where prosthetic material or pericardial patches have been used require antibiotic cover. The child found to have a murmur as an incidental finding on preoperative examination must have this investigated further before being passed as fit for day care. Paediatric cardiological advice and further investigations such as ultrasound and electrocardiogram (ECG) may be required.

Absolute contraindications to paediatric day-case anaesthesia and surgery (Table 19.2) include metabolic disorders and diabetes mellitus because of the problems of blood glucose and fluid control during the perioperative fasting period.

Any child with a known or suspected difficult airway should be excluded [6]. A family history of malignant hyperthermia or sudden infant death syndrome precludes day care. Children from populations known to be at risk of having a significant haemoglobinopathy should be screened by haemoglobin electrophoresis [7].

The child with an active infection is not suitable for day care for at least 2 weeks after symptoms have resolved. This delay should be extended to 4 weeks for a child with a lower respiratory tract infection and 6 weeks for children with pertussis or measles as respiratory tract irritability is a recognized feature of these disorders [8]. An increased incidence of laryngospasm and bronchospasm is seen during induction, maintenance and recovery in children with active upper or lower respiratory tract infections. Features such as purulent crusting around the nose, pyrexia, lethargy, productive cough and chest signs should alert the anaesthetist [9]. Many children have chronic nasal discharge due to allergic rhinitis or adenoid infection or hypertrophy and there is no benefit in delaying their procedure provided they are otherwise suitable for day care.

Table 19.2 Exclusion criteria for paediatric day-case anaesthesia

Surgical and anaesthetic factors
Duration more than 1 h
Junior unsupervised staff
Opening of body cavities
Significant bleeding risk
Prolonged postoperative pain
Age
Premature or ex-premature baby less than 60 weeks postconceptual age
The term neonate in a centre with no access to inpatient neonatal care
The 'occasional' term neonate: surgeon and anaesthetist must be senior, suitably trained and carrying out such cases regularly
Intercurrent and familial medical disorders
Poorly controlled systemic disease: epilepsy, asthma, uncorrected congenital heart disease
Uninvestigated heart murmur
Metabolic disorders
Diabetes mellitus
Difficult airway
Malignant hyperthermia
SIDS
Haemoglobinopathy
Active infection especially of upper/lower respiratory tract, pertussis, respiratory syncytial virus, measles
Psychosocial factors
Parent unable/unwilling to care for child at home
Single parent family with many siblings and no help
Poor housing
No telephone
Inadequate personal transport
Long distance from hospital

SIDS, sudden infant death syndrome.

Psychosocial factors

Parents have to be assessed as being capable of caring for their child after a day-case procedure. There may be other siblings who require care and this may present particular problems for the single parent. Poor housing conditions, lack of a telephone, inadequate transport or long distance from the hospital may preclude day care. Support from and easy access to a community nurse, health visitor and general practitioner help greatly in instilling confidence in the anxious parent.

The avoidance of separation from their child, a feeling of involvement in the care of their child and the lesser disruption to daily routine are persuasive arguments in favour of paediatric day care. Financial savings are often used in promoting day care but should not pressurize staff into inappropriate case selection.

Facilities for day care

The ideal facility should be specifically modified or designed for the purpose of managing the paediatric day-case patient. The ward area should be separate from an adult facility and dedicated to paediatric surgery and segregated from bedbound ill children.

Since the majority of children will come in well and leave in a similar state it should possess a major emphasis on play and freedom of movement.

It should have sufficiently trained, paediatrically qualified nursing staff. Depending on the throughput of cases this may approximate to one nurse per patient. The theatre should be close to but out of earshot of the paediatric unit.

The operating theatre requires to be technically equipped for paediatric anaesthesia with a separate paediatric temporary holding area. If the children's unit is part of an adult hospital, where possible a theatre should be set aside, decorated and equipped as a paediatric theatre. Nursing and technical staff should be experienced in paediatric care.

The recovery unit. The recovery unit should be staffed with paediatrically trained staff and the facility should be large enough to accommodate unconscious recovering children with a larger area for newly recovered children and their parents.

Anaesthetic staff. The management of largely unpremedicated small children and their parents requires a great deal of training and continual practice. Although the surgical procedures are of a relatively minor type, the anaesthesia is just as demanding as that of major cases and is worthy of the most senior anaesthesiologists. Outside major paediatric centres it is recommended that in each major district hospital one or two consultant anaesthetists should have a special interest and training in paediatric anaesthesia and take a major interest in paediatric day-care and including continuing education [10, 11].

Recovery from anaesthesia

The rate of recovery is influenced by premedication, the induction and maintenance techniques, the analgesic technique and its efficacy, the age of the patient, the duration of the surgery and the method of assessment of recovery.

Premedication

Sedative premedication is only occasionally required in modern practice. Midazolam (orally or intranasally), ketamine (intramuscularly) or methohexitone (rectally) do not significantly prolong recovery provided the dose is limited.

Induction and maintenance technique

Inhalational induction and maintenance produce the most rapid recovery. Halothane remains the agent of choice for paediatric inhalational induction with its relatively pleasant odour. Its relative lack of adverse respiratory effects means that the rate of induction is faster than the newer compounds, even though these should produce more rapid induction as judged by their physicochemical properties. The only potential rival to halothane so far in terms of ease of induction is sevoflurane [12]. Of the three agents in current common use (halothane, enflurane and isoflurane), enflurane has been shown to produce the most rapid recovery [13]. It has been suggested that the best of both worlds can be gained from a halothane induction and isoflurane maintenance [14]. Of the new agents, sevoflurane induction and maintenance has been shown to produce more rapid recovery than halothane induction and maintenance [15]. Desflurane maintenance produces particularly rapid recovery [16].

Recovery after intravenous induction of anaesthesia with propofol is quicker than after thiopentone when used for induction followed by a volatile agent to maintain anaesthesia for brief procedures with an appropriate regional block for postoperative analgesia [17]. Propofol induction and maintenance by infusion gives comparable recovery times to propofol induction and halothane maintenance [18]. Interestingly, inhalational induction with halothane followed by a propofol infusion for maintenance is associated with a more rapid recovery than the use of halothane for both induction and maintenance.

Analgesia

The child in severe pain will awaken sooner and will have a poor quality of recovery. Pain may well be an important confounding variable in many of the studies of recovery after paediatric surgery and there is a need for standardization of operation type and analgesic method in future studies. Opioids will tend to delay recovery and have other adverse effects, particularly emesis. A child with 'perfect' analgesia from a regional block may also be slow to recover due to lack of sensory stimulation from the operative site, but will have a much better quality of recovery. A potential disadvantage of very rapid reawakening after very quick surgery is that regional blockade with bupivacaine with its slow onset time (10–20 min) may not have had time to take effect.

Assessment of recovery

Techniques such as psychometric testing cannot be applied to young children to assess recovery. It has been demonstrated clearly that the time taken to reach predetermined milestones such as eye opening or giving the correct name are sensitive enough indices for comparing anaesthetic techniques in children [17, 19]. The Steward Score [20] is an alternative. It assesses the safe return of protective reflexes by assigning a score to each of three variables: wakefulness, ventilation and movement.

Postoperative care and discharge criteria

Recovery is usually swift and uncomplicated if the principles of balanced anaesthesia and analgesia and pre-emptive analgesia are followed. Postoperative pain, nausea and vomiting, bleeding, failure to ambulate and unexpected perioperative complications may all have to be taken into account when deciding whether the child is ready to be discharged [21, 22].

Postoperative pain

Failure of intraoperative local analgesia can lead to problems in re-establishing pain control. In a recent clinical audit of paediatric day-cases, an appropriate local anaesthetic technique was used in 73% of cases. This provided good analgesia for most patients: 74% of children had no pain or only mild pain during their time in the day surgery unit. However, 25% were assessed as having moderate pain and 1% had severe pain during their stay [23]. The assessment of postoperative pain can be difficult in paediatrics particularly in young children. A variety of scoring systems have been described and validated and there is no reason why these should not be used in the day surgery unit [24–26]. Correct diagnosis of the cause of apparent pain and distress is important. Parental presence at the time of awakening, the presence of a familiar toy, the early establishment of oral fluid intake and the avoidance of overrestrictive garments may all help to minimize anxiety and distress [22]. Analgesic drugs and techniques should be introduced early to children in pain (Chapter 21). If these fail in the recovery area consideration must be given to inpatient admission for pain control by opioids either in repeated doses or using infusion techniques.

Postoperative nausea and vomiting

The incidence of nausea and vomiting is considerably reduced when opioids and endotracheal intubation are avoided and when good local analgesia is established before the child reawakens.

Emesis can be troublesome after squint surgery, orchidopexy, herniotomy and upper gastrointestinal endoscopy. However, the use of propofol for the induction and maintenance of anaesthesia has been shown to minimize the incidence of nausea and vomiting after paediatric squint surgery [27]. In our practice the incidence of emesis after squint surgery is 10% when a technique comprising propofol induction, spontaneous respiration via an LMA, rectal diclofenac and amethocaine eye drops are used (personal observations). Nitrous oxide may contribute to emesis in children as in adults. Other preventative measures include droperidol in low dosage, 0·075 mg kg^{-1}, metoclopramide, 0·15 mg kg^{-1} or ondansetron, 0·01 mg kg^{-1} [28–31]. There are concerns about using droperidol and metoclopramide in paediatric day-care because of their sedative effects and propensity for producing extrapyramidal side effects. Ondansetron has a very good safety profile and may find a role in the prevention of postoperative nausea and vomiting despite its expense. Some advocate emptying the stomach of the anaesthetized child and avoid oral fluids immediately following surgery. Correction of fluid deficits caused by preoperative fasting may also be helpful.

Bleeding

Bleeding may occur after circumcision, frenulectomy, adenoidectomy or adeno-tonsillectomy and may require reoperation and/or inpatient admission.

Failure to ambulate

Motor loss after caudal epidural block is rare when 0·125% or 0·25% bupivacaine is used [32]. Indeed, motor blockade may be more of a problem after ilioinguinal/iliohypogastric blocks due to involvement of femoral nerve branches to the quadriceps thigh muscles [33, 34].

Unexpected perioperative complications

Regurgitation and aspiration of gastric contents, bronchospasm, hypersensitivity reactions, suxamethonium apnoea, suspected malignant hyperthermia and post-extubation stridor warrant inpatient observation, further investigation and treatment. This may best be conducted in an intensive care area.

Discharge criteria

Discharge criteria must take into account the age of the child, the preoperative assessment, surgical and social factors.

Vital signs and conscious level should be normal for the child's age and preoperative medical condition. There should be no respiratory distress or stridor and protective reflexes should be fully regained. The child should be able to move appropriately for his age although residual motor blockade due to local anaesthetic should not necessarily preclude discharge in the smaller child. The ability to drink and tolerate clear fluids is desirable but adequately hydrated children who have not been subjected to a prolonged preoperative fasting period can be allowed home prior to drinking if they meet the other discharge criteria. Nausea and vomiting, bleeding and pain must be controlled and assessed prior to discharge. Patients requiring and receiving opioids should not be sent home.

All paediatric day cases must be escorted home by a responsible parent or guardian. Travel should be by private transport or taxi rather than public transport. Full verbal and written instructions should be given to the parent regarding postoperative wound care, activities and whom to contact in the event of problems with bleeding, pain, emesis and wound disruption. This contact may be via the family doctor, community nurse or the day surgery unit itself. Many units arrange follow-up visits by a district or community nurse who will call at the home within 24 h. This nurse performs a useful audit function informing the day surgery unit staff of the clinical data on patients with complications [35, 36].

References

1 Capper JWR, Randall C. Post-operative haemorrhage in tonsillectomy and adenoidectomy in children. *J Laryngol Otol* 1984; 98: 363–5.

2 Koka BV, Jeon IS, Andre JM. Post-intubation croup in children. *Anesth Analg* 1977; 56: 501.

3 Haynes SR, McGinn G, Morton NS. The laryngeal mask airway in paediatric anaesthesia: a review. *Paediatr Anaesth*; in press.

4 Campling EA, Devlin HB, Lunn JN. Report of the *National Confidential Enquiry into Perioperative Deaths*, 1989. London: NCEPOD.

5 Steward DJ. Preterm infants are more prone to complications following minor surgery than are term infants. *Anesthesiology* 1982; 56: 304–6.

6 Ward CF. Pediatric head and neck syndromes. In: Katz J, Steward D, eds. *Anesthesia and Uncommon Pediatric Diseases*. Philadelphia: WB Saunders.

7 British Society of Haematology. Guidelines for haemoglobinopathy screening. *Clin Lab Haematol* 1988; 10: 87–94.

8 Keneally JP. Day stay surgery in paediatrics. *Clin Anesth* 1985; 3: 679–96.

9 Berry F. The child with the runny nose. In: Berry FA, ed. *Anesthetic Management of the Difficult and Routine Pediatric Patient*, 2nd edn. New York: Churchill Livingstone, 1990: 267–83.

10 Hatch DJ. Anaesthesia for children (Editorial). *Anaesthesia* 1984; 39 (5): 405–6.

11 Morris SP. Paediatric day-case anaesthesia. *Br J Anaesth* 1992;' 68: 3–4.

12 Kleinman S, Lerman J, Yentis S, Sikich N. Induction and emergence characteristics of and haemodynamic responses to sevoflurane in children. *Can J Anaesth* 1992; 39: A100.

13 Simmons M, Miller CD, Cummings GC, Todd JG. Outpatient paediatric dental anaesthesia. A comparison of halothane, enflurane and isoflurane. *Anaesthesia* 1989; 44: 735–8.

14 Pandit UA, Steude GM, Leach AB. Induction and recovery characteristics of isoflurane and halothane anaesthesia for short outpatient procedures in children. *Anaesthesia* 1985; 40: 1226–30.

15 Naito Y, Tamai S, Shingu K, Fujimori R, Mori K. Comparison between sevoflurane and halothane for paediatric ambulatory anaesthesia. *Br J Anaesth* 1991; 67: 387–9.

16 Taylor R, Lerman J. Induction and recovery characteristics of desflurane in infants and children. *Can J Anaesth* 1992; 39: 6–13.

17 Runcie CJ, MacKenzie S, Arthur DS. Morton NS. Comparison of recovery from anaesthesia induced in children with either propofol or thiopentone. *Br J Anaesth* 1993; 70: 192–5.
18 Doyle E, McFadzean W, Morton NS. I.V. anaesthesia with propofol using a target-controlled infusion system: comparison with inhalation anaesthesia for general surgical procedures in children. *Br J Anaesth* 1993; 70: 542–5.
19 Puttick SN, Rosen M. Propofol induction and maintenance with nitrous oxide in paediatric outpatient dental anaesthesia. *Anaesthesia* 1988; 43: 646–9.
20 Steward DJ. A simplified scoring system for the post-operative recovery room. *Canad Anaesth Soc J* 1975; 22: 111–13.
21 Thornes R. *Just for the Day. Caring for Children in the Health Services.* London: NAWCH, 1991.
22 McConachie IW, Day A, Morris P. Recovery from anaesthesia in children. *Anaesthesia* 1989; 44: 986–90.
23 Stuart JC, Morton NS. A clinical audit of day case surgery for children. *J One-Day Surg* 1991; 1: 15–18.
24 Tarbell S, Cohen I, Marsh J. The toddler–preschooler postoperative pain scale: an observational scale for measuring postoperative pain in children aged 1–5. *Pain* 1992; 50: 273–80.
25 Norden J, Hannallah R, Getson P, O'Donnell R, Kelliher G, Walker N. Reliability of an objective pain scale in children. *J Pain Sympt Manage* 1991; 6: 196.
26 Broadman L, Rice L, Hannallah R. Comparison of a physiological and visual analogue scale in children. *Can J Anaesth* 1988; 35: S137–8.
27 Watcha MF, Simeon RM, White PF, Stevens JL. Effect of propofol on the incidence of postoperative vomiting after strabismus surgery in pediatric outpatients. *Anesthesiology* 1991; 75: 204–9.
28 Abramowitz MD, Oh Th, Epstein BS. The antiemetic effect of droperidol following outpatient strabismus surgery in children. *Anesthesiology* 1983; 59: 579–83.
29 Lerman J, Eustis S, Smith DR. Effect of droperidol pretreatment of postanesthetic vomiting in children undergoing strabismus surgery. *Anesthesiology* 1986; 65: 322–5.
30 Broadman LM, Ceruzzi W, Patane PS. Metoclopramide reduces the incidence of vomiting following strabismus surgery in children. *Anesthesiology* 1990; 72: 245–8.
31 Vassallo SA, Ferrari L. Anesthesia for Ophthalmology. In: Cote CJ, Ryan JF, Todres ID, Goudsouzian NG, eds. *A Practice of Anesthesia for Infants and Children*, 2nd edn. Philadelphia: WB Saunders.
32 Wolf A, Valley RD, Fear DW. Bupivacaine for caudal analgesia in infants and children: The optimal effective concentration. *Anesthesiology* 1988; 69: 102–6.
33 Hannallah RS, Broadman LM, Belman AB. Comparison of caudal and ilioinguinal/iliohypogastric nerve blocks for control of postorchiopexy pain in pediatric ambulatory surgery. *Anesthesiology* 1987; 66: 832–4.
34 Stuart JC, Morton NS. A clinical audit of day case surgery for children. *J One-Day Surg* 1991; 1: 15–18.
35 Atwell JD, Gow MA. Paediatric trained district nurse in the community: expensive luxury or economic necessity? *Br Med J* 1985; 291: 227–9.
36 Anon. Following up day case anaesthesia in general practice. *Drugs Ther Bull* 1990; 28: 81–2.

Chapter 20
General Anaesthesia for Paediatric Day-Case Surgery

D. Lord

Quantitatively a great deal of paediatric surgery is for minor ear, nose and throat (ENT) or urological surgery. Hitherto many of these children were subjected to prolonged preoperative and postoperative admission. The reasons, undoubtedly well intentioned, were to ensure optimum conditions preoperatively and to guarantee the availability of medical and nursing care postoperatively should it be required.

Children by definition come with a built in carer/minder or parent. Paediatric patients are far more portable than adults and provided that early discharge is as safe as inpatient treatment, the child and parents prefer to be in their own home.

The limitations to surgical treatment within a day are essentially the requirement for continued skilled medical or nursing observation or the provision of continued potent postoperative analgesia. A difficult area is that case, for example tonsillectomy, which does not usually require potent postoperative analgesia and although the required level of postoperative supervision is minimal, the child may be much better being left to sleep overnight. Health-care managers see day-care as an answer to growing waiting lists and limited resources. This increasing pressure leads to confusion and conflict between that which is surgically and anaesthetically possible and humane management, and this is true for paediatric surgery, a fruitful area for mediation by health economists.

If preparation, treatment and discharge are to be condensed into such a short time great care should be taken to ensure that not only is the practice safe, but also that the child and parents do not have the feeling that they are being processed. The most acceptable phraseology to use is 'quality of patient care' or 'quality control and assurance'.

Psychological preparation

Preparation for day-case admission should begin with a visit to the day-ward straight from the outpatient clinic or alternatively at an arranged 'Saturday club' or special introductory visit. The parents can be advised of procedures and given information booklets and advice. A contact is made where questions can be answered directly or support given over the telephone if requested. The child can be shown his or her bed area or 'personal space', where the child's name will be displayed and is shown the range of toys, games and facilities available for the next visit. He or she is encouraged to bring personal effects, e.g. toothbrush, toys or comforter. Video presentations, and colouring books aimed specifically at the child provide more information.

A conducted tour of the anaesthetic and recovery rooms allays preconceived impressions and fears. The children are encouraged to handle anaesthetic circuits and ask questions. Simple badges and certificates of achievement to be gained when they are admitted impress younger children. Adolescents are not impressed by such things but will respond to praise of their 'adult' manner and behaviour. At no time should the child be deceived.

Preadmission clinics shortly before the day of admission reduce the non-attender rate and give the opportunity for any preoperative laboratory or diagnostic investigation. The parents should telephone the ward within 2 days of the proposed admission date to confirm attendance and may receive further counselling if required.

Preoperative fasting

There are two major conflicting concerns, hypoglycaemia and the regurgitation of solid and fluid gastric contents. The period of fasting that can be tolerated without danger of hypoglycaemia depends on the age, and the medical and nutritional state [1] and hypoglycaemia is unlikely in the routine preoperative child [2, 3].

The need for prolonged deprivation of fluids has been questioned [4, 5]. Several studies have demonstrated that the volume and pH of gastric contents is unchanged if sugar containing fluids are given up to 2 h before surgery [6, 7].

Solid food including milk should be withheld for a period of 6 h but fruit juices containing sugar may be given on demand up to 3 h and should be encouraged in the young child. (Some anaesthetists would advocate oral fluids up to 2 h before surgery [6].)

Preoperative investigations

The scale of investigation depends on the presenting condition [8]. Routine investigation is restricted to urine analysis and sometimes a haemoglobin investigation but this should be avoided unless there is a specific medical indication. Chest X-rays are only required in the investigation of a suspected cardiac or respiratory condition.

The day of surgery

Staggered admission should ensure that timing of admission and subsequent surgery are matched. Long periods of waiting are distressing particularly for the parents [9]. Although the child will usually be well occupied with a range of toys, games, computers and videos, a play leader can be particularly helpful during this phrase of preparation.

Medical and nursing assessment

The presenting complaint will already be well documented and any coincidental illness or condition should have been elicited in the outpatient clinic. A well-prepared simple questionnaire should limit the need for an extensive preoperative history and the examination can be confined to the cardiorespiratory system, unless the child has a potential muscular problem or other serious congenital disorder which could affect the conduct of anaesthesia.

Preparation for theatre

Young children find it abnormal to undress in the middle of the day. The children may wear their own nightwear or select their gown from a collection of designer theatre wear with motifs, cartoons or captions. If distressed by undressing, clothes can be removed in theatre once the child is anaesthetized. On no account should underpants, knickers or socks be surrendered before anaesthesia either for reasons of modesty or warm feet.

The child may walk, be carried or piggybacked to theatre. Trolleys are rarely necessary and reminiscent of tumbrels and threatening to the unsedated patient.

Parental involvement

This has been a matter of controversy for some years. Parents have argued the right to accompany their child during their waking moments at induction and recovery and this has been strongly supported by nurses [10] and individual anaesthetists [11, 12].

Parents can be of great help in encouraging a smooth passage to theatre and unconsciousness. A little mentioned advantage of parental presence is that the young child is far more likely to accept a situation if it is sanctioned by parental presence, thus transferring responsibility for the procedure from the anaesthetist to the parent in the child's eyes, i.e. 'mum wouldn't let anything nasty happen to me therefore it must be alright'.

One or both parents, or a parent and supporter (grandparent or friend) should be encouraged to accompany their child during the induction of anaesthesia. This is associated with an improvement in the disposition of the child with parents remaining calm and supportive [12, 13] even if they become upset on leaving the child. The majority of parents believe their presence to be of benefit to their child and anaesthetist [14]. However, as yet while most anaesthetists will accept one parent who leaves immediately after induction, not every parent wishes to come to theatre [15]. Also very anxious parents should be advised that their anxiety may be transmitted to the child [16], which is undesirable and perhaps they should not be present during induction and their role taken over by a member of the nursing team. Concerns about being watched by the parents, of parents interfering with the conduct of anaesthesia or of adverse parental behaviour are usually dispelled by experience [17]. Whilst some anaesthetists insist on a minimum age others allow parents of children of all ages into the anaesthetic room. Similarly parents are unfortunately often restricted from accompanying their child in the emergency situation when, for example, it is often relatively easy to establish a local anaesthetic block, e.g. infiltration or Bier block with the child sitting on the parental lap. Counselling by the anaesthesiologist and day-unit staff is essential so that the parents know exactly what is to be expected and allowed. An invitation to leave, accompanied by thanks and encouragement and a skilled escort nurse ensure that the parents leave as soon as consciousness is lost and before any airway manipulation is necessary.

A more contentious point is the role of parents in the recovery room. Parents can be of help in comforting a child whilst semi-conscious, but are a positive disadvantage prior to the return of protective reflexes. A satisfactory compromise is an immediate recovery area and a separate recovery ward to which children are returned as soon as the child is stable and can support his or her own airway.

It should be remembered that the quality of service depends just as much on parental satisfaction as well as the result. Adequate communication with the parents will prevent most misunderstandings.

Premedication

The main benefits of effective premedication are the predictable production of sedation, anxiolysis, amnesia and possible analgesia and anticholinergic activity (Table 20.1). Whilst it is desirable to produce some or all of these effects in the inpatient for major surgery it is questionable whether this is necessary for minor surgery, since effective premedication is likely to be associated with a delayed recovery and prolonged admission.

The majority of anaesthesiologists would agree that with careful preparation the support of parents in the anaesthetic room and a sympathetic anaesthetic approach, premedication provides little advantage to the child or anaesthetist. It is therefore unfortunate that the ability of a premedication technique to improve the response to separation from a parent is so frequently quoted. A further problem is insufficient time between the administration of the premedication and induction of anaesthesia for the development of adequate action and the variability of effect between individuals.

Booker and Chapman [18] compared the routine use of intramuscular morphine and atropine with an orally administered preparation of dichloralphenazone, paracetamol and atropine and found no difference in preoperative demeanour. This study conducted by postal questionnaire confirmed the unacceptability of the intramuscular premedication, which was associated with a high incidence of nausea and vomiting, and the finding that following morphine the children were significantly more drowsy at home.

Oral premedication has been shown to be as effective as the intramuscular route [19] and although a combination of narcotic and benzodiazepine mixtures have been

Table 20.1 Drug administration sites and doses

Drugs used for premedication of day-case children	
Diazepam	
Oral	0·2 mg kg^{-1}
Midazolam	
Oral	0·4 mg kg^{-1}
Nasal	0·2 mg kg^{-1}
Rectal	0·5 mg kg^{-1}
Atropine	
Oral	0·02 mg kg^{-1}
Drugs used for preinduction of anaesthesia	
Ketamine	
Oral	6 mg kg^{-1}
Nasal	3 mg kg^{-1}
Rectal	10 mg kg^{-1}
Methohexitone	
Rectal	25 mg kg^{-1}
Intravenous induction agents	
Thiopentone	5–6 mg kg^{-1}
Methohexitone	1–2 mg kg^{-1}
Propofol	3–4 mg kg^{-1}
Neuromuscular blocking agents	
Suxamethonium	1–2 mg kg^{-1}
Increment	0·1–0·2 mg kg^{-1}
Mivacurium	0·1–0·2 mg kg^{-1}
Increment	0·05 mg kg^{-1}
Vecuronium	0·1 mg kg^{-1}
Increment	0·02 mg kg^{-1}
Atracurium	0·3 mg kg^{-1}
Increment	0·1 mg kg^{-1}

used [20], benzodiazepines on their own or in combination with atropine are more commonly prescribed in day-case patients. Recent interest has concentrated on oral midazolam; in a dose of 0·5–0·75 mg kg^{-1} midazolam produced significant sedation at 30 min without prolongation of recovery [21]. Payne *et al.* [22] found that oral midazolam 0·45 mg kg^{-1} produced a greater incidence of amnesia than a combination of trimeprazine, methadone and droperidol. However Anderson *et al.* [23] in a comparison of chloral hydrate, diazepam, alprazolam and midazolam 0·3 mg kg^{-1} found chloral hydrate to be superior in the under 4 age group and that midazolam conferred no advantage over placebo in children over 4 years.

The variability of absorption, unpalatable taste and difficulty of correctly timing administration has prompted the exploration of alternative routes of administration.

Midazolam instilled intranasally develops a peak plasma concentration of 0·57 of the intravenous dose within 10·2 $\pm$ 2 min of administration [24]. A dose of 0·2 mg kg^{-1} would seem to be most appropriate [25] and is effective in producing anterograde but not retrograde amnesia [26]. There is little advantage in increasing the dose to 0·4 or 0·6 mg kg^{-1}.

The rectal route of administration of drugs has been practised for many years mainly when the oral route cannot be used or when the drug is unsuitable for parenteral administration. Midazolam 1 mg kg^{-1} administered rectally gives a peak plasma concentration of between 0·4 and 0·5 of the level following intravenous administration within 16 min [27]. It is questionable whether rectal administration when used for routine sedation produces less distress or confers any advantage over gentle but firmly applied intravenous or inhalational induction of anaesthesia in the presence and with the support of parents.

The inconsolable child

Occasionally a child presents for anaesthesia in a very distressed state in spite of rational argument from parents, nursing staff and anaesthetist. The choice is then between hospital admission and heavy sedation, forced induction which is distressing for the child and all concerned or the adoption of an alternative approach.

Techniques of heavy sedation must be practised within the theatre facility itself ideally in a preanaesthetic holding area with adequate monitoring and resuscitation equipment.

Rectal methohexitone 20–30 mg kg^{-1} in a 10% solution induces sleep in 6·7–7·8 min in 87–93% of patients depending on dosage, with a slightly faster onset time at the higher dose [28]. The cardiovascular parameters remain stable [29, 30] and oxygen saturation is maintained [31]. Induction is continued by spontaneous inhalation of halothane.

The advantages are: (a) heavy sedation is produced without a painful injection at a site removed from the anaesthetic room; (b) decreased parental anxiety with the child falling asleep on parents lap; and (c) rapid induction with immediate acceptance of a face mask. Although immediate recovery is longer than after intravenous induction with thiopentone [32], discharge from hospital is not delayed.

The disadvantages include: (a) more staff to monitor the child from administration to the commencement of anaesthesia; (b) the procedure whilst not painful still commits an intrusion which is unacceptable to older children and arguably undesirable at any age; (c) expulsion of the drug before it has had effect is some cases; (d) delayed recovery for very short procedures; and (e) if the technique is used frequently a special preinduction holding room is required.

Ketamine has also been administered rectally as a preinduction agent [33–35]. Intramuscular induction with a 5% solution of methohexitone 6 mg kg^{-1} [36] or low dose ketamine 2 mg kg^{-1} [37] has been used to facilitate inhalational induction but since these injections are very painful they should rarely be used.

Ketamine can also be administered by the oral route [38] in a dose of 6 mg kg^{-1} or intranasally [39] at 3 mg kg^{-1}. When given as a premedicant there is said to be no incidence of dysphoric reactions.

Anticholinergic agents

Atropine and glycopyrrolate are the only anticholinergic agents suitable for day-surgery since scopolamine can produce oversedation. They are used to reduce secretions, to diminish or block parasympathetic effects including laryngeal reflexes and to prevent bradycardia secondary to the administration of suxamethonium, halothane, opioids and propofol.

Preoperative oral administration of atropine is more effective against secretions but its routine administration is unnecessary and it produces unpleasant tachycardia and may produce central excitement and hyperpyrexia.

The intravenous administration of atropine 0·02 mg kg^{-1} is rapidly effective and routine administration should be considered in the following situations:

1 In children under 1 year where secretions cause more problems particularly during stimulation of the oropharynx.

2 Always preceding suxamethonium.

3 Before eye surgery.

4 In response to bradycardia which is producing a fall in blood pressure, SaO_2 or peripheral perfusion.

5 Atropine may also be given intramuscularly or via an endotracheal tube [40, 41] when it is rapidly effective at twice the intravenous dose.

6 Glycopyrrolate 0·01 mg kg^{-1} may have some advantages over atropine because it has minimal central excitatory effects, produces less tachycardia and arrhythmias and its effect outlasts neostigmine [42, 43].

Induction of anaesthesia

Anaesthesia may be induced by inhalation of volatile agents or intravenously (see Table 20.1). An individual anaesthetist may have a preference for one method over another but both techniques have their place depending on the child, the situation and the type of surgery proposed. Because of previous experience either good or bad, a child may prefer one technique over another and rarely a mother may transfer her preference to the child. Adequate preanaesthetic counselling by the anaesthesiologist and day-ward staff are essential in the preparation of the child.

It is inadvisable to offer the child a choice immediately prior to induction as chaos usually ensues as the child refuses first one and then the other. Care should be taken to pursue the agreed technique in a sympathetic yet firm manner. The child should be anaesthetized in the position in which it is happiest. If unwilling to leave parental contact anaesthesia may be induced by either the intravenous or inhalational routes with the child in its parent's arms or sitting on his or her knee.

Intravenous induction

As in adult patients intravenous induction is the preferred technique for infants and children of all ages in many paediatric centres since it ensures rapid anaesthesia, with a shortened period in which the child may object, thus reducing the opportunities for loss of control. Intravenous access for the administration of emergency as well as anaesthetic drugs, and for fluid infusion is secured before any intervention. Rapid induction is followed by rapid control of the airway and ability to quickly adjust the depth of anaesthesia throughout the surgical procedure.

Very small needles, high quality cannulae in small sizes and the introduction of a eutectic mixture of local anaesthetic (EMLA) cream for skin anaesthesia have improved the acceptance of the technique.

A limiting factor is the availability of satisfactory veins and the ability of the anaesthetist to cannulate them.

The best sites for venipuncture are in order: (a) the dorsum of the hand; (b) the 'fan' of superficial veins on the inner aspect of the wrist; and (c) the dorsum of the foot. Scalp veins and deeper veins should be avoided as a routine. Similarly the antecubital veins are frequently shrouded in adipose tissue and close to the brachial artery.

Suitable veins may be difficult to find in the 'chubby' infant, a frightened child, in cold weather with insufficient time to warm up, in children having frequent anaesthesia, e.g. chemotherapy or radiotherapy, and the child who has had extensive neonatal care.

EMLA cream should be applied at two sites selected preferably by the anaesthetist. Whilst not mandatory the application of EMLA cream is expected and allows the introduction of a small intravenous cannula where previously a needle or butterfly was used.

The efficacy of EMLA cream will be improved if:

1 The anaesthetist personally marks the places for application in biro or felt tip (preferably with a funny face).

2 Infants and young children have the occlusive dressing protected by an 'important' light bandage to prevent premature 'squidging' or eating by the patient.

3 At least 30 min and preferably 1 h is allowed before venepuncture.

4 Only the central non-adherent part of the occlusive dressing is removed prior to venepuncture thus avoiding pulling hairs.

Drugs should be prepared and syringes filled prior to the child entering the anaesthetic room. Since the procedure has already been explained there is no benefit in repeating that he or she is going to experience 'just a little scratch'.

Agents for intravenous induction (see Table 20.1)

Thiopentone is the most commonly used agent in hospital practice. Propofol has advantages of earlier and pleasant recovery in the older child but its use is not accompanied by earlier discharge times unless it is the sole agent. Methohexitone has many of the advantages of propofol at substantially smaller cost. The relative merits of the various agents are more fully discussed in Chapters 2 and 3.

Inhalational induction

Inhalational induction in the day-case patient is appropriate if a preference is indicated by the child or if there are no obvious veins for intravenous induction. An infant will usually accept a face mask if it is introduced slowly so that the child is semi-conscious when a seal with the face is made. If not already established, intravenous access must be secured immediately consciousness is lost since, although atropine and suxamethonium, the two drugs most likely to be needed, can be given intramuscularly albeit at twice the intravenous dose, their onset of action is delayed. When inhalational induction is planned in older children, their co-operation should be obtained since forced induction, although relatively rapid, is unpleasant for all concerned and will leave more of a lasting adverse impression on the child than a rapid intravenous induction.

Several techniques have been described to facilitate inhalational induction:

1 Removing the mask from the anaesthetic circuit and using the hands, moving slowly from a position a few inches from the face progressively nearer until the child is sufficiently sedated to accept the mask.

2 The use of lightweight transparent silicone rubber masks which are less intimidating.

3 Distraction by continuous conversation and praise or by telling a story.

4 Disguising the gaseous exit in a soft toy or as part of a personal stereo which also distracts the child whilst going to sleep.

5 Allowing the child to hold the mask and circuit only giving assistance as consciousness is lost.

6 The smell of the vapour can be camouflaged with an inexpensive cologne sprayed into the anaesthetic mask.

Before the face mask touches the face a high concentration of volatile agent should be administered in nitrous oxide with at least 30% oxygen. When a seal is made the concentration should be reduced, e.g. for halothane down to 0·5% and then increased slowly thereby reducing the incidence of coughing and breath holding. Once a concentration of 4% has been reached it can again be reduced this time to just above the minimum anaesthetic concentration for the agent.

Single breath induction

This technique can provide more rapid induction in children who will co-operate with the technique [44, 45]. The child is asked to breathe out as far as possible and then takes a deep breath from a circuit primed with 50% nitrous oxide in oxygen and, for example, 5% halothane thus receiving a vital capacity of anaesthetic gases. The child is then asked to breathe normally and the halothane concentration is reduced to 3%. Loss of eyelash reflex occurs considerably faster than with a conventional incremental increase in concentration. Similar techniques using isoflurane have been described [46–48].

Volatile agents for induction

Halothane remains the most suitable agent for the induction of anaesthesia. Its more acceptable odour and lower incidence of airway irritation give it advantages over isoflurane and enflurane which in spite of theoretical advantages, produce a slower induction due to breathholding, increased secretions and a higher incidence of laryngospasm. The new agent desflurane also has this problem (see Chapter 2).

Maintenance of anaesthesia

Following induction, anaesthesia is continued with either muscle relaxation, intubation and positive pressure ventilation or the inhalation of volatile agents. Ventilation will usually be controlled when:

1 Endotracheal intubation is required, thus reducing the work of inspiration.

2 For all but the shortest procedures in the infant.

3 When the child has a pre-existing cardiac or respiratory condition which might be adversely effected by the underventilation caused by respiratory or myocardial depression secondary to volatile agents.

The combination of supplementary local or regional analgesia reduces the concentration of volatile agent required and minimizes the risk of alveolar hypoventilation during spontaneous breathing [49].

Intraoperative narcotics

Narcotics can be used in the management of day-case patients either to supplement nitrous oxide and relaxant anaesthesia or to reduce the amount of volatile anaesthetic required with spontaneous ventilation. Narcotics can smooth induction and recovery and provide supplementary analgesia when a regional block is used for postoperative pain relief.

Care should be taken in the choice and dose of narcotic. Morphine and pethidine are associated with a prolonged period of drowsiness and postoperative nausea outlasting the analgesic effect. The intraoperative administration of fentanyl 0·001–0·002 mg kg^{-1} or alfentanil 0·03–0·05 mg kg^{-1} [50] do not increase the recovery time or prolong the time to discharge in comparison with halothane, and reduce the requirements for postoperative narcotics.

Securing the airway

The laryngeal mask (LM)

The Brain laryngeal mask [51] is an innovative device which provides a more secure airway than conventional airways (e.g. Guedel). It offers many of the advantages of endotracheal intubation without the disadvantage of laryngeal cannulation and possible irritation. After an initially cautious reception from the paediatric anaesthetic community, the device has established itself as a major development in anaesthetic technique.

The LM has been used to advantage in the control of the difficult airway [52–56] and as a guide for minimally invasive fibreoptic laryngoscopy and bronchoscopy [53, 58, 59].

Thorough technical instruction is provided [60] although modifications to the technique of insertion such as partial inflation of the cuff [61] and rotation in the oropharynx [62, 63] have been described.

The advantages of the device are:

1 A low resistance, low dead space airway requiring less inspiratory work in comparison with a tracheal tube to suit a child of comparable age [64]. This does not apply to the reinforced versions which have a reduced diameter and the same resistance as appropriate comparable tracheal tubes.

2 The airway is well tolerated at light planes of anaesthesia and is therefore suitable for sedative techniques in diagnostic and therapeutic radiology [65] and magnetic resonance imaging [66], and can be inserted under propofol alone. The mask maintains a good airway until return of protective reflexes if the patient is not disturbed [60] although some authors report a smoother transition to consciousness if the LM is removed during deeper anaesthesia [67].

3 Avoidance of intubating the larynx and possible trauma to the glottis or cricoid ring. This is especially important in diagnostic laryngoscopy.

Its principal disadvantages are:

1 The LM does not protect the airway from passive or active regurgitation although oropharyngeal secretions are excluded from the larynx.

2 The paediatric sizes of LM are derived from the adult versions and do not take into account the anatomical differences in children which may account for the higher incidence of abnormal positioning [68] compared with adults [69]. However the incidence of problems [70] approximates to the anaesthesiologist's paediatric experience [67, 71]. Position should only be accepted if unobstructed. Positive pressure ventilation can be practised without a leak at inflation pressures up to 15 cmH_2O.

3 The LM may be more easily displaced than a tracheal tube or Guedel airway during surgery. Continuous monitoring of the end tidal CO_2 concentration is essential to ensure continued correct positioning.

4 The LM has been associated with possible trauma to the pharyngeal wall with repeated use [72] and cuff pressure monitoring is recommended [60, 73].

5 There is a tendency for junior anaesthetists to rely on the LM rather than develop experience with the face mask or endotracheal intubation [74].

The mask can be introduced directly after propofol but if thiopentone or methohexitone have been used the anaesthetic should be deepened for example with an inhalational agent before insertion, to avoid airway problems such as laryngospasm and airway obstruction. Alternatively, a muscle relaxant may be used.

Tracheal intubation

Originally children were anaesthetized by inhalation of various mixtures of vapours during spontaneous breathing. From the 1960s this was replaced in several paediatric centres by intravenous induction, muscle relaxation, tracheal intubation and the maintenance of light anaesthesia with nitrous oxide and oxygen and opioid supplements during intermittent positive pressure ventilation. Tracheal intubation has been practised routinely for all day-care patients with few complications. With more modern volatile anaesthetics, better monitoring and the use of balanced anaesthesia, combining general with local anaesthetic, techniques have turned full circle and spontaneous respiration is again more popular and tracheal intubation is seldom required for the majority of day-case patients.

Reasons for avoiding routine tracheal intubation are:

1 Most procedures performed on children as day-cases do not require significant muscle relaxation and neither relaxants nor deep inhalational anaesthesia are indicated since in addition the majority of procedures are of short or very short duration.

2 Postextubation croup is avoided. The two main causative factors, traumatic intubation and chemical irritation can be avoided by careful technique and the use of disposable implant tested tubes [75]. However, when it occurs stridor is usually evident either at extubation or will usually develop within 1 h of extubation [76] but patients are usually observed over a longer period. Persistent stridor is an indication for admission and specific treatment with humidification, steroids and if necessary nebulized adrenaline.

3 The development of the LM which avoids intubation in procedures on the head and neck.

4 The avoidance of extubation laryngospasm creating a smoother transition from anaesthesia to consciousness.

The major advantage of tracheal intubation with ventilatory support is that the airway is secured and unaffected by surgical stimulation and will remain so until the procedure is completed.

Specific indications for tracheal intubation and positive pressure ventilation are emergency induction, an airway shared with the surgeon, any respiratory or cardiac condition which may be compromised by spontaneous inhalation of volatile agents, and infants who are more susceptible to the adverse respiratory effects of anaesthesia [49].

Technique of intubation. Modern disposable tubes in addition to being non-irritant have a thinner wall for a given internal diameter and thus have a lower resistance. An indication of the appropriate diameter is gained from the formula age divided by 4 plus 4·5 mm and approximating to the smaller size calculated. The tube should be lightly held between finger and thumb and no resistance should be felt at the cricoid ring after the glottis has been negotiated. Confirmation of correct size is achieved by the detection of a slight leak of gas when the airway is pressurized to approximately 25 cmH_2O. Larger leaks can be controlled by a throat pack rather than reintubation. Over the age of 10 years the size and shape of the cricoid ring becomes more unpredictable and a low pressure cuffed tracheal tube will avoid excessive leak or the selection of a tube which is unexpectedly too large.

Most tubes carry length markings from the tip. They should be passed according to the formula age divided by 2 plus 13 cm from the teeth. The absence of endobronchial intubation should always be confirmed by auscultation.

Primary dentition can be deceptively loose especially around 6 years and in addition to taking exceptional care, a 'tooth count' should be performed before and after intubation.

Muscle relaxants

As in adults, suxamethonium is usually avoided in children who are going to be active postoperatively. The incidence of muscle pains increases with age from up to 4% for 4 year olds to 23% for 14 year olds [77–79]. Its use is restricted to emergency control of the airway in severe laryngospasm or for short periods where the airway must be controlled in infants.

Pancuronium, alcuronium and D-tubocurare have been used routinely in day-case patients but their use has been superseded by atracurium and vecuronium which have an intermediate duration of action.

The low incidence of adverse effects, the cardiovascular stability and their prompt and complete reversal make atracurium and vecuronium equally suitable for day-cases of intermediate length. Atracurium 0·3 mg kg^{-1} i.v. or vecuronium 0·1 mg kg^{-1} i.v. can be completely reversed within 15 min or less depending on the return of a post-tetanic count of 2–6 when a peripheral nerve is stimulated. Incomplete spontaneous reversal should be antagonized by 0·035–0·07 mg kg^{-1} of neostigmine i.v. with 0·015–0·030 mg kg^{-1} of atropine i.v. [80].

Mivacurium has a duration of action between suxamethonium and vecuronium. Its fast recovery characteristics even after infusion should displace suxamethonium from use with the exception of the emergency situation. A dose of 0·1–0·2 mg kg^{-1} i.v. is recommended for children from 2 to 12 years with 95% recovery of block in 14–19 min [81, 82].

The duration of day-case procedures are too short to warrant infusions with the exception of mivacurium where 0·6–1·0 mg kg^{-1} h^{-1} i.v. will maintain 89–99% blockade. The degree of blockade is increased by the addition of any volatile agent.

Monitoring

Although many of the procedures may be of short duration there is a minimum acceptable standard of monitoring. This will include:

1 Pulse oximetry.
2 End tidal carbon dioxide concentration.
3 Electrocardiogram.
4 Non-invasive blood pressure.
5 Temperature monitoring.
6 Nerve stimulator for use with muscle relaxants.

The routine use of an oesophageal or precordial stethoscope has much to recommend it since it allows continued monitoring of heart and breath sounds and maintains vigilance when filling in records, is not affected by diathermy and is inexpensive.

Analgesia

Local anaesthesia can be used to provide the most effective analgesia lasting well into the postoperative period in the majority of patients. This may consist of local anaesthetic creams, instillation of local anaesthetic into the wound, infiltration, regional block or central or caudal block.

Non-steroidal anti-inflammatory drugs (NSAIDs) may be used to provide analgesia postoperatively, to supplement intraoperative narcotics or to provide analgesia when local analgesia wears off. They work by inhibiting prostaglandin synthesis thus minimizing the activation and sensitization of peripheral nociception. Ideally they should be started prior to the 'noxious' stimulus and continued until healing begins. Indomethacin has been used intravenously [83, 84], and diclofenac has been used rectally [85, 86]. Current interest is focused on the intravenous use of ketorolac 0·9 mg kg^{-1} during surgery [87, 88]. All these agents have been shown to provide improved analgesia with reduction of requirement for narcotic analgesia, without respiratory depression and an increased incidence of nausea and vomiting. It is likely, given the mode of action, that all these agents have a 'ceiling' effect and that their main use is in supplementing analgesia provided by regional local techniques or central narcotic action. All NSAIDs prolong bleeding time by blocking prostaglandin synthetase and inhibiting platelet aggregation. Increased perioperative bleeding has not been demonstrated with either diclofenac or ketorolac and their other complications are discussed in Chapter 2.

Paracetamol 15–20 mg kg^{-1} orally is most commonly used in a syrup base although suppositories can be introduced intraoperatively.

Short-acting opiates may be administered intraoperatively when a local block cannot be performed. Should a child require opiate analgesia postoperatively, admission will be required.

Anaesthetic equipment

A full range of face masks, oropharyngeal airways and tracheal tubes and straight bladed paediatric laryngoscopes are essential. Confusion sometimes occurs as to the type and size of anaesthetic circuit which should be used.

The Jackson Rees modification of Ayres T-piece has become the standard circuit for both controlled and spontaneous respiration. In young children, a hooded valve is necessary for effective scavenging of expired gasses and the Bain circuit is a convenient modification for all but the smallest child. The fresh gas flow should be adjusted to produce normocarbia for intermittent positive pressure ventilation which will involve a degree of rebreathing. Rebreathing should be avoided during spontaneous respiration. A capnograph is essential for adequate monitoring since the many formulae available provide no more than a guide [89].

The following recommendation will provide a starting point. Spontaneous breathing fresh gas flow (FGF) ml min^{-1}:

$$FGF = 3 \times (1000 + 100 \times kg)\ [90].$$

Controlled breathing:

$$FGF = (200 \times kg + 1000)\ [91].$$

Tidal volumes for controlled ventilation should be roughly twice normal at 12–15 ml kg^{-1}. At these volumes most adult ventilators can be adjusted to deliver volumes suitable for children of 10 kg or over. Pressure limited ventilators will ventilate patients of all sizes but are sensitive to changes in compliance.

The use of expensive volatile agents and the necessity for waste gas scavenging has encouraged the reintroduction and modification of the circle system with or without soda–lime. This is acceptable provided that the tubes have a low compliance, and smaller gauge. Resistance is greater than with the T-piece but much lower than that of a tracheal tube [92, 93]. End tidal carbon dioxide concentration, inspired oxygen concentration and vapour concentration monitoring are essential for the safe use of a circle system.

References

1 Watson BG. Blood glucose levels in children during surgery. *Br J Anaesth* 1972; 44: 712–15.
2 Jensen BH, Wernberg M, Anderson M. Preoperative starvation and blood glucose concentrations in children undergoing inpatient and outpatient anaesthesia. *Br J Anaesth* 1972; 54: 1071–4.
3 Aun CST, Panesar NS. Paediatric glucose homeostasis during anaesthesia. *Br J Anaesth* 1990; 64: 413–18.
4 Miller DC. Why are children starved? (Editorial). *Br J Anaesth* 1990; 64: 409–10.
5 Strunin L. How long should patients fast before surgery? Time for new guidelines (Editorial). *Br J Anaesth* 1993; 70: 1–3.
6 Splinter WM, Stewart JA, Muir JG. Effect of preoperative apple juice on gastric contents, thirst and hunger in children. *Can J Anaesth* 1989; 36: 55–8.

7 Splinter WM, Stewart JA, Muir JG. Large volumes of apple juice preoperatively do not affect gastric pH and volume in children. *Can J Anaesth* 1990; 37: 36–9.
8 Schweizer P, Warth H, Leriche C. Studies to be conducted before projected operations from the pediatric surgeon's point of view. *Eur J Pediatr Surg* 1991; 1: 135–8.
9 Astfalk W, Warth H, Leriche C. Day case surgery in childhood from the parents' point of view. *Eur J Pediatr Surg* 1991; 1: 323–7.
10 Coulson D. A proper place for parents. *Nursing Times* 1988; 84: 26–8.
11 Davenport HT, Valman B. Parents in the anaesthetic room (Letter). *Lancet* 1987; i: 45–6.
12 Hannallah RS, Rosales JK. Experience with parents' presence during anaesthesia induction in children. *Canad Anaesth Soc J* 1983; 30: 286–9.
13 Hickmott KC, Shaw EA, Goodyer I, Baker RD. Anaesthetic induction in children: the effects of maternal presence on mood and subsequent behaviour. *Eur J Anaesth* 1989; 6: 145–55.
14 Ryder IG, Spargo PM. Parents in the anaesthetic room. A questionnaire survey of parents' reactions. *Anaesthesia* 1991; 46: 977–9.
15 Kellow NH. Parents do not always want to be present at induction of anaesthesia of their children (Letter). *Anaesthesia* 1991; 46: 993.
16 Bevan JC, Johnston C, Haig MJ *et al.* Preoperative parental anxiety predicts behavioural and emotional responses to induction of anaesthesia in children. *Can J Anaesth* 1990; 37: 177–82.
17 Hannallah RS, Abramowitz MD, Oh TH, Ruttimann UE. Residents' attitudes toward parents' presence during anesthesia induction in children: does experience make a difference? *Anesthesiology* 1984; 60: 598–601.
18 Booker PD, Chapman DH. Premedication in children undergoing day-care surgery. *Br J Anaesth* 1979; 51: 1083.
19 Nicholson AC, Betts EK, Jobes DR *et al.* Comparison of oral and intramuscular preanaesthetic medication for pediatric inpatient surgery. *Anesthesiology* 1989; 71: 8.
20 Brustowicz RM, Nelson DA, Betts EK *et al.* Efficacy of oral premedication for pediatric outpatient surgery. *Anesthesiology* 1984; 60: 475.
21 Feld LH, Negus JB, White PF. Oral midazolam preanesthetic medication in pediatric outpatients. *Anesthesiology* 1990; 73: 831–4.
22 Payne KA, Coetzee AR, Mattheyse FJ. Midazolam and amnesia in pediatric premedication. *Acta Anaesth Belg* 1991; 42: 101–5.
23 Anderson BJ, Exarchos H, Lee K, Brown TC. Oral premedication in children: a comparison of chloral hydrate, diazepam, alprazolam, midazolam and placebo for day surgery. *Anaesth Intens Care* 1990; 18: 185–93.
24 Walbergh EJ, Wills RJ, Eckhert J. Plasma concentrations of midazolam in children following intranasal administration. *Anesthesiology* 1991; 74: 233–5.
25 Wilton NCT, Leigh J, Rosen DR, Pandit UA. Preanesthetic sedation of preschool children using intranasal midazolam. *Anesthesiology* 1988; 69: 972–5.
26 Twersky RS, Hartung J, Berger B, McClain J, Beaton C. Midazolam enhances anterograde but not retrograde amnesia in pediatric patients. *Anesthesiology* 1993; 78: 51–5.
27 Saint-Maurice C, Meistelman C, Rey E, Esteve C, de Lauture D, Olive G. The pharmacokinetics of rectal midazolam for premedication in children. *Anesthesiology* 1986; 65: 536–8.
28 Liu LMP, Goudsouzian NG, Liu PL. Rectal methohexital premedication in children: A dose-comparison study. *Anesthesiology* 1980; 53: 343–5.
29 Forbes RB, Murray DJ, Dull DL, Mahoney LT. Haemodynamic effects of rectal methohexitone for induction of anaesthesia in children. *Can J Anaesth* 1989; 36: 526–9.
30 Audenaert SM, Lock RL, Johnson GL, Pedigo NW Jr. Cardiovascular effects of rectal methohexital in children. *J Clin Anesth* 1992; 4: 116–19.

31 Daniels AL, Cote CJ, Polaner DM. Continuous oxygen saturation monitoring following rectal methohexitone induction in paediatric patients. *Can J Anaesth* 1992; 39: 27–30.
32 Goresky GV, Steward DJ. Rectal methohexitone for induction of anaesthesia in children. *Canad Anaesth Soc J* 1979; 26: 213–15.
33 Maltby JR, Watkins DM. Repeat ketamine anaesthesia of a child for radiotherapy in the prone position. *Can Anaesth Soc J* 1983; 30: 526–30.
34 Pedraz JL, Calvo MB, Lanao JM, Muriel C, Santos Lamas J, Dominguez-Gil A. Pharmacokinetics of rectal ketamine in children. *Br J Anaesth* 1989; 63: 671–4.
35 Holm-Knudsen R, Nygard E, Laub M. Rectal induction of anaesthesia in children. A comparison between ketamine–midazolam and halothane for induction and maintenance of anaesthesia. *Acta Anaesth Scand* 1989; 33: 518–21.
36 Khazzam A, Karkas A. Intramuscular methohexital as a sole pediatric anesthetic–analgesic agent. *Anesth Analg* 1972; 51: 895.
37 Hannallah RS, Patel RI. Low-dose intramuscular ketamine for anesthesia pre-induction in young children undergoing brief outpatient procedures. *Anesthesiology* 1989; 70: 598–600.
38 Gutstein HB, Johnson KL, Heard MB, Gregory GA. Oral ketamine preanesthetic medication in children. *Anesthesiology* 1992; 76: 28–33.
39 Lin SM, Liu K, Tsai SK, Lee TY. Rectal ketamine versus intranasal ketamine as premedicant in children. *Ma Tsui Hsueh Tsa Chi* 1990; 28: 177–83.
40 Bray BM, Jones HM, Grundy EM. Tracheal versus intravenous atropine. A comparison of the effects on heart rate. *Anaesthesia* 1987; 42: 1188–90.
41 Saarnivaara L, Kautto UM, Iisalo E, Pihlajamaki K. Comparison of pharmacokinetic and pharmacodynamic parameters following oral or intramuscular atropine in children. Atropine overdose in two small children. *Acta Anaesth Scand* 1985; 29: 529–36.
42 Ali-Melkkilä T, Kaila T, Kanto J. Glycopyrrolate, Pharmacokinetics and some pharmacodynamic findings. *Acta Anaesth Scand* 1989; 33: 513–17.
43 Warran P, Radford P, Manford MLM. Glycopyrrolate in children. *Br J Anaesth* 1981; 53: 1273–6.
44 Ruffle JM, Snider MT. Comparison of rapid and conventional inhalation inductions of halothane in healthy men and women. *Anesthesiology* 1987; 67: 584–7.
45 Liu LMP, Ryan JF. Modified single breath induction of anesthesia in children with halothane with and without nitrous oxide. *Anesthesiology* 1989; 71: A1008.
46 Lamberty JM, Wilson IH. Single breath induction of anaesthesia with isoflurane. *Br J Anaesth* 1987; 59: 1214–18.
47 Loper K, Reitan J, Benthuysen J, Snook L. Comparison of halothane and isoflurane for rapid anesthetic induction. *Anesth Analg* 1987; 66: 766–8.
48 Mackenzie JW. Rapid inhalational induction using isoflurane in children (Letter). *Anaesthesia* 1990; 45: 256.
49 Hatch D, Fletcher M. Anaesthesia and the ventilatory system in infants and young children. *Br J Anaesth* 1992; 68: 398–410.
50 Youngberg JA, Subaiya C, Graybar GB. Alfentanil for day-stay surgery in children: An evaluation. *Anesth Analg* 1984; 63: 213.
51 Brain AIJ. The laryngeal mask—a new concept in airway management. *Br J Anaesth* 1983; 55: 801–5.
52 Chadd GD, Crane DL, Phillips RM, Tunell WP. Extubation and reintubation guided by the laryngeal mask airway in a child with the Pierre-Robin syndrome. *Anesthesiology* 1992; 76: 640–1.
53 Brimacombe J. The laryngeal mask airway and flexible bronchoscopy. *Thorax* 1991; 46: 740.
54 Ebata T, Nishiki S, Masuda A, Amaha K. Anaesthesia for Treacher Collins syndrome using a laryngeal mask airway. *Can J Anaesth* 1991; 38: 1043–5.

55 Walker RW, Murrell D. Yet another use for the laryngeal mask airway (Letter). *Anaesthesia* 1991; 46: 591.
56 Ravalia A, Goddard JM. The laryngeal mask and difficult tracheal intubation (Letter). *Anaesthesia* 1990; 45: 168.
57 Beveridge ME. Laryngeal mask anaesthesia for repair of cleft palate. *Anaesthesia* 1989; 44: 656–7.
58 Maekawa H, Mikawa K, Tanaka O, Goto R, Obara H. The laryngeal mask may be a useful device for fiberoptic airway endoscopy in pediatric anesthesia (Letter). *Anesthesiology* 1991; 75: 169–70.
59 McNamee CJ, Meyns B, Pagliero KM. Flexible bronchoscopy via the laryngeal mask: a new technique. *Thorax* 1991; 46: 141–2.
60 Brain AIJ. *The Intavent Laryngeal Mask Instruction Manual*, 2nd edn. Intavent, 1991.
61 Newman PTF. Insertion of a partially inflated laryngeal mask airway. *Anaesthesia* 1991; 46: 235.
62 Chow BFM, Lewis M, Jones SEF. Laryngeal mask airway in children: insertion technique (Letter). *Anaesthesia* 1991; 46: 590–1.
63 McNicol LR. Insertion of laryngeal mask airway in children (Letter; comment). *Anaesthesia* 1991; 46: 330.
64 Bhatt SB, Kendall AP, Lin ES, Oh TE. Resistance and additional inspiratory work imposed by the laryngeal mask airway. *Anaesthesia* 1992; 47: 343–7.
65 Grebenick CR, Ferguson C, White A. The laryngeal mask airway in paediatric radiotherapy. *Anesthesiology* 1990; 72: 474–7.
66 Langton JA, Wilson IG, Fell D. Use of the laryngeal mask airway during magnetic resonance imaging. *Anaesthesia* 1992; 47: 532.
67 McGinn G, Haynes SR, Morton NS. An evaluation of the laryngeal mask airway during routine paediatric anaesthesia. *Paediatr Anaesth* 1993; 3: 23–8.
68 Rowbottom SJ, Simpson DL, Grubb D. The laryngeal mask in children. A fibreoptic assessment of positioning. *Anaesthesia* 1991; 46: 489–91.
69 Payne J. The use of the fibreoptic laryngoscope to confirm the position of the laryngeal mask. *Anaesthesia* 1989; 44: 865.
70 Mason DG, Bingham RM. The laryngeal mask airway in children. *Anaesthesia* 1990; 45: 760–3.
71 Bailie R, Barnett MB, Fraser JF. The Brain laryngeal mask. A comparative study with the nasal mask in paediatric dental outpatient anaesthesia. *Anaesthesia* 1991; 46: 358–60.
72 Marjot R. Trauma to the posterior pharyngeal wall caused by a laryngeal mask airway. *Anaesthesia* 1991; 46: 589–90.
73 Marjot R. Pressure exerted by the laryngeal mask airway cuff upon the pharyngeal mucosa. *Br J Anaesth* 1993; 70: 25–9.
74 Wilson IG. The laryngeal mask airway in paediatric practice. *Br J Anaesth* 1993; 70: 124–5.
75 Koka BV, Jeon IS, Andre JM *et al.* Postintubation croup in children. *Anesth Analg* 1977; 56: 501.
76 Steward DJ. Outpatient paediatric anesthesia. *Anesthesiology* 1975; 43: 268.
77 Bush GH, Roth F. Muscle pains after suxamethonium in children. *Br J Anaesth* 1961; 33: 151–5.
78 Lyle DJR. Suxamethonium pains in outpatient children. *Anaesthesia* 1982; 37: 774–5.
79 Morton NS. Modern paediatric day case anaesthesia: a review. *Paediatr Anaesth* 1992; 2: 235–44.
80 Meakin G, Sweet PT, Bevan JC *et al.* Neostigmine and edrophonium as antagonists of pancuronium in infants and children. *Anesthesiology* 1983; 59: 316–21.
81 Basta SJ. Clinical pharmacology of mivacurium chloride: a review. *J Clin Anesth* 1992; 4: 153–63.
82 Goudsouzian NG, Alifimoff JK, Eberly C *et al.* Neuromuscular and cardiovascular effects of mivacurium in children. *Anesthesiology* 1989; 70: 237–42.
83 Maunuksela EL, Olkkola KT, Korpela R. Does prophylactic intravenous infusion of indomethacin improve the management of postoperative pain in children? *Can J Anaesth* 1988; 35: 123–7.
84 Maunuksela EL, Olkkola KT, Korpela R. Intravenous indomethacin as postoperative analgesic in children: acute effects on blood pressure, heart rate, body temperature and bleeding. *Ann Clin Res* 1987; 19: 359–63.

85 Bone ME, Fell D. A comparison of rectal diclofenac with intramuscular papaveretum or placebo for pain relief following tonsillectomy. *Anaesthesia* 1988; 43: 277–80.
86 Moores MA, Wandless JG, Fell D. Paediatric postoperative analgesia. A comparison of rectal diclofenac with caudal bupivacaine after inguinal herniotomy. *Anaesthesia* 1990; 45: 156–8.
87 Watcha MF, Jones MB, Lagueruela RG, Schweiger C, White PF. Comparison of ketorolac and morphine as adjuvants during pediatric surgery. *Anesthesiology* 1992; 76: 368–72.
88 Olkkola KT, Maunuksela EL. The pharmacokinetics of postoperative intravenous ketorolac tromethamine in children. *Br J Clin Pharmacol* 1991; 31: 182–4.
89 Badgwell JM, Wolf AR, McEvedy BA, Lerman J, Creighton RE. Fresh gas formulae do not accurately predict end-tidal Pco_2 in paediatric patients. *Can J Anaesth* 1988; 35: 581–6.
90 Lindahl SG, Charlton AJ, Hatch DJ. Accuracy of prediction of fresh gas flow requirements during spontaneous breathing with the T-piece. *Eur J Anaesth* 1984; 1: 269–74.
91 Hatch DJ, Yates AP, Lindahl SG. Flow requirements and rebreathing during mechanically controlled ventilation in a T-piece (Mapleson E) system. *Br J Anaesth* 1987; 59: 1533–40.
92 Rasch DK, Bunegin L, Ledbetter J, Kaminskas D. Comparison of circle absorber and Jackson Rees systems for paediatric anaesthesia. *Can J Anaesth* 1988; 35: 25–30.
93 Conterato JP, Lindahl SG, Meyer DM, Bires JA. Assessment of spontaneous ventilation in anesthetized children with use of a pediatric circle or a Jackson Rees system. *Anesth Analg* 1989; 69: 484–90.

Chapter 21
Local Anaesthesia for Paediatric Day-Case Surgery

N. S. Morton

The mainstay of perioperative analgesia in modern paediatric day-case practice is provided by techniques involving local anaesthesia. These give reliable pain relief and avoid the need for opioids with their potential for inducing sedation and emesis [1]. During balanced anaesthesia the depth of general anaesthesia may be reduced as the local anaesthetic block takes effect which may subsequently hasten the recovery of consciousness and reduce side effects. When local anaesthetics are used to pre-empt pain in this way, the general quality of recovery is much improved.

Surface anaesthesia can be provided for the skin, conjunctiva, urethra, eardrum and oral mucosa by local anaesthetics formulated as creams, drops, gels or sprays (Table 21.1). Simply instilling local anaesthetic solution into small superficial surgical wounds provides acceptable analgesia [2]. Infiltrating local anaesthetic around superficial lesions or into wound edges is also very effective [3, 4].

Peripheral nerve blocks with the long acting amide local anaesthetic bupivacaine give excellent results (Table 21.2), and are relatively non-invasive and free of serious complications. Caudal epidural block can safely be used for paediatric day-case surgery but is more invasive and can have more serious complications [5].

Surface anaesthesia

Skin

The formulation of lignocaine and prilocaine as a eutectic mixture of local anaesthetics (EMLA cream, Astra Pharmaceuticals) has revolutionized the management of painful surface procedures in children. When applied to the skin for 1 h under an occlusive dressing, excellent analgesia is produced for venepuncture and venous cannulation [6]. Small surface lesions such as naevi may be excised using EMLA or, alternatively, prepreparation of a lesion with EMLA may be preferred prior to local infiltration with bupivacaine. If this is carried out using a very fine needle, 27 or 30 G, with warmed local anaesthetic solution and a slow rate of injection, stinging and discomfort on injection will be minimized. A similar procedure can be used, for example, for muscle biopsies, arthrograms, lumbar puncture and injection into implanted subcutaneous reservoirs for venous access [7].

Alternatives to EMLA are being actively researched, because EMLA requires a

Table 21.1 Surface anaesthesia

Site	Formulation
Skin	EMLA cream Amethocaine gel Amethocaine patch Liposomal amethocaine Lignocaine + GAMPh
Eardrum	EMLA cream
Prepuce	EMLA cream Lignocaine gel Lignocaine ointment Lignocaine spray
Conjunctiva	Amethocaine drops
Urethra	Lignocaine gel
Anus	Lignocaine gel
Surface wounds	Bupivacaine instillation Bupivacaine infiltration

EMLA, eutectic mixture of local anaesthetics.

Table 21.2 Peripheral nerve blocks for paediatric day-cases

Penile block
Ilioinguinal/iliohypogastric nerve block
Digital nerve block
Metacarpal block
Metatarsal block
Great auricular nerve block
Dental blocks

prolonged application time and tends to produce vasoconstriction unless it has been in place for more than 2 h [6]. The most promising to date are amethocaine, in a gel, patch or liposomal formulation, and lignocaine with the absorption promoter GAMPh (Table 21.1) [6]. Amethocaine has a quicker onset of action, produces more prolonged analgesia at the site of application and tends to produce vasodilation.

Eardrum

Myringotomies have also been performed in older co-operative children after the application of EMLA [8]. Concern has been expressed about ototoxicity of prilocaine should it enter the middle ear [9]. However, no clinical or audiogram evidence of toxicity was found in a recent study [8].

Prepuce

Preputial adhesions may be divided after EMLA has been placed under the foreskin for 1 h [10]. The application of lignocaine as a spray, ointment or gel to the circumcision site while the child is still anaesthetized provides remarkably good postoperative analgesia [11] (Table 21.1). Pain relief is equivalent to that provided by morphine or penile block. Applications can be repeated, for example by the parents at home. The spray may be more useful, in that direct contact with the operation site is not required to apply the local anaesthetic. However, the spray is more concentrated (100 mg ml^{-1}; 10 mg per metered dose) and more expensive than the ointment (50 mg ml^{-1}) or the gel (20 mg ml^{-1}).

Conjunctiva

Amethocaine drops (0·5 or 1·0%) provide excellent surface analgesia of the eye after surgery for strabismus [12]. The drops should be instilled in divided doses at the start and at the end of surgery to achieve better 'pre-emptive' analgesia. The child should awaken pain free and pain relief will last about 3 h. Paracetamol, diclofenac, ketorolac or dihydrocodeine should be started before the local anaesthetic wears off. An alternative is to teach the parents how to instil amethocaine drops and give them enough for use at home to cover the first 12–24 h period. When this approach is used, particularly with propofol induction and/or maintenance of anaesthesia and the use of a laryngeal mask airway instead of tracheal intubation, the incidence of troublesome postoperative emesis is less than 10% (personal observations).

Surface wounds

Instillation of bupivacaine into small open surgical wounds is as effective as peripheral nerve blockade [2] but probably provides a shorter period of effective postoperative analgesia.

Infiltration of inguinal wounds with bupivacaine is as effective as peripheral nerve or caudal epidural blockade [4, 13] and does not produce excessive systemic blood concentrations of local anaesthetic [3]. Many other surface wounds are amenable to local infiltration at the time of wound closure.

For correction of prominent ears, the pinna can be readily infiltrated with bupivacaine, adrenaline and hyaluronidase *prior* to the surgical incision and this produces both excellent analgesia and haemostasis.

Peripheral nerve blockade

Dorsal nerve of penis block (penile block)

The dorsal nerves of the penis are terminal branches of the pudendal nerve which has contributions from spinal levels S2, S3 and S4. The dorsal nerves are blocked during their passage through a triangular fascial compartment formed by the division of the suspensory ligament of the penis where it fuses with Buck's fascia, the circumferential sheath which envelopes the shaft of the penis. The corpora cavernosa form the base of this triangle and the symphysis pubis its 'apex'. The nerves lie lateral to the dorsal artery and veins and give off a ventral branch within the fascial triangle [14].

Two main techniques of penile block are used, namely midline or paramedian. Both techniques rely on deposition of plain, non-adrenaline containing 0·5% bupivacaine (0·5–4 ml) in the fascial compartment where the dorsal nerves lie. This subfascial plane may have septae within it which prevent even spread. The midline technique (Fig. 21.1) is a single injection method but carries the risks of (a) damage to the dorsal vessels with haematoma formation; and (b) intravascular injection with the possibility of failed block and local anaesthetic toxicity. The paramedian technique (Fig. 21.2) [15] reduces these risks and can be performed bilaterally to ensure complete circumferential spread deep to Buck's fascia. A neglected sign of circumferential spread is simple visual inspection of the root of the penile shaft which shows a 'fullness' and slight pallor immediately after the block has been performed (Fig. 21.3). If this is noted all the way round the base of the penis then the block is invariably excellent and long lasting (N. S. Morton, personal observation).

The commonest mistake when attempting penile blocks is to inject the local anaesthetic too superficially. This should be detected at the time of injection as a superficial swelling which does not spread circumferentially. If the local anaesthetic is not within the previously described fascial plane, the block will be ineffective. The younger infant and neonate often have up to 1 cm of subcutaneous fat overlying the symphysis pubis and this may make appreciation of the depth of needle placement more difficult. The 'click' described by many authors on passing through the fascial plane is not so obvious in small children, especially with modern very sharp disposable needles.

Other common causes of failure of this block are intravascular injection and too deep injection into the corpora cavernosa. Gentle aspiration prior to injection should help to detect these.

It is important to stress that adrenaline should *not* be used in the local anaesthetic solution for penile blocks as tissue necrosis could result from constriction of end arteries. The volume injected should be matched to the size of the child so that the tension within the fascial compartment does not cause venous obstruction and subsequent oedema and swelling of the operation site.

Penile blocks are difficult to learn and should be taught under the close supervision of an experienced member of the senior staff. They are however more effective than caudal epidural blockade [5].

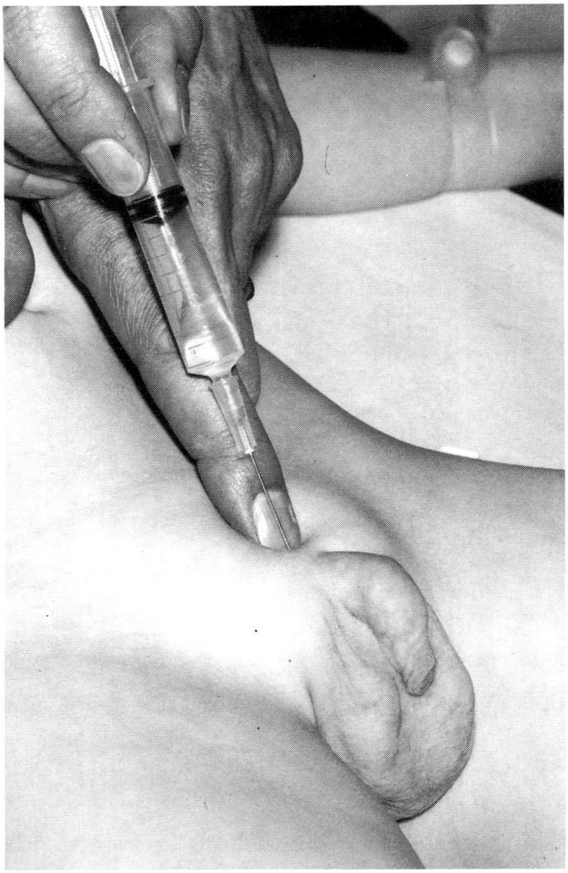

Fig. 21.1 Midline technique for penile block.

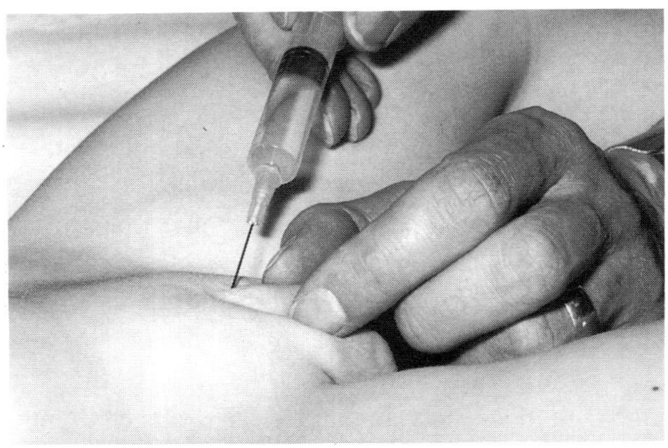

Fig. 21.2 Paramedian technique for penile block.

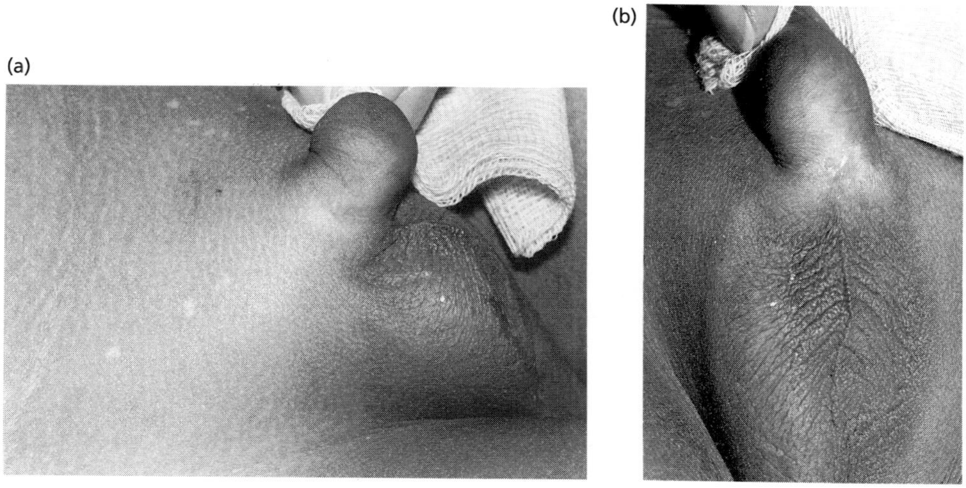

Fig. 21.3 (a) Circumferential fullness and slight pallor after injection at the base of the shaft of the penis (b) indicate that the local anaesthetic has been deposited in the correct plane deep to Buck's fascia.

Ilioinguinal/iliohypogastric nerve block (inguinal block)

For operations in the inguinal region, the ilioinguinal/iliohypogastric combined block is as effective as caudal epidural block [16]. These nerves are conveniently blocked together using a single injection technique in anaesthetized children. A short bevelled needle is inserted through the skin and subcutaneous tissues at a distance equivalent to one patient-finger's breadth medial to the anterior superior iliac spine (Fig. 21.4). The tip of the needle will now rest on the external oblique aponeurosis and with gentle pressure will 'pop' through into the subaponeurotic plane which can then be filled up with 0·25% bupivacaine. The terminal branches of the ilioinguinal, iliohypogastric and subcostal nerves run in this plane and are readily blocked by a volume of 0·3 ml kg^{-1} without fanwise injections as some authors recommend [17]. A further 0·1 ml kg^{-1} injected as the needle is withdrawn (from a redirected position deep to the internal oblique muscle on the inner aspect of the ilium) to the subcutaneous tissues will improve the success of this block because of variations in the pattern of terminal branching.

This block is very suitable for inguinal herniotomy incisions and also the inguinal incision for orchidopexy. The scrotal incision, however, may not be covered by this block. The ilioinguinal nerve supplies the upper anterior part of the scrotum which can be used for siting the incision to create a dartos pouch. Many surgeons, however, use a more distal incision which must be separately infiltrated with bupivacaine.

This block will fail if the injection is made too superficially. Care must be taken to avoid penetrating the peritoneal cavity and to avoid injection too near to the inguinal ligament as this risks blockade of branches of the femoral nerve supplying the quadriceps with resultant leg weakness.

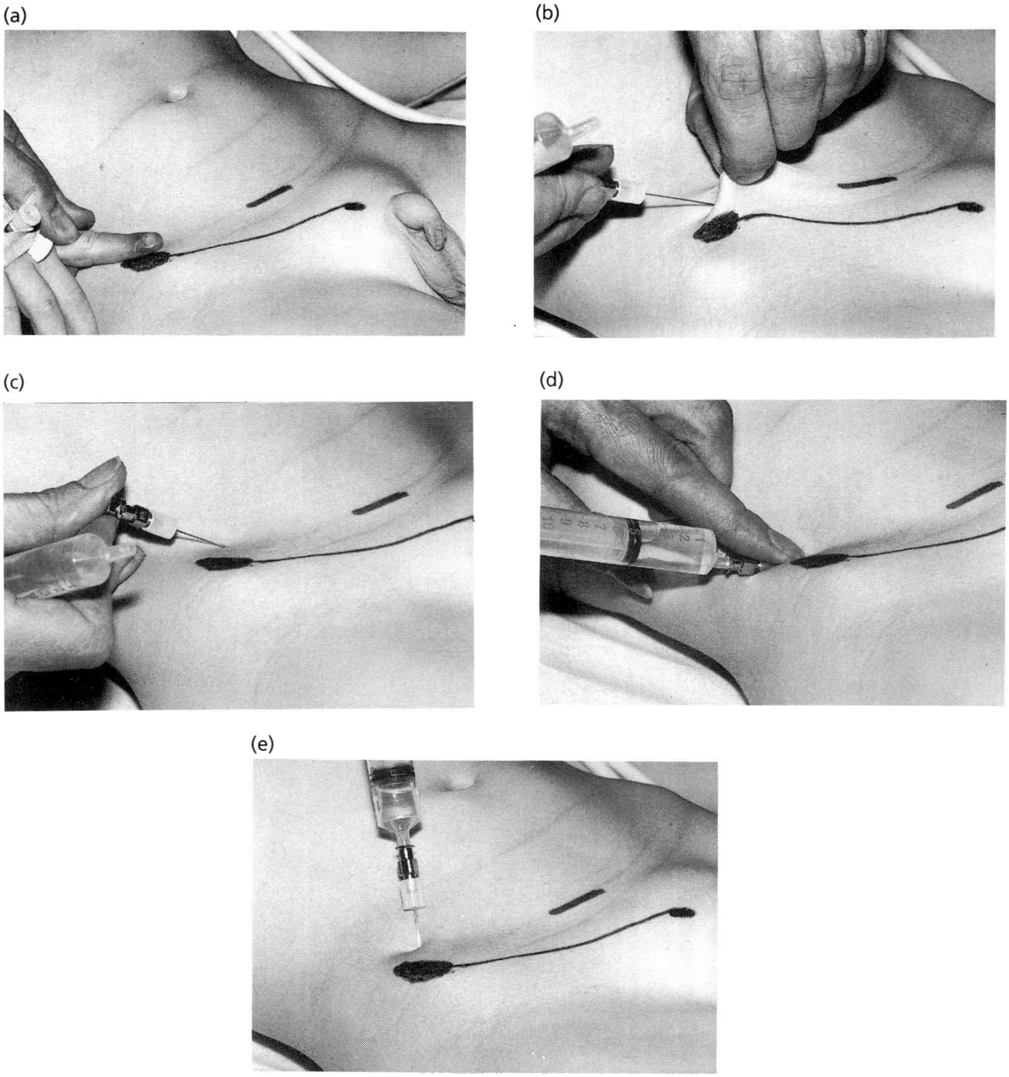

Fig. 21.4 Ilioinguinal/iliohypogastric blocks (a) the anterior superior iliac spine is identified and the injection is made one patient-finger's breadth medial to it; (b) a fold of skin is lifted to help insertion of a short bevelled local block needle; (c) the needle is advanced through the external oblique aponeurosis; (d) two-thirds of the local anaesthetic dose is given; and (e) the remainder placed on the inner aspect of the iliac crest.

Digital nerve block

Toes and fingers may be blocked in older children using the ring block technique (Fig. 21.5). Care must be taken not to use too large a volume of local anaesthetic as this may cause circumferential constriction of the venous drainage or arterial blood supply to the digit. Adrenaline should *not* be used in the local anaesthetic solution because of the

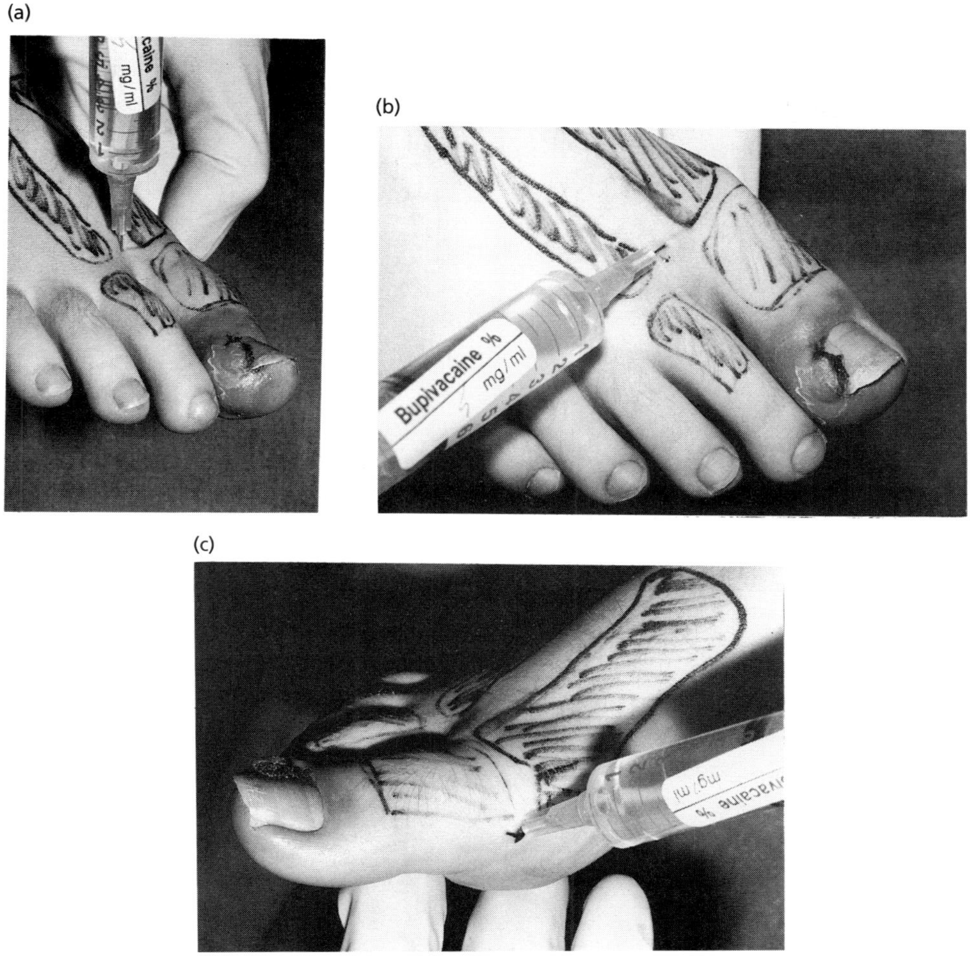

Fig. 21.5 (a–c) Digital nerve block (ring block) of great toe.

risk of severe vasoconstriction with ischaemic damage to the tissues and possibly the innervation.

Metatarsal or metacarpal blocks using plain bupicavaine solutions are an alternative and are to be preferred in younger children to avoid digital compression noted above (Fig. 21.6).

Great auricular nerve block

This nerve is readily blocked by a subcutaneous infiltration of 2–5 ml of bupivacaine 0·25 or 0·5% to raise a bleb between the posterior border of the base of the mastoid process and the angle of the mandible (Fig. 21.7). This will produce anaesthesia of the posterior surface of the ear for otoplasty which will last for several hours. With this

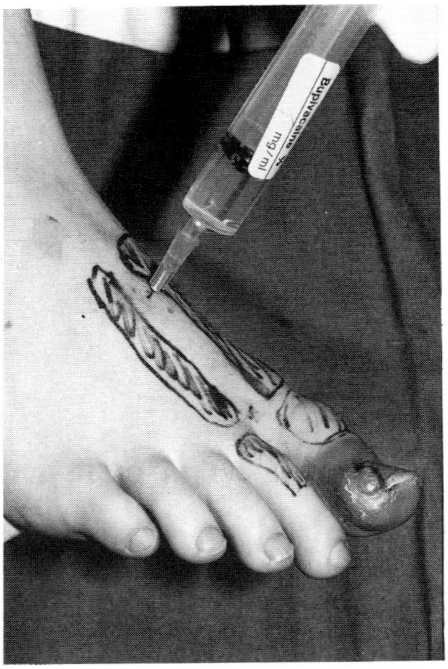

Fig. 21.6 Metatarsal block.

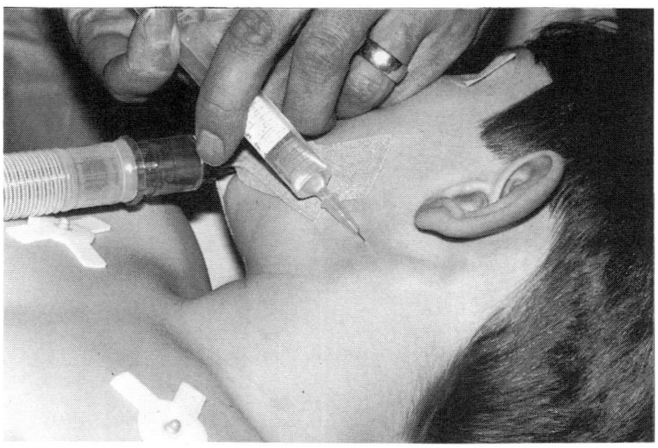

Fig. 21.7 Great auricular nerve blockade for otoplasty.

block for postoperative analgesia, opioids are not required and nausea and vomiting will be minimized.

Caudal epidural block

Access to the caudal epidural space via the sacrococcygeal membrane is often easier in children than in adults. The landmarks for the sacral hiatus, the sacral cornua, may be visible in thinner children (Fig. 21.8). They are usually palpable as the apex of an equilateral triangle whose base is formed by the posterior inferior iliac spines. The hiatus itself is usually approximately the size and shape of the child's thumbnail but considerably anatomical variation occurs including absence of a hiatus, a long thin slit

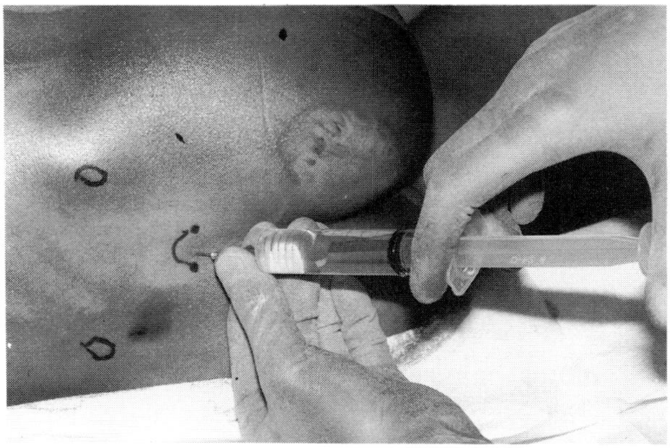

Fig. 21.8 A caudal epidural block in a child.

or a broad defect. In younger infants the dural sac may extend distally to the level of the body of the second or third sacral vertebrae and care must be taken to avoid dural puncture.

An aseptic technique is advisable even for single shot caudal epidural blocks. A maximum dose of 2 mg kg^{-1} of bupivacaine should be used and the volume may be reasonably calculated as 0·05 ml kg^{-1} per segment to be blocked [18]. Thus for a circumcision (S1–S5) 0·25 ml kg^{-1} is adequate while for an orchidopexy (T8–S5) 0·75 ml kg^{-1} will be required.

Many anaesthetists use larger volumes with the aim of spreading the solution higher and thereby perhaps prolonging the block [19]. Thus a simplified volume schedule would be 0·5 ml kg^{-1} for a circumcision, 1·0 ml kg^{-1} for a herniotomy and 1·25 ml kg^{-1} for an orchidopexy. Care must be taken with these larger volumes to check that the maximum allowable mass of bupivacaine is not exceeded, namely 2 mg kg^{-1}. Some authors are now suggesting that 3 mg kg^{-1} is safe in the anaesthetized child because general anaesthesia raises the threshold for local anaesthetic toxicity. It should be remembered, however, that the systemic uptake from the caudal epidural space is large and rapid, second only to intercostal nerve blockade. It may be prudent therefore to either add adrenaline to limit the peak plasma concentration or to limit the total mass of drug. Wolf *et al.* [20] found no benefit in terms of analgesic efficacy and duration, from using solutions more concentrated than 0·125% bupivacaine for single shot caudal epidural blocks. Indeed the incidence of motor blockade was significantly less when 0·125% bupivacaine was compared with 0·25% solution. This is particularly relevant to day-case surgery where ability to ambulate is one of the criteria for discharge. Problems with caudal epidural analgesia therefore include technical difficulty in finding the sacral hiatus, subarachnoid injection in small infants, intravascular injection, motor blockade, urinary retention and nausea and vomiting. The latter may be induced by a rise in cerebrospinal fluid pressure. Epidural haematoma, abscess and implantation dermoid tumours are also possible complications. Many anaesthetists now favour the less invasive peripheral nerve blocks for paediatric day-case work because they have been shown in most comparative studies to be equally effective if not superior to caudal epidural blockade [5, 16].

Systemic analgesics for paediatric day-cases

It is important to anticipate the local anaesthetic wearing off and prevent severe pain breaking through. Systemic analgesics should be given regularly prophylactically and parents need clear instructions on this point. These can be continued for 24–48 h at home.

For mild pain and as an adjunct, paracetamol (15–20 mg kg^{-1}, 4–6-hourly, orally or rectally) is well tolerated by most children and at least the oral route is familiar to most parents.

For moderate pain, as an adjunct, for pre-emptive analgesia and as part of a balanced analgesic technique, the non-steroidal anti-inflammatory drugs are very useful. Diclofenac (1 mg kg^{-1}, 6-hourly, rectally), ketorolac (0·5 mg kg^{-1}, 6-hourly, i.m. or i.v.) or ibuprofen (2·5–10 mg kg^{-1}, 6-hourly, orally) are convenient for children. (See Chapter 2 for recent recommendations regarding the reduction of the adult dose of ketorolac by 66%.)

For severe breakthrough pain or failed local analgesia, opioids may have to be considered. Codeine (0·5–1·0 mg kg^{-1}, 4–6-hourly, orally, rectally or i.m.), dihydrocodeine (0·5 mg kg^{-1}, 4–6-hourly, orally) or morphine (0·1–0·2 mg kg^{-1}, titrated i.v. or i.m.) may be required. This latter group may require inpatient admission for pain control and access to such care must be available.

Conclusions

Appropriate use of local anaesthetic techniques is an essential part of modern paediatric day-case anaesthesia. The provision of excellent analgesia on awakening considerably simplifies postoperative care and the quality of recovery is greatly enhanced. There is a need for these techniques to be more widely taught and used as paediatric day-case surgery expands. Training under consultant supervision in day-surgery units must be organized so that children are not subjected to the vagaries of the trainees' learning curves.

References

1 Cohen MM, Cameron CB, Duncan PG. Paediatric anaesthesia morbidity and mortality in the perioperative period. *Anesth Analg* 1990; 70: 160–7.

2 Casey WF, Rice LJ, Hannallah RS, Broadman L, Norden JM, Guzzetta P. A comparison between bupivacaine instillation versus ilioinguinal/iliohypogastric nerve block for postoperative analgesia following inguinal herniorrhaphy in children. *Anesthesiology* 1990; 72: 637–9.

3 Mobley KA, Wandless JG, Fell D. Serum bupivacaine concentrations following wound infiltration in children undergoing inguinal herniotomy. *Anaesthesia* 1991; 46: 500–1.

4 Reid MF, Harris R, Phillips PD, Barker I, Pereira NH, Bennett NR. Day case herniotomy in children. A comparison of ilioinguinal nerve block and wound infiltration for postoperative analgesia. *Anaesthesia* 1987; 42: 658–61.
5 Vater M, Wandless J. Caudal or dorsal nerve block? A comparison of two local anaesthetic techniques for post-operative analgesia following day case circumcision. *Acta Anaesth Scand* 1985; 29: 175–9.
6 Freeman JA, Doyle E, Ng TI, Morton NS. Topical anaesthesia of the skin: a review. *Paediatr Anaesth* 1993; in press.
7 Halperin DL, Koren G, Attias D, Pellegrini E, Greenberg ML, Wyss M. Topical skin anaesthesia for venous, subcutaneous drug reservoir and lumbar punctures in children. *Pediatrics* 1989; 84: 281–4.
8 Bingham B, Hawke M, Halik J. The safety and efficacy of EMLA cream topical anaesthesia for myringotomy and ventilation tube insertion. *J Otolaryngol* 1991; 20: 193–5.
9 Anniko M, Schmidt S. The ototoxic potential of EMLA. *Acta Otolaryngol* 1988; 105: 255–65.
10 MacKinlay GA. Save the prepuce. Painless separation of preputial adhesions in the outpatient clinic. *Br Med J* 1988; 297: 590–1.
11 Tree-Trakarn T, Piryavaraporn S. Post-operative pain relief for circumcision in children: a comparison among morphine, nerve block and topical analgesia. *Anesthesiology* 1985; 62: 519–22.
12 Watson DM. Topical amethocaine in strabismus surgery. *Anaesthesia* 1991; 46: 368–70.
13 Fell D, Derrington MC, Taylor E, Wandless JG. Paediatric post-operative analgesia. *Anaesthesia* 1988; 43: 107–10.
14 Brown TCK, Weidner NJ, Bouwmeester J. Dorsal nerve of penis block—anatomical and radiological studies. *Anaesth Intens Care* 1989; 17: 34–8.
15 Soliman MG, Tremblay NA. Nerve block of the penis for post-operative pain relief in children. *Anesth Analg* 1978; 57: 495.
16 Hannallah RS, Broadman LM, Belman AB. Comparison of caudal and ilioinguinal/iliohypogastric nerve blocks for control of postorchiopexy pain in pediatric ambulatory surgery. *Anesthesiology* 1987; 66: 832–4.
17 Alifimoff JK, Cote CJ. Pediatric regional anesthesia. In: Cote CJ, Ryan JF, Todres ID, Goudsouzian NG, eds *A Practice of Anesthesia for Infants and Children*, 2nd edn. Philadelphia: WB Saunders, 1993; 429–50.
18 Takasaki M, Dohi S, Kawabata Y. Dosage of lidocaine for caudal anesthesia in infants and children. *Anesthesiology* 1977; 47: 527–9.
19 Armitage EN. Caudal block in children. *Anaesthesia* 1979; 34: 396.
20 Wolf A, Valley RD, Fear DW. Bupivacaine for caudal analgesia in infants and children: the optimal effective concentration. *Anesthesiology* 1988; 69: 102–6.

Part 3:
Procedural Safety

Chapter 22
Issues Involved in Safe Practice

D. M. Nolan

This review of procedural safety will identify those factors which may reduce the overall safety and effectiveness of anaesthesia administered for day-case surgical procedures.

A surgical day-case may be defined as a patient who is admitted for investigation or operation as a planned procedure on a non-resident basis who none the less requires facilities for recovery [1]. Technically, this definition excludes minor operative procedures undertaken in outpatient or accident and emergency departments but a short review of the special problems associated with this group of patients will be included (see Appendix 1).

The established rationale behind the development of day-care surgical units is convenience for the patient and also benefits in costs not only for the patient but also for the institutions providing surgical services and the health-care system as a whole. Benefits to the patient include:

1 Reduced disruption of personal life.

2 Reduced risk of postoperative infection.

3 Reduced family costs in terms of travelling and extra needs imposed by an inpatient stay.

4 Reduced cancellation risk compared to 'inpatients' who not infrequently lose their beds to emergency patients.

Benefits to the institution include:

1 Increased patient throughput.

2 Easing of pressure on some acute surgical specialties.

3 Reduction of waiting lists.

4 Saving in hospital 'hotel' costs.

5 Easier recruitment and retention of nursing staff due to lack of night duties and weekend working.

Organizational and clinical standards must be of the highest order at each stage of the progression of the patient through day-case surgery if the benefits for both the patient and institution are not to be outweighed by problems arising as a result of this process.

Between 1990 and 1991 a series of reports were published which emphasized the importance of day-case surgery. The Value for Money Unit of the National Health Service Management Executive produced recommendations in 1989 within the Bevan

Table 22.1 The Audit Commission's basket of procedure

Inguinal hernia repair	Orchidopexy
Excision of breast lump	Cataract extraction
Anal fissure excision	Correction of squint
Varicose vein stripping or excision	Myringotomy
Cystoscopy, diagnostic and operative	Submucous resection
Circumcision	Reduction of nasal fracture
Excision of Dupuytren's contracture	Operation for bat ears
Carpal tunnel decompression	Dilatation and currettage
Arthroscopy, diagnostic and operative	Laparoscopy
Excision of ganglion	Termination of pregnancy

report [2] on the subject of day-case surgery. The same unit subsequently expanded the recommendations in 1991 with the publication of *Day Surgery: Making it Happen* [3]. This document attempts to assist those individuals involved in setting up day-case units. It recommended development of protocols for patient selection, that only suitably qualified surgeons and anaesthetists should undertake the work and that the organizational support mechanism, e.g. clerical staff, should be the best available to ensure the smooth running of such units.

The Audit Commission became responsible for auditing the Health Service in the UK in October 1990. During that month it published *A Short Cut to Better Services* [4]. It commented that despite the clear advantages of day-case surgery and the documented reduction in costs of approximately 30% compared with equivalent inpatient surgery, that the percentage of patients treated as day cases in England and Wales remained below the level achieved in other countries. It lists a 'basket' of 20 procedures which are feasible as day cases and which should be used as a means of performance assessment (Table 22.1). The suggestion is not that these are the only cases which should be performed as day cases, but that if all health authorities performed day-case surgery on the listed group that an extra 186 000 patients could be treated per annum at no additional cost to the National Health Service in the UK.

Monitoring and evaluation process

1 Responsibility assignment: the director of the department should be responsible overall for monitoring and evaluation activities.
2 Delineation of the scope of care: the identification of the range of surgical procedures and patients served is not difficult.
3 Identification of important aspects of care.
Particular attention should be paid to those aspects of care which occur frequently, or those affecting large numbers of patients and in addition those which pose serious risks or are less beneficial if not provided correctly, and those which are historically prone to problems.

Indicators related to these aspects of care can be identified. An indicator is a defined measurable event, complication or outcome which enables an assessment of an incidence, which, in turn, permits comparison with results in other units or health-care systems.

Characteristics of a good indicator include: clear precise definitions, measurability, reproducibility and reliability, together with relevance to clinical practice.

The range of reviewed indicators in an outpatient setting may include:

1 Unplanned hospital admission.
2 Unplanned intensive care unit (ICU) admission.
3 Failure to recover from a general anaesthetic in a specified time.
4 Peripheral nerve injury.
5 Brain and spinal cord injury.
6 Myocardial infarction.
7 Cardiac arrest.
8 Respiratory arrest.
9 Pulmonary aspiration of gastric contents.
10 Dental trauma.
11 Postoperative nausea and vomiting.
12 Excessive pain.
13 Excessive bleeding.
14 Patient satisfaction.

Thresholds should be established below which the level of performance of the unit in relation to the given indicator is unacceptable and about which further evaluation and remedial action will be taken. When the incidence of indicated events exceeds threshold values, a plan of corrective action should be implemented which specifies precisely what remedial action is being taken and by whom. After sufficient time has elapsed ongoing data collection should indicate whether the action taken has resolved the problem, i.e. audit.

Continuous quality improvement (CQI) is an approach to maximizing the application of professional practice standards in anaesthesia delivery. There is a stronger direction towards feedback and practice modification than occurs in conventional quality assurance. It has been comprehensively reviewed by Tinker and Jensen [5]. Suggested examples of CQI relevant to anaesthesia include multicentre trials in order to assess the efficacy of various anaesthetic and monitoring practices.

Procedural issues

1 Patient selection: issues to be considered include: (a) age; (b) home circumstances; (c) nature and length of procedure; (d) preoperative evaluation; and (e) disease screening.

2 Staff: level of training and experience of surgeon and anaesthetist; training and experience of nursing personnel.

3 Day-case surgery environment: (a) preoperative facilities; (b) theatre facilities; and (c) recovery area.
4 Monitoring equipment—adequacy of monitoring facilities.
5 Quality control and critical incidents—methods of ensuring high quality care and identification of critical incidents.
6 Recovery and discharge: consideration of: (a) adequate recovery; and (b) home circumstances.

Some of the factors governing safety in a day-case situation are unalterable, e.g. nature of procedure, whilst others vary, e.g. level of experience of staff, home circumstances, and so on. This chapter provides an overview of those factors which govern safe practice of procedures undertaken on a day-case basis.

Patient selection

Successful organization of a day-surgery programme requires careful selection and preparation of the patient. Controversy exists concerning which patients are fit for day-surgery procedures. In most units it is impracticable for an anaesthetic opinion on suitability for day-case anaesthesia to be available at surgical outpatient clinics at which the decision to embark on surgery is taken. The surgeons involved therefore require to have available a set of criteria which influence anaesthesiologists and of the contraindications to day-case anaesthesia. Examples of this include:
1 Age limits: generally 6 months to 70 years but these are by no means exclusive.
2 American Society of Anesthesiologists classification of risk restricted to ASA I and II and controlled III.
3 Home circumstances: all such patients require continued presence of a responsible adult for the first postoperative night.
4 Surgical factors: procedures lasting more than 1 h should be excluded, as should those where significant postoperative pain or bleeding may be a problem.

Clearly most of the listed factors do not vary.

There is controversy concerning which patients are to be considered fit for day-case anaesthesia but it is generally felt that only those patients who are fit and healthy, ASA I or II are suitable. In certain instances those patients who are ASA III and whose systemic disease is well controlled may be suitable but should not be listed without prior consultation with an anaesthetist or evaluation by an assessment unit. Preoperative evaluation should involve an assessment of the patient's medical and social conditions. It is an opportunity to obtain informed consent for the surgical procedure, and an occasion upon which the patient may be acquainted with the personnel, geographical location, environment and method of organization of the unit concerned. Inevitably the detailed assessment of each patient being considered for day-case surgery may cause delays in a busy outpatient clinic. To facilitate the process most units have an assessment clinic to which the patients are referred directly from the outpatient area. Initial evaluation will be undertaken by the nursing staff supported by an anaesthesiologist. To complete the assessment a questionnaire is used by the examining nurse (see Chapters 11 and 23).

Relatively recently the use of a computerized health quiz has been reported [6]. Using this system the patient answers 'yes', 'no', or 'don't know' to a series of screening questions. In a series of 239 patients the same answers were given 97% of the time when asked identical questions, either by the computer or in a traditional interview setting. An example of an algorithm for assessing the type of investigation required and the fitness for day-case surgery is illustrated in Chapter 11.

History, physical examination and laboratory tests

Many studies have demonstrated that the most effective way of screening for disease is a thorough history and examination. Laboratory tests including haemoglobin and urea and electrolyte assessment performed without indication appear to have little predictive value on outcome. In a retrospective review of 803 patients undergoing surgery for varicose vein stripping or inguinal herniorrhaphy 1972 preoperative tests were performed [7]. Only 63 abnormalities were revealed in patients in whom history and physical examination had not revealed a requirement for testing. No change in subsequent patient management occurred as a result of identifying these abnormalities.

Other studies have drawn attention to the doubtful value of laboratory screening tests. Durbridge *et al.* [8] in a review of 1500 individuals randomly assigned to groups which were or were not subjected to testing, on admission to hospital, identified no benefit to patients in terms of length of hospital stay or eventual outcome.

The cost of routine preoperative testing is extremely high. Furthermore, in healthy individuals most abnormal results will represent false positives and current evidence suggests that there is little predictive value in preoperative investigation. The literature suggests that usually laboratory tests are unnecessary except for medicolegal purposes and inferior to history and physical examination as a disease screening method. They are regarded as an inefficient way of screening for asymptomatic diseases, and furthermore, most abnormalities which are occasionally uncovered frequently are not pursued [9]. The patient should be booked within 4 weeks of laboratory tests if they are to be considered valid.

Electrocardiogram (ECG)

A recent editorial by Paraskos [10] in response to an original article by Gold *et al.* [11] reviews retrospectively 751 consecutive adult patients under 60 years of age undergoing day-case surgery. Increasing age and lower ASA grades were associated with an increased incidence of abnormal preoperative ECGs. Twelve patients out of the total exhibited an adverse cardiovascular event but it was concluded that a preoperative ECG may have been of use in only six of these.

The author's opinion was that the preoperative ECG is not a useful predictor of adverse cardiovascular events.

Blood pressure, heart rate and SaO_2

If the assessment unit is equipped with a small portable monitor then measurement of these three are easily obtained together with a display of the ECG. Arguably the SaO_2 should now be part of routine preoperative evaluation. In addition, in patients with known active inflammatory disease, e.g. rheumatoid arthritis or human immunodeficiency virus (HIV) related infections, a single measurement of *C-reactive protein* will give a clue as to the likely level of activity of the disease process (see Chapter 11 and Appendix 7). Alternatively, the value will be high following recent thrombosis or infarctive episodes, e.g. deep venous thrombosis (DVT) or myocardial infarction.

Chest X-ray

Examples of abnormalities seen on X-rays which may influence anaesthetic management are tracheal deviation, mediastinal masses, pulmonary nodules, pulmonary oedema and cardiomegaly. However, a chest X-ray is no better a predictor of chronic lung disease requiring altered anaesthetic technique than history and physical examination [12]. A recent French study [13] reviewed the use of chest X-rays with respect to preoperative risk factors including age, smoking, emergency surgery, significant past respiratory or cardiovascular history, abnormal respiratory or cardiovascular findings on examination, and a chest X-ray within the preceding year. Of the preoperative films 22% were regarded as abnormal, although the surgical and/or anaesthetic procedures were modified as a result in only 0·5% of cases overall.

In summary, therefore, the selection procedure for day-case surgery should be meticulous. If inadequate history taking occurs at the time of listing it is likely that problems which ought to have been anticipated lead to delays on the day of scheduled surgery and may even result in cancellation. Merely subjecting the patient to a battery of routine tests is not a substitute for history and examination. Nor should it be assumed that the condition of the patient is necessarily unchanged from the occasion upon which he or she was listed. All patients require to be re-evaluated prior to surgery particularly to exclude upper respiratory tract infections, since viral infections may exacerbate asthma and chronic obstructive airways as a result of an increase in vagal reflex bronchoconstriction and exaggerated response to tachykinins [14].

Staff

Medical staff

The standards required in a day-case unit demand that both operator and anaesthetist should be experienced personnel. This applies at every stage, since arguably it is as inappropriate for junior trainees to be given responsibility for the listing of patients for day-case surgery as it is for them to be immediately responsible for perioperative management. Clearly, it is important for the purposes of training that junior surgical and anaesthetic trainees should have exposure to day-case surgery but their supervision should be close and personal [1]. Once adopted the practice of day surgery involves a transfer of consultant commitment from inpatient to day care of sessions [1].

Non-medical personnel

Delivery of high quality day-surgical care requires co-ordination of patient management. This is most effectively achieved by employing staff dedicated solely to the unit. Recruitment to day-case units is generally found to be easier than ward and theatre recruitment since the better defined hours, and lack of weekend work, make such units attractive to female and other staff with domestic commitments.

Nursing personnel

All nurses involved in day-case work should be trained to work in theatre, the recovery area, and on the day ward. The most efficient way of ensuring that the varying demands of these locations can be met is the organization of rotations through each area of the unit. As a result of this diverse range of ability the day-case unit nurse should acquire a high status which has been shown to improve morale.

Theatre staffing. The nursing establishment for day-case theatres should not differ from that required for an inpatient theatre. A minimum of three trained staff, one of whom should be anaesthetically trained, should be allocated to each theatre for scrubbing, circulating and providing assistance to the anaesthetist. In addition, one health-care assistant or operating department orderly is necessary, particularly where a rapid turnover of patients occurs. The safe administration of anaesthesia requires skilled and exclusive trained assistance [15].

Recovery room staffing. This area must have sufficient trained nursing personnel. For the effective servicing of one theatre two trained staff, i.e. one per patient recovering, would be required. In the UK the nurse in charge of a recovery room should have received basic training equivalent to the ENB course 182 in anaesthesia and similar standards exist in many other countries.

Day ward. For a unit of, for example, 10 beds, two or more full-time equivalent trained staff are required to ensure constant ward supervision and to enable checking of controlled drugs. In addition, one health-care assistant should be available. This individual's duties would include assisting in admission and preparation of patients and for health assistance after they are downgraded from first stage recovery and also preparation for their return home.

Secretarial staff. The safe processing of large numbers of patients requires a well equipped and staffed office. Without this facility generation of theatre lists, admission lists and maintenance of patient records becomes impossible and may lead to errors in patient management.

The unit nurse manager should establish safe codes of practice relating to three main areas:

1 The patient—admission, intraoperative management, recovery and discharge.
2 The anaesthetist—providing adequate levels of trained assistance.
3 The environment—particularly preparation and recovery.

Ideally it should be possible for all members of the nursing personnel to undertake all the above tasks. It has been established that the staff morale in such units is higher and staff turnover is substantially less than in most operating health environments.

Working environment

The design and management of a day-case unit should be such that patient flow is optimal. This requires free unrestricted movement of patients in and out of the facility with separation of pre- and postoperative areas.

Size. A ward with 20 beds or trolley spaces is becoming normal but the relationship between theatre capacity and the size of the recovery area depends to some extent on the case mix [1]. Operating theatre capacity will depend upon the specialty. Minor gynaecological and urological procedures will have a faster and greater turnover than, for example, hernia repairs and laparoscopic procedures. Ten to 12 cases per theatre day is a safe calculation. A 20-bedded unit would cope with two dedicated operating theatres during normal working hours.

A throughput of 1·5 patients per bed for 240 days per annum is possible in an integrated day surgery unit with an 80% bed occupancy and the annual turnover of a 20-bedded unit should be in excess of 7500 patients [1] although some units achieve a higher turnover with fewer beds.

Location. An integrated day surgery unit should have its own ward and theatre units forming a dedicated unit. The advantages of this are efficient management, reduced porterage and development of a distinct ambience. Ideally it should be located on the ground floor and be easily accessible to car parking and transport facilities in order to avoid the use of elevators for postoperative patients and long walks on discharge. If an integrated unit is not possible, the day ward should be as close to theatres as possible, and specific theatres should be allocated to the practice of day surgery. However, the level of technology may modify this approach in the future as is already the case for interventional radiology, endoscopic procedures and *in vitro* fertilization.

Specifications. The design specification and levels of equipment of the operating theatres, anaesthetic rooms and recovery ward should be no different to that required for inpatient units.

The anaesthetic room. This should allow free access around a trolley, will require adequate drug cupboard space, working surfaces and hand basins. The risks of general anaesthesia per se in day-case patients are identical to those in inpatients. The same basic essential services will therefore be required. These will include piped gases and suction, gas scavenging devices, modern anaesthetic machines and internationally recommended monitoring.

Operating theatre. The day-case surgery theatre should not differ from the inpatient theatre in terms of its specification. It needs to comfortably accommodate the necessary surgical equipment and also the anaesthetic machine together with monitoring equipment. Good lighting, air conditioning, piped gases and gas scavenging devices are required.

It may be possible to allocate a specific area in which regional blockade may be performed. This should be an area immediately adjacent to the operating theatre allowing close supervision by anaesthetic and nursing staff and immediate access to resuscitation equipment if required.

Recovery area. This must be located immediately adjacent to the theatres in order to facilitate prompt attendance by surgeons and/or anaesthetists. Turnover is high in the day-case unit and it is usually necessary to allow four spaces per theatre. Equipment should be at the same level as any high dependency area with full services including monitoring equipment and a means of ventilating patients, i.e. a conventional ventilator to deal with emergency situations, e.g. respiratory arrest and abnormal response to muscle relaxants.

Reception area. A reception area adjacent to the ward is crucial for the organization of patients as they arrive and while awaiting collection after recovery. The arrangement of ward and waiting areas should permit separation of preoperative from postoperative patients. Day-case management not only for surgery but also for other procedures (e.g. endoscopy, interventional radiology) is becoming an increasingly attractive option for patients. The reception areas, design of the unit and attitudes of the staff should create an atmosphere which is friendly and welcoming to both patients and their relatives or friends.

Monitoring

The effective and safe use of monitoring devices depend upon both the device and user. Safe monitoring should allow prompt and early detection of adverse events and critical incidents enabling therapeutic intervention, which may avert potentially disastrous consequences. Both the anaesthesia delivery system and the patient should be monitored.

The nature of surgical procedures and level of fitness dealt with in the day surgery unit would rarely demand the use of the more invasive modalities, e.g. central venous pressure, pulmonary artery flotation catheters and arterial lines.

Circuit monitoring

Ideally all components of the patient circuit should be monitored. This includes oxygen, carbon dioxide, nitrous oxide and anaesthetic vapours (halogenated hydrocarbons). Most gas analysers utilize the principle of non-dispersive infrared absorption [15, 16]. Instruments are currently available which measure and display the concentration of carbon dioxide, oxygen, nitrous oxide and all the anaesthetic vapours. Measurement of the concentrations of these circuit constituents yields the following information [16, 17].

Oxygen. Readings:
1 Verify fractional inspired oxygen concentration from flow meters.
2 Track oxygen values in low flow circuits.
3 Can assist in the evaluation of oxygen uptake.

Carbon dioxide. Readings verify
1 Correct endotracheal tube placement.
2 Adequacy of ventilation.
3 Maintenance of cardiac output.

End tidal carbon dioxide concentration. In patients with relatively normal lungs and cardiovascular function, end tidal carbon dioxide measurement indicates correct placement of a tracheal tube or laryngeal mask and permits the assessment of the correct level of alveolar ventilation. It indicates disconnection of the breathing duct from the patient or other serious leaks in the circuit, and also obstruction of the airway. It also assists in the diagnosis of cardiac arrest, pulmonary embolism and gas embolism.

Airway pressure. This should be measured with a pressure gauge incorporated into the anaesthesia breathing circuit [18]. Low circuit pressure alarms are mandatory if mechanical ventilation is used to detect disconnection immediately.

Nitrous oxide. Readings:
1 Verify inspired concentration from flow meters.
2 Can assist the measurement of nitrous oxide uptake during anaesthesia.
3 Monitors washout during emergence and recovery.

Halogenated hydrocarbon. Measurement can
1 Identify inspired concentration of anaesthetic vapour.
2 Confirm accurate vaporizer calibration.
3 Assist the evaluation of uptake during anaesthesia and washout during emergence and recovery.

Patient monitoring. This is divided into central nervous system and cardiovascular system monitoring
1 Central nervous system. The ultimate central nervous system monitor would be one which would assess the depth of anaesthesia. There is at present no consistently accurate and widely available measure of depth of anaesthesia, which is simple, easy to use and stabilizes rapidly. Because of the use of short-acting drugs in day-case anaesthesia and hence the possibility of awareness of the patient, continuous diligence by the anaesthetist is required to prevent this occurrence which has serious medicolegal implications. There is a real need for a monitor of depth of anaesthesia, or automated anaesthesia using a cerebral signal which is quick and easy to apply with a rapid response time*.
2 Cardiovascular system. Blood pressure measurement is achievable by auscultation, palpation or oscillotonometry. The latter principle is used in most automatic blood pressure measuring devices [19, 20]. Automatic blood pressure measurement allows regular recordings to be made whilst the anaesthetist may be engaged in other tasks, and should be available in all locations in which anaesthesia is administered. A recording device incorporated in the blood pressure monitor enables a permanent record of measurements made to be attached to the anaesthetic record sheet.

Electrocardiography. Monitoring electrical activity of the heart is routine practice. The principle abnormalities recognized are cardiac arrythmias, and myocardial ischaemia. The standard leads I and II are the most useful for arrythmia detection while a modified V_5 lead configuration is most appropriate for detection of ischaemia [21].

Neuromuscular junction. Many patients undergoing day-case surgery will be anaesthetized using techniques which do not involve the use of muscle relaxants. Modern standards dictate that facilities to monitor the neuromuscular junction should be available at any location where anaesthesia is administered. The capacity to monitor the level of neuromuscular blockade is important, particularly in relation to the new relaxant mivacurium with its short duration of action and extremely rapid recovery profile.

* Dr Gavin Kenny at the Western Infirmary, Glasgow, seems to have developed an easy to apply, reliable system using auditory evoked potentials to maintain a constant level of anaesthesia automatically during the administration of a propofol infusion.

Multisystem monitoring. The ability to measure arterial oxygenation is critical. There is a continuing trend towards the universal adoption of minimum monitoring standards. Standards in Australia, New Zealand and South Africa now demand that pulse oximetry must be available for every anaesthetized patient [22, 23]. In the USA only in extenuating circumstances may a similar requirement be waived [24].

Pulse oximetry. Despite the undoubted value of measuring arterial saturation few data demonstrate any advantageous effect on ultimate patient outcome. However, a recent retrospective study of 17 000 cases [25] showed that the introduction of pulse oximetry was associated with a reduced number of admissions to the intensive care unit.

Temperature. Temperature monitoring facilities should be available at all locations in which anaesthesia is administered particularly during laparoscopic and urological surgery. Although hypothermia is the more common temperature disorder, arising from anaesthesia and surgery, the anaesthetist must be aware of the potential for development of malignant hyperpyrexia (Appendix 2).

The importance of thorough preoperative checking of equipment by the anaesthetist cannot be overemphasized. The Association of Anaesthetists of Great Britain and Ireland recommended in 1990 a procedure for the checking of anaesthetic machines incorporating an oxygen analyser [26].

Critical incidents

Human error remains the most common factor causing a critical incident. Cooper *et al.* [27] reviewed 1089 preventable critical incidents. Of those described 4% had a 'substantive negative outcome' involving failure of equipment. The most common associated factor was failure to check. A smaller UK study [28] identified that human error was more common than failure of equipment and in 27 out of 81 incidents failure to perform a basic check was the most commonly associated factor. Possibly the most dangerous hazard in anaesthesia is its relative safety which may frequently induce a sense of complacency, which requires constant diligence and meticulous attention to detail for its prevention.

Quality control

The problems of quality control are of the utmost importance in any organization. In a day-case surgery unit the issue is particularly relevant because of the high turnover of patients and the premise that the service operates on a reduced expenditure basis which may, in the current harsh economic climate, imply cost cutting of essential support services.

The term 'quality' remains a somewhat abstract concept which expresses the capacity of the delivered health care to meet most medical and non-medical goals

Table 22.2 Attributes used to monitor quality control and assurance

Effectiveness: the ability of a procedure or treatment to improve health status
Efficiency: the delivery of a maximal number of comparable units of care for a given health care expenditure
Accessibility: the ease with which care is obtainable in the face of various potential barriers of financial, cultural or psychological types
Acceptability: the degree to which the health care delivered satisfies the patient
Provider competence: the technical and interpersonal skills of an individual
Risk management: refers to programmes designed to reduce or eliminate mishaps, and their associated costs, to patients

which are shaped by patients' values and expectations [29]. The standard of quality achieved is determined by variables which relate to the patient, his or her medical and other attendants and the physical environment. Much research is currently being undertaken into quality assurance. Much quality control in the clinical setting relates principally to detection and subsequent management of lapses in quality [30, 31].

All health-care professionals have a prime responsibility to provide high quality care which involves continuing education. The rationale for developing programmes to maintain quality is strengthened by the recognition of the fact that the bulk of anaesthetic related adverse incidents are preventable and potentially costly.

Terminology

The attributes which may be monitored [32] as we seek to maintain quality of care in the outpatient setting [33] are presented in Table 22.2.

Quality assurance

This is a programme which provides an organized procedure for the evaluation of the care provided and the forming of mechanisms for its improvement. Deficiencies in quality of care delivered may be identified by tracking trends by audit, corrective measures may be instituted and subsequent documentation of their successful outcome should occur.

Special problems of emergency anaesthesia in accident and emergency departments

Patients who are undergoing general anaesthesia for minor ambulatory surgery for such procedures as suturing of lacerations, fracture manipulations and drainage of abscesses are not technically classified as day-case surgery patients, i.e. booked 'inpatients for a day' or for a period thereof, but as outpatients.

The level of fitness of these patients will be similar to that of the day-case surgery patient, i.e. categories ASA I and II. As this group is however unselected, patients in ASA categories III and IV may present. They may be suitable for short and relatively minor surgery providing their medical condition is well controlled, and that their home circumstances are satisfactory.

It should be remembered that patients requiring anaesthesia in the accident and emergency department are more likely to have a history of alcohol and drug abuse, concurrent infections and most importantly, a full stomach. Fear, pain, recent alcohol consumption and injury occurring soon after food ingestion are all associated with delayed stomach emptying. It is recommended that precautions to prevent pulmonary aspiration of gastric contents should be taken for 12 h after even minor or moderate injuries.

Children who require anaesthesia in the accident and emergency department require all the facilities, expertise and facilities for the presence of parents that inpatient care demands [34].

Standards of anaesthetic care and safety in the accident and emergency department must be equally as high as in other theatre suites [35]. A trained anaesthetic nurse or operating department assistant must be assigned solely to help the anaesthetist when anaesthesia is to be undertaken in the accident department. The danger of pulmonary aspiration of gastric contents is ever present in this situation.

If staffing and facilities are not available to the same level as those available in the main operating suite then the work should be transferred to the latter facility. Anaesthesia for the procedures commonly undertaken in the accident department may be provided by general or regional techniques, or perhaps less frequently by sedation.

Local analgesic infiltration and peripheral nerve blocks

Safe use of local anaesthesia requires knowledge of the toxic dose of the drug to be administered. If safety measures are adopted it is acceptable for the operator to administer the local anaesthetic and also to perform the operation provided he or she is trained in advanced resuscitation and intubation and supported by an assistant who is familiar with methods of oxygen therapy and monitoring, and also trained in cardiopulmonary resuscitation. Clearly all necessary equipment, including a defibrillator and means of automatic ventilation of the lungs, and drugs for life support should be available (see Chapter 5).

Intravenous regional analgesia (IVRA) and major regional anaesthesia should only be undertaken when one individual performs the surgery while a second attendant, either an anaesthetist or a trained nurse, monitors the patient and has immediate access to full resuscitation equipment including a defibrillator.

Sedation techniques. Should only be used by doctors with suitable experience and training. The conditions and prerequisites for the practice of safe sedation are outlined in Chapter 16. Venous access, the use of pulse oximetry, trained assistance and immediate access to oxygen therapy, suction equipment, drugs and resuscitative equipment, are all mandatory. Recovery facilities should be available and patients should have fully recovered before being handed over to other staff. If the facilities and staffing levels are less than adequate the patient should be transferred to the main theatre recovery area.

Safety issues in anaesthesia for laser surgery

Many surgical subspecialities now utilize lasers. The applications continue to widen and include ophthalmology, gynaecology, endoscopy, ENT and dermatology amongst others [36].

Lasers of particular interest to the anaesthetist are those currently widely used in the patient's airway, carbon dioxide (CO_2) and neodymium–yttrium aluminium garnet (Nd–Yag) lasers. The carbon dioxide laser is particularly useful in the treatment of laryngeal and tracheal pathology. It has shallow penetration and produces localized tissue damage extending to less than 0·5 mm around the site of injury.

The Nd–Yag laser has much greater penetration than the carbon dioxide laser and may cause much more severe tissue damage. The UK Department of Health guidance on the safe use of lasers in medical practice is one of the best available safety documents [37]. Eye protection should be worn by all staff. The wavelength of the laser, degree of protection and type of laser for which they are intended should be indicated on the eyewear. Eye protection for the surgeon is built into the viewing optics, e.g. a microscope or endoscope. Ordinary spectacles are protective against the carbon dioxide laser but do not have side protectors. The patient also requires protection from stray laser radiation, especially to the skin and eyes.

The carbon dioxide laser is the most commonly used. The damage produced is thermal and protection of a tracheal tube during procedures in and around the airway is required; the use of metal foil wrapped around tracheal tubes is an inexpensive way of achieving protection but the cuff remains difficult to protect. Filling the cuffs with water or saline coloured with methylene blue, as an indicator of damage causing a leak, may reduce the risk.

Metal flexible tracheal tubes may be useful but have their own set of disadvantages including gas leakage around the tube and reduced visibility for the surgeon. In addition although not flammable they can be heated by continuous exposure to the laser beam producing the risk of mucosal burns.

Jet and cuirass ventilation for laser surgery of the larynx and trachea are described briefly in Chapter 18.

Radiology departments

Problems encountered by the anaesthesiologist in peripheral units, such as radiology departments, include difficulties associated with poor lighting, access to the patient and often less than satisfactory recovery facilities.

For interventional radiological procedures such as revascularization of the lower limbs effective patient selection and counselling processes are clearly important. Patients may have painful orthopaedic conditions, which may make lying still for relatively prolonged procedures difficult, or they may have neurological conditions which make imaging difficult because the patient is unable to control involuntary movement. In both these instances general anaesthesia may be preferable to the more common practice of local anaesthesia and sedation.

For preoperative preparation in patients who are to undergo sedation, many units now place no restriction on the intake of oral fluids, whilst other authorities would argue that because of the small but finite risk of anaphylaxis, due to the local anaesthetic or contrast medium, and the depressant effect of sedative drugs a patient should always be prepared as if full resuscitative measures will be applied. In many units patients may leave the department and hospital environment within 1 h. As with all patients undergoing day-case procedures, they should be accompanied by a responsible adult and should be given clear instructions concerning requirements for resting at home in order to avoid complications such as a haematoma for example at the site of a femoral arterial puncture.

For patients who have undergone general anaesthesia for radiological procedures recovery may take place in the X-ray department itself, and increasingly larger units are equipped to a level which allows this. In smaller units, or in most which do not possess adequate physical facilities or sufficient nursing support, transfer to a 'parent' day-case recovery ward or to a main theatre recovery area may be appropriate, once the patient has recovered protective laryngeal reflexes and an adequate level of consciousness.

The problem of peripheral units such as X-ray departments are logistical. Safety issues which need to be addressed include the servicing of anaesthetic machines, which may not be utilized with as great a frequency as in the past, the provision of full monitoring facilities which should include a facility to monitor patients being transferred to a longer term recovery unit, or to an intensive care unit if a serious critical incident has occurred.

In the development of any new radiology unit, an anaesthesiologist of suitable experience should be involved at the planning stage.

Magnetic resonance departments

Involvement of anaesthetists with patients undergoing magnetic resonance imaging (MRI) is increasing. Examples of patients which they may be required to manage on a day-case basis include infants and small children or intellectually subnormal adults, who would not otherwise remain still during the investigation, and also adults who exhibit excessive levels of anxiety or who may be claustrophobic. Fortunately the new generation of scanners function rapidly, removing the need for anaesthesia, since most patients can manage with little or no sedation.

Problems with provision of anaesthesia in an MRI unit include the requirement to exclude ferromagnetic equipment from the magnetic field, limited access to the patient, malfunctioning of monitoring equipment produced by changing magnetic field gradients and degradation of image and spectral quality arising from stray radio-frequency currents produced by the monitoring equipment and leads [38].

The major danger from working in strong magnetic fields is the danger to staff, patients and equipment from metallic objects accelerating towards the magnet. This includes anything from small pens to oxygen cylinders. In addition, a smaller hazard under some circumstances is the removal of magnetic bar coding from personal and other documents, e.g. credit cards.

The main issue is the decision to place anaesthetic equipment including a machine and monitoring close to or outside the magnetic field. If placed close to the magnet the anaesthetic machine and components must be non-ferromagnetic.

The machine should not be moved once examination has commenced as reduced magnetic field homogeneity may result if a large metallic mass is repositioned. If placed outside the magnetic field long monitoring leads and ventilation tubing are required. Ideally two anaesthetists or an anaesthetist accompanied by a trained assistant should be available to manage the patient and equipment. Clearly the same problems and remarks apply when critically ill patients are presented for MRI scanning but that is not within the range of this book.

A non-magnetic version of the Ohmeda XL 210 anaesthetic machine is now available.

Breathing systems which have been successfully utilized in MRI units include 10 m long non-coaxial Mapleson D systems and Bain systems (coxial Mapleson D). At 10 m from the magnet, gas cylinders may be changed if piped gases are unavailable.

Should cardiopulmonary resuscitation be required the panels must be removed from the electromagnetic field. Defibrillators should be kept at a safe distance from the magnet. An episode of defibrillator failure has been described in a situation in which a defibrillator was kept at the edge of a magnetic field [39]. Long leads are required.

Standard laryngoscopes are metallic, not ferromagnetic, and undergo torque in high magnetic fields, and batteries are highly magnetic. It has been suggested that a plastic laryngoscope with a 3 V lithium battery and an aluminium 'filler' is a simple solution [38].

Monitoring. Many MRI manufacturers produce ECG and respiratory monitors compatible with their own systems.

ECG. Faraday's law states that a voltage is induced across a column of conducting fluid flowing through a magnetic field, and is maximal when the fluid flow is at 90° to the field, producing, for example, ECG changes in leads I, II, V and V_2 when blood flows through the transverse aorta [40]. They may mimic the ECG changes of conditions such as pericarditis and hyperkalaemia.

Careful placement of electrodes can minimize such ECG changes produced by static and changing magnetic fields. Dimick's recommendations [40] are that:

1 Leads should be twisted to reduce loops across which potential differences can be generated.

2 Placement of the ECG electrodes as close as possible to the centre of the magnetic field.

3 Keep limb electrodes in the same plane and close together.

4 V_5 and V_6 chest leads are least likely to develop and record artifacts because they are close to the QRS axis.

Pulse oximetry. This has proved the most difficult monitor to use within magnetic fields. The Nellcor N-200 consistently performed best in a review of four pulse oximeters in an MRI unit [38]. Standard Nellcor probes have no magnetic components and do not require modification. Purpose designed instruments are now available from several manufacturers.

Capnography. Because of the long gas pathways involved the end tidal carbon dioxide concentrations may not be accurate but trends can be followed and the respiratory rate estimated.

Non-invasive blood pressure. Provided the ferrous connections on a standard automated cuff are changed to nylon and the tubing is lengthened satisfactory readings can be obtained.

Pacemakers. The changes in field current in an MR scanner can induce current flow in pacemaker connections and wires, which, since they are in contact with cardiac muscle, can cause microshock and ventricular fibrillation. *Under no circumstances* should a patient fitted with a pacemaker be placed in an MR scanner unless it can be rendered safe by disconnection and, for example, insulation of the external leads of an epicardial pacemaker. Expert guidance should always be sought and one person should be dedicated to supervision of the patient [41]. With present technology, patients with permanent internal pacemakers *cannot be placed* in an MR scanner.

Recovery and discharge

However simple the surgical procedure undertaken, any area in which anaesthesia is undertaken must have facilities in which the patient can be allowed to make a full recovery to a point where consciousness is regained and protective reflexes are restored.

Facilities should include full resuscitation equipment, easy access to drugs for pharmacological support, full monitoring equipment and some means of ventilatory support. A recovery room should always be included in the planning stage when a day-case unit is being designed.

The recovery ward specifically serving the needs of a day-case unit is generally termed a 'step-down' unit. Patients are transferred to this area having made a degree of recovery in the main recovery area to a point at which they are able to sit and are mentally alert. Oral fluids are offered, patients are permitted to become ambulatory and are frequently required to remain in the area until they are able to void urine.

Precise discharge criteria may vary between units but it is essential that a formal assessment is made of the patient's general fitness to return home and that he or she is reviewed by a senior member of the surgical team, preferably the surgeon who performed the procedure.

Factors which may preclude discharge from hospital or cause delay include excessive pain, bleeding, fatigue and postoperative nausea and vomiting. Patients who have impaired psychomotor function have an increased risk of accidents occurring either during the journey or at home.

Stages of recovery may be divided into early, intermediate and late. Early recovery in this context is taken to imply readiness for discharge home from hospital but until the patient has fully returned to normal daily activities he or she is considered to be in a recovery phase. Intermediate recovery refers to the first four days and late recovery thereafter.

There are a number of psychomotor tests which can be undertaken to assess full return of cognitive function (see Chapter 6). Clearly these tests are complex to perform and are of little value in the immediate clinical setting in helping to determine whether the patient is fit to be discharged home [42].

The success of a day-case surgery programme depends to a great extent on a safe approach to the discharge of the patient to the home environment. If patients are discharged home before they are ready an unacceptably high rate of readmission may occur. Patients should be escorted home by a competent person.

Common side effects

Postoperative nausea and vomiting

Delay in discharge from hospital may be prolonged because of protracted nausea and vomiting although this problem is rarely a reason for admission [43]. Nausea and vomiting are the most common side effects of anaesthesia observed in the recovery room. Factors contributing to this problem include opioid analgesics, pain, the anaesthetic agent or technique, sudden positional changes, history of motion sickness, hypotension, obesity, site of the surgical operation and day of menstrual cycle [44]. Admission to hospital from a day-case unit may result not only from uncontrolled nausea and vomiting but also from protracted somnolence after treatment with potent anti-emetics [45].

Postoperative pain

Excessive postoperative pain is a further reason for admission to hospital or for a delay in discharge. Pain should be controllable by oral analgesics or by non-steroidal anti-inflammatory agents. Consideration should be given intraoperatively to the use of local anaesthetic blocks as an adjunct to general anaesthesia, if appropriate.

If large doses of opioid analgesics are required it is inappropriate for a patient to be discharged to a home environment.

Natof [46] reviewed some of the causes of hospitalization after ambulatory surgery.

Driving after general anaesthesia

There have been several studies using psychomotor tests related to driving after exposure to different analgesics, sedatives and anaesthetics [42, 43]. Many drugs have been shown to impair psychomotor and cognitive skills for as long as 10–12 h after general anaesthesia. Bed rest alone has also been demonstrated to produce impairment of cognitive and psychomotor function [47].

Kortilla [42] recommends that if the duration of anaesthesia has been less than 30 min driving should be avoided for 24 h. If the duration of anaesthesia is greater than 2 h a 48 h restriction on driving is probably more appropriate.

Conclusion

The increase in provision for day-case surgery has created new roles for the anaesthetist extending beyond the normal operation theatre. The anaesthetist is the medical attendant often most directly involved with the procedural care of the patient and with whom responsibility rests to ensure adequate screening and evaluation has occurred before the day of surgery. Many units are now recognizing the central role of the anaesthetist as the co-ordinator of such a facility.

The modern day-case unit differs fundamentally from a conventional hospital operating theatre environment. It should be an independent facility requiring effective communication between surgeon, anaesthetist and dedicated nursing staff, with meticulous attention to detail at every stage of the process of patient care.

References

1 Commission on the Provision of Surgical Services. *Guidelines for Day Case Surgery*. London: Royal College of Surgeons of England, 1992.

2 Bevan PG. *The Management and Utilisation of Operating Departments*. London: NHS Management Executive Value for Money Unit, 1989.
3 Value for Money Unit, NHS Management. *Day Surgery: Making it Happen*. London: HMSO, 1991.
4 The Audit Commission for Local Authorities and the National Health Service in England and Wales. *A Short Cut to Better Services. Day Surgery in England and Wales*. London: HMSO, 1990.
5 Tinker JH, Jensen NF. *Quality—a Lesson from the Japanese*. International Anaesthetic Research Society: Review Course Lectures, 1992.
6 Lutner RE, Roizen MF, Stocking CB, Thisted RA, Kim S, Duke PC *et al*. The automated interview vs. the personal interview. *Anaesthesiology* 1991; 75: 394–400.
7 Delahunt B, Turnbull PRG. How cost effective are routine preoperative investigations? *N Z Med J* 92: 431.
8 Durbridge TC, Edwards F, Edwards RG *et al*. Evaluation of benefits of screening tests done immediately on admission to hospital. *Clin Chem* 1976; 22: 968.
9 Roizen MF, Rupani G. Preoperative assessment of adult outpatients. In: White PF, ed. *Outpatient Anaesthesia*. Edinburgh: Churchill Livingstone, 1990: 183.
10 Paraskos JA. Who needs a preoperative electrocardiogram? *Arch Intern Med* 1992; 152: 261–3.
11 Gold BS, Young ML, Kinman JL, Kitz DS, Berlin J, Schwartz JS. The utility of preoperative electrocardiograms in the ambulatory surgical patient. *Arch Int Med* 1992; 152: 301–5.
12 Roizen MR, Rupani G. Preoperative assessment of adult outpatients. In: White PF, ed. *Outpatient Anaesthesia*. Edinburgh: Churchill Livingstone, 1990: 187–8.
13 ACAPEM. La radiographique thoracique préopératoire systématique en chirgurie génerale est-elle utile? *Ann Fr Anesth Réanim* 1992; 11: 88–95.
14 Jacoby RE, Hirschmann CA. General anaesthesia in patients with viral respiratory infections: An unsound sleep? *Anaesthesiology* 1991; 75: 27–31.
15 Association of Anaesthetists of Great Britain and Ireland. *Assistance for the Anaesthetist*. London: Association of Anaesthetists of Great Britain and Ireland, 1988.
16 Severinghaus JW. Monitoring anaesthetic and respiratory gases. In: Blitt CD, ed. *Monitoring in Anaesthesia and Critical Care Medicine*, 1st edn. New York: Churchill Livingstone, 1985: 265.
17 Swerdlow DB. Mass spectrometry and respiratory gas monitoring. In: Barash PG, ed. *American Society of Anesthesiologists Annual Refresher Courses*. Philadelphia: JB Lippincott, 1985: 205.
18 Fairley HB. Respiratory monitoring. In: Blitt CD, ed. *Monitoring in Anaesthesia and Critical Care Medicine*, 2nd edn. New York: Churchill Livingstone, 1990: 339–40.
19 Maier WR. Non invasive blood pressure monitoring. In: Blitt CD, ed. *Monitoring in Anaesthesia and Critical Care Medicine*, 2nd edn. New York: Churchill Livingstone, 1990: 81.
20 Geddes LA, Voel ZM, Combs C. Characterisation of the oscillometric method for measuring blood pressure. *Ann Biomed Eng* 1982; 10: 271.
21 Stevenson RL, Rogers MC. Electrocardiographic monitoring and dysrhthymia analysis. In: Blitt CD, ed. *Monitoring in Anaesthesia and Critical Care Medicine*, 2nd edn. New York: Churchill Livingstone, 1990: 135.
22 Australian and New Zealand College of Anaesthetists. *Monitoring During Anaesthesia*. Policy Document, 1990: 18.
23 Rocke DA, Murray WB, Osborn IJS. Towards safer anaesthesia—implementing practice standards. *S Afr Med J* 1990; 78: 501–2.
24 American Society of Anesthesiologists. Standards for basic intraoperative monitoring. *ASA Directory of Members* 1992: 675–6.
25 Cullen DJ, Nemeskal AR, Cooper JB, Zaslavsky A, Dwyer MJ. Effect of oximetry, age and ASA physical status on the frequency of patients admitted unexpectedly to a postoperative intensive care unit and the severity of their anaesthesia related complications. *Anesth Analg* 1992; 74: 181–8.

26 Association of Anaesthetists of Great Britain and Ireland. *Checklist for Anaesthetic Machines.* London: Association of Anaesthetists of Great Britain and Ireland, 1988.
27 Cooper B, Newbower RS, Kitz RS. An analysis of major errors and equipment failures in anaesthesia management: considerations for protection and detection. *Anaesthesiology* 1984; 60: 34–42.
28 Craig J, Wilson ME. A survey of anaesthetic misadventures. *Anaesthesia* 1981; 36: 933–6.
29 Steffen GF. Quality medical care: a definition. *J Am Med Ass.* 1988; 260: 56.
30 Orkin FK. Risk management and quality assurance in outpatient anaesthesia care. *Probl Anesth* 1988; 2: 152.
31 Brown EM. Quality assurance in anesthesiology. *Adv Anesth* 1989; 6: 1.
32 Institute of Medicine. Advancing the quality of health care: key issues and fundamental principles. *Natl Acad Sci* Washington DC, 1974.
33 Fromberg R. *Monitoring and Evaluation: Anesthesia Services.* Chicago: Joint Commission on Healthcare Organisations, 1987.
34 Thornes R. *Just for the Day. Caring for Children in the Health Service.* London: NAWCH, 1991.
35 Association of Anaesthetists of Great Britain and Ireland. *The Role of the Anaesthetist in the Emergency Service.* London: Association of Anaesthetists of Great Britain and Ireland, 1991.
36 Padfield A, Stamp JM. Anaesthesia for laser surgery. *Eur J Anaesth* 1992; 9: 353–66.
37 Department of Health. *Guidance on the Safe Use of Lasers in Medical Practice.* London: HMSO, 1984.
38 Peden CJ, Menon DK, Hall AS, Sargentoni J, Whitwam JG. Magnetic resonance for the anaesthetist. Part II: anaesthesia and monitoring in MR units. *Anaesthesia* 1992; 47: 508–17.
39 Snowdon SL. Defibrillator failure in a magnetic resonance unit. *Anaesthesia* 1989; 44: 359.
40 Dimick RN, Hedlund LW, Herfrens RJ, Fram EK, Utz J. Optimising electrocardiographs. Electrode placement for cardiac-gated magnetic resonance imaging. *Invest Radiol* 1987; 22: 17–22.
41 Peden CJ, Collins AG, Butson PC, Whitwam JG, Young IR. Induction of microcurrents in critically ill patients in magnetic resonance systems. *Crit Care Med* 1993; in press.
42 Kortilla K. Recovery and driving after brief anaesthesia. *Anaesthetist* 1982; 30: 377–82.
43 Kortilla K. Practical discharge criteria. *Probl Anaesth* 1988; 2: 144–52.
44 Wetchler BV. Postoperative nausea and vomiting in day case surgery. *Br J Anaesth* 1992; 69 (suppl 1): 33S–39S.
45 Wetchler BV. Problem solving in the postanaesthesia care unit. In: Wetchler BV, ed. *Anaesthesia for Ambulatory Surgery,* 2nd edn. Philadelphia: JB Lippincott, 1991: 375–436.
46 Natof H. Complications. In: Wetchler BV, ed. *Anaesthesia for Ambulatory Surgery.* Philadelphia: JB Lippincott, 1985: 321–56.
47 Edward H, Rose EA, Schorow M, King TC. Postoperative deterioration in psychomotor function. *J Am Med Ass* 1981; 245: 1342–3.

Chapter 23
Nursing and Unit Organization

S. Penn

Competent management is essential for a surgical day unit to achieve quality care, safety, economy and reduction in waiting lists. This was established in the recent reports on day surgery from The Audit Commission [1] and The Value for Money Unit of The National Health Service Executive [2].

To superintend the overall use of the service, a multidisciplinary 'users' committee should be established, headed by a consultant who has an active role in the unit, and should include surgeons, anaesthetists, nurses and managers. Initially this committee needs to approve an operational policy and should meet not less than quarterly to agree strategies and to update the policies (Table 23.1).

With a comprehensive operational policy and the committee for support, a clinical nurse manager is the most suitable person to co-ordinate the everyday management of the service. Apart from managerial expertise the clinical nurse manager requires leadership qualities in order to co-ordinate the team and to liaise between surgeons, anaesthetists, administrators and the patients.

Facilities

The unit organization depends on the available facilities. Fortunately, dedicated self-contained day-surgery units are now the usual type being constructed. The critical consideration is the physical location of the unit and it is generally felt that in order to ensure a safe level of practice, it should be located within the grounds of a parent hospital.

The siting of the unit within the hospital is important. As day surgery undergoes expansion it will incorporate more intermediate surgery and minimally invasive procedures. Furthermore, the anaesthetic criteria may extend to include not only ASA I and II patients, but ASA III and the elderly. Complications may occur, such as bowel perforation during laparoscopic investigations or perforation of the uterus during termination of pregnancy, and so full backup facilities such as access to blood transfusion laboratories and admission facilities should be available.

Self-contained day units are easier to control and organize by the clinical nurse manager, who should have authority over both the operating theatres and the ward area for maximum efficiency.

Information technology is needed to assist in monitoring performance, quality,

Table 23.1 Contents of operational policy

Definition of a day case
Clear lines of responsibility
Details of accommodation and facilities
Preadmission patient selection and assessment
Details of appointment systems and session allocation
Patient activity—treatment and movement
Admission procedures
Operating theatre policies
Recovery, discharge and aftercare
Paediatric day surgery/other specialist groups
Patient information
Financial provisions/targets

costs and other important aspects of patient care. Audit is important in all key issues of the unit and can only help to enhance the service. Resources must be allocated to provide software packages to facilitate this and to provide training, so that the information collected is accurate and meaningful.

Administration

Buildings and facilities

The unit fabric must be maintained and kept in good decorative order. A large number of the local community pass through the unit, either as a patient or as an escort, and so the decor and atmosphere are important to the impression that their local hospital creates.

Maintenance of equipment

The maintenance of equipment is of paramount importance, not least for the high daily usage and the inordinate waste of resources that results from down time. A good working relationship with equipment suppliers should be established, to encourage a prompt and efficient service. This may facilitate arrangement of short term loans of equipment when it is sent away for repair.

Supplies

With the rapid turnover of patients, supplies need to be ordered frequently. It is uneconomical to hold vast quantities of capital in stock, rather than working capital and invariably there is a shortage of storage space.

Staffing and skill mix

It is both efficient and economical to employ staff who are competent to work in any area of a day-surgery unit. This creates a team spirit which is crucial to the smooth running of the service. Nurses appreciate the concept of providing total patient care in its real sense as they are able to become involved in patient education and counselling as well as the critical care aspect of the theatre environment.

At present, the 'normal' hours of work are attractive but as day surgery expands, longer days and weekends will inevitably be considered thereby making full use of expensive facilities.

Nationally, the number of people entering nurse training is decreasing, and nurses with theatre skills are becoming difficult to recruit. However, day-case units are finding recruitment of these skilled nurses easier than other areas within the hospital, due to a high level of job satisfaction and the regular hours of employment. It is an ideal area in which to employ part-time nurses or those who wish to share a full time position, rendering the posts attractive to nurses with family commitments.

There needs to be a change of culture and managers must recognize the move from inpatient to day-care treatment and recruit staff for day-care units accordingly. The establishment should consist of a majority of highly skilled nurses, backed up by operating department assistants or practitioners, health-care assistants and clerical assistance.

Health-care assistants have an important role to play as part of the team. They are able, with training, to work in most areas within the unit. They can help to physically prepare the patients for surgery, can assist the trained staff in theatre, and in the ward area are capable of doing many of the routine tasks. The most important factor to instill into them, is that they must communicate with the trained staff. A patient may divulge a concern or problem to the health-care assistant, which may in fact be of considerable significance in the patients treatment.

Clerical help in the unit is of paramount importance because the function of the reception area is one of the keys to success. The patients bookings are made by reception staff, in liaison with the clinical nurse manager. Unless there are competent staff in this area, the operating lists will never run to their maximum potential and surgical sessions can easily either overrun or be underutilized.

The receptionists are also responsible for ensuring that notes, X-rays and the results of investigations are available. They answer telephones including relatives enquiries, book outpatient appointments, and generate discharge letters to the patients general practitioners. They must also have a knowledge of the computer systems within the unit and be able to communicate with the hospital administration system.

Adequate clerical staff should be allocated to day-care units, to ensure that skilled nurses do not have to perform these clerical duties.

The unit can be cleaned by domestic staff during the evening after the unit has closed. However, a housekeeper is a useful member of staff, who can help by preparing

Table 23.2 Ideal staffing levels in an integrated day-care unit with two theatres

Grade	Title	Number
H	Clinical nurse manager	1
G	Senior sister/sister	1
F	Junior sister/senior S/N	2
E	Staff nurse	5
D	Staff nurse/enrolled nurse	5
A/B/C	Health-care assistant/auxiliary	2
ODA	Operating department assistant	2
ODO	Operating department orderly	2
	Clerical staff	3
	Housekeeper	1

patients refreshments, organize various supplies and generally undertake non-nursing tasks and errands during the working day.

The figures in Table 23.2 show the ideal staffing levels for a day-care unit, which has a separate preoperative area, two theatres, a four-bedded immediate postoperative recovery area and an 18-bedded ward area. The patients are screened by nursing staff at their outpatient visit.

Stress

The pressure of working in a day surgery unit should be recognized. Although there is a high level of job satisfaction and the hours of work are attractive, there is a continued high turnover of patients. All of these patients have to be admitted, operated on and discharged within a short time, and there will also be those attending for screening and advice. It is recognized that patients need reassurance throughout their treatment. There are rarely quiet periods as theatre sessions need to be fully utilized, and with the demand for day surgery increasing, the hours units are open may well extend.

The senior nurses must recognize signs of stress amongst the individual members of their staff which, if ignored, can lead to the potential problem of 'burn out'. This is a specific and destructive physical and emotional exhaustion and will result in lack of self-esteem and confidence, negative attitudes and indifference to patient care.

Managers have a responsibility to ensure that the patients receive safe standards of care and that there are enough nurses to cope with the workload. Senior staff must have enough time to supervise the less experienced nurses performing their tasks, be supportive and sensitive to the needs of nurses striving for excellence in their professional field.

Training and education

In order to facilitate nurse rotation throughout the unit, they must be adequately trained. They need to acquire all of the skills of a theatre nurse, have knowledge of anaesthetic techniques, be capable of caring for the unconscious patient, as well as having excellent communication skills and a sympathetic manner.

The surgical experience that nurses gain at present during their training will be reduced as the more complicated surgery is concentrated in specialist units and much of the inpatient work is transferred to the day surgery unit. Therefore student nurses need to be introduced to this field at an early stage in their training so that they become familiarized with the concept of total patient care.

The national reports on day surgery from The Royal College of Surgeons [3], and the Audit Commission and The Value for Money Unit [2] acknowledged the training needs of surgeons, anaesthetists and nurses. Specialist post-basic training is available which specifically addresses the needs of nurses working in this area.

Nurses need to be offered the opportunity to gain a high level of understanding of the psychological and sociological processes which will contribute to excellence in the nursing care of patients in the day surgery setting. They need to develop their skills to assess the individual, to plan holistic care and to carry out and evaluate the complex nursing skills required by these patients.

The English National Board have approved two courses, ENB A21 and ENB N33. The former is a 6-month course called 'Perioperative and day care nursing practice'. It is a specialist branch of a common core high dependency/critical care course. This means that parts of the curriculum are shared with participants on branches of other critical care ENB courses, but the remainder of the curriculum is specific to day surgery. The course is intended for nurses who have little day surgery experience but who wish to further their career in this specialty.

The short course, ENB N33 entails only 10 days in college with assessment over 3 months. It has been set up for experienced day surgery nurses to ensure that theoretical knowledge is sufficient to underpin practical experience.

There is a large demand for these educational opportunities and hopefully, the availability of these courses will become more widespread as units undergo certification. Managers must maintain an educational budget and allow for training needs within the establishment to enable nurses to enhance their knowledge and skills.

Patient activity

Preoperative patient assessment

The success of day surgery is largely dependent on the correct selection of suitable patients. Units need to work in close liaison with general practitioners who, having a better insight into the patient's medical and social history, should ideally indicate on their hospital referral letters, if the patient is a suitable candidate for day surgery.

In outpatients the surgeon decides whether the procedure required can be suitably undertaken on a day-care basis. However, assessing a day case takes longer than assessing a patient for inpatient admission. With the pressure of time in a busy outpatient clinic, the surgeon may not have time to give the patient a full explanation of the process, nor a thorough medical examination. Furthermore, patients do not always understand all of the information that they have been given during the consultation, or may have omitted to impart some significant drug history or social reason which could make day surgery a doubtful option.

Here the nurses have an important role. After the initial outpatient visit, the patient should be directed to the day unit for assessment by competent day-surgery nurses. Using criteria which have been agreed by the Day-Surgery Unit Users Committee, the nurses help the patient to complete a questionnaire asking about past medical history (see Appendix B, Chapter 11). The patient is weighed and the blood pressure recorded. A simple monitor will also allow a basic ECG and measurement of SaO_2. The nurses also check that any relevant investigations, such as haemoglobin levels or X-rays, have been completed. If the patient does not meet the necessary criteria, there should be a system available for obtaining an anaesthetic opinion and the presence of an interested consultant anaesthetist with overall responsibility for the unit can be a decided advantage.

Socially, the nurse ensures that the patient will arrange transport home, has somebody to look after them, and that their social circumstances are appropriate for the nature of the procedure, e.g. that they will not have several flights of stairs to climb if they are having a hernia repair. An understanding of why driving should not be undertaken, the importance of fasting preoperatively and other rules and regulations must be instilled so that the patients understand their responsibilities.

This system means that it is not the nurse who makes decisions on each patient, but that it is the nurse who highlights potential problems and refers the patients for specific medical opinions.

The above selection process gives an opportunity to commence the 'named nurse process', as the interview nurse for each particular patient can be that patient's named nurse on the day of operation. However, some units may feel that, for the number of patients attending the unit for the initial assessment, an assessment nurse post should be created. This nurse could be based in the day-care surgery unit as a member of the team, and not in the outpatient department as the former gives an opportunity for the patient to see the unit and to meet the staff.

For children, the explanations may be extended if it is considered necessary. For units with a high paediatric turnover, the possibility of running a session, perhaps on a Saturday when the unit is closed, should be investigated. This 'Saturday club' would address the specific needs of reducing the anxiety levels of children on the day of their admission (see also Chapter 20).

At this initial visit, all patients should be given a time and date for their admission for operation, along with relevant written instructions.

This selection process by nurses, giving the patients full explanations and the opportunity to ask questions, cuts down the non-attendance of patients, especially when they are given a say in their admission date.

Day of admission

Having passed through the comprehensive preoperative assessment, the patients should arrive on the day of operation properly prepared both mentally and physically. They should be greeted by a friendly receptionist, who checks their administrative details and introduces them to a nurse.

Using the same care plan containing the initial selection questionnaire, the immediate preoperative preparation is completed (Appendix A). The patients are then seen individually by the surgeon and the anaesthetist, who ascertain that the recent medical history is satisfactory. The consent form has to be signed if this was not done in the outpatient clinic.

Immediately prior to surgery all patients change into appropriate theatre clothing. As premedication is not routinely administered, the patient is able to walk into the operating theatre to be anaesthetized. Many units have now adopted this procedure and have found the use of an anaesthetic room unnecessary.

After the operation the patients can be transferred to a trolley using a 'pat-slide' so that there is no lifting involved. Operating trolleys are now available and some units are using these instead of conventional operating tables (see also Chapter 11).

The patients are then moved to the recovery area and closely monitored until awake, when they can be transferred to the ward. Refreshments are given when the patients have sufficiently recovered.

The assessment of the patient's fitness for discharge is usually delegated to the discretion of the nursing staff, using criteria which have been laid down in the operational policy (see Appendix B). If there is a problem, a senior member of the medical staff, anaesthesiologist or surgeon must be available to return to the unit to examine the patient.

The patients are discharged from the unit with a follow-up appointment for the outpatient clinic, any medication that may have been prescribed, including analgesics, and a discharge letter to deliver to the general practitioner. This ensures that, if the patient needs to contact the general practitioner because of complications they have the relevant information.

Appointments for family planning, counselling and other follow-up services in the community are made before the patient leaves the unit.

Patient information

Comprehensive written information for the patient, to endorse verbal instructions, is essential both pre- and postoperatively. For the day-surgical operation to be successful, the patients are required to participate in their own care. Full co-operation cannot be expected unless they understand the instructions. By providing written information, the patients can refer to it when necessary, as they may well have forgotten some of the details given verbally.

Individual information sheets for specific procedures performed in the unit should be available and given to each patient at the initial preassessment visit, and also the preoperative requirements such as the necessary fasting time. Compiling this information takes time and it is ideal if all of the surgeons can agree on the pre- and postoperative regimen for their particular procedures. This minimizes confusion for the patients and ensures that all members of the unit's staff give the same advice to the patient.

This written information needs updating regularly and it may be necessary to provide it in different languages.

Quality

Those of us involved in day surgery feel that the standards are high and that the care the patients receive is excellent, but this needs to be demonstrated. Quality plans are required to provide a formal guarantee of the degree of excellence in the services we provide. These plans should include not only aspects of care from the patient's point of view but also the need to support and develop staff.

Often our attention is only drawn to a particular problem when either a patient does not understand an aspect of their care, or when a member of staff makes a mistake. We then attempt to correct the problem. This is obviously not the best way to enhance quality issues. Quality audits should be carried out on a 6- or 12-monthly basis to provide the purchasers of health care with the concrete evidence that the quality of care we claim to deliver is actually being provided. Quality standards ought to be developed in conjunction with general practitioners.

Figure 23.1 gives a broad outline of areas for assessment that should be included in quality plans.

Organization of lists

Due to increasing demand for use of the service, the Day Unit Users Committee should frequently review its utilization and reallocate sessions as necessary to ensure that the throughput which has been contracted by each specialty is met.

Specialist groups of patients, for example children, require individual attention. The ideal way to deal with them is to allocate dedicated sessions when they can be

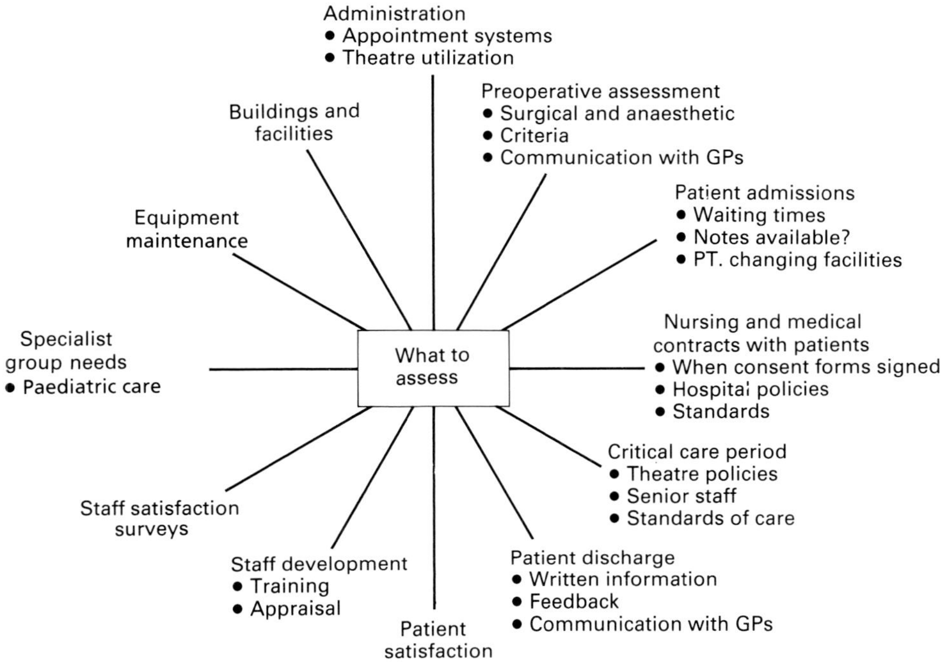

Fig. 23.1 Quality issues for audit.

accommodated together. For children, this would enable units to comply with the recommendations in the report *Just for the Day* [4].

Staggered admission times for patients can improve the quality of the service but can also slow down the throughput, as the surgeon and anaesthetist have to leave the theatre to see patients between cases. However, the sessions can be split into two, so that not all of the morning patients have to arrive at 8 a.m. Some can arrive at 10.30 a.m., causing a natural break in the operating list. This helps to keep the staff motivated as, after a list of rapid procedures, either the surgeon, the anaesthetist or the nursing staff have lost concentration and mistakes can occur.

Community involvement

At present, the day surgery being performed calls for little involvement from community nurses. However, if day surgery is to expand, the service may need to rely on their help a little more, perhaps having community nurses involved with the day-surgery team. General practitioners and community nurses need to be included in the development of the service locally. They should be given copies of all the information leaflets, so that they are aware of the instructions being given to their patients both pre- and postoperatively. Specific information, such as discharge summaries, need to be delivered to the general practitioners as quickly as possible, perhaps by facsimile or computer link. Whichever way the communication channels are improved, great care must be taken to maintain confidentiality.

A close liaison with general practitioners and community nurses must be maintained so that they do not become sceptical of day surgery in the future, and have no reason to believe that it has been developed solely for economic reasons.

'Patient hotels'

With the possibility of achieving more than 50% of all surgery within a day surgery environment, the future has to be considered. The concept of the 'patient hotel' on hospital premises is developing and becoming a reality, enabling an increase in the amount and complexity of surgery carried out in the day unit. The hotel solves the problem of patients who are unsuitable for day surgery for social reasons, because of travelling distance or because they are elderly and lack support at home. For more complicated procedures, such as laparoscopic cholecystectomies, the hotel has the advantage of giving the patients and the medical staff the security of having help and being on hand respectively.

This idea is far more acceptable to patients who do not relish the idea of a night in a busy, noisy, impersonal inpatient ward. It is also economical as most of a hospital budget is spent on personnel. By accommodating patients in hotel facilities, with the backup of medical staff and emergency services, the patients have their independence but are secure in the knowledge that help is available if necessary, e.g. via a nurse stationed at the hotel reception.

The future

The changes that are occurring in the health service must lead to more pressure for the expansion of day surgery. A well organized and managed service offers high quality, reduced waiting lists and financial efficiency. The purchasers of health care will wish to treat as many patients as possible from scarce resources.

The manager, in order to maintain a service of excellence, needs to ensure that all members of the multidisciplinary team address the issues of training and education, audit, quality and communication. With a commitment to these key issues, day surgery will continue to be a major element in the surgical care of the population in the future.

References

1 Audit Commission. *A Short Cut to Better Services: Day Surgery in England and Wales*. London: HMSO, 1990.
2 NHS Management Executive Value for Money Unit. *Day Surgery: Making it Happen*. London: HMSO, 1991.
3 Commission on the Provision of Surgical Services. *Revision of Guidelines for Day Surgery*. London: Royal College of Surgeons of England, 1992.
4. Thornes R. *Just for the Day. Caring for Children in the Health Services*. London: NAWCH, 1991.

Appendix A. Example of a care plan

Day Surgery Care Plan

Date: / /

Primary Nurse

1. Admission Procedure Time: :	Refer to relevant Protocol	
2. Preparation for Surgery	Refer to health status questionnaire	
3. Surgical Intervention Time: :	Wholly compensatory nursing care Maintain sterile field	
4. Recovery Time: :	Airway Circulation Vital signs Nausea/Vomiting Pain Partly compensatory nursing care Fully concious Homeostasis restored	
5. Post-operative care Time: :	Pain Blood Loss Nausea/Vomiting Dizziness/Postural-hypotension Voided Taking Fluids	
6. Discharge Time: :	Refer to discharge Criteria	

Continued on p. 380.

Appendix A *Contd.*

PREFERRED NAME ____________________

NEXT OF KIN ____________________ Tel. __________

____________________ Tel. __________

PERSON COLLECTING ____________________ Tel. __________

SURGERY PROPOSED ____________________

SURGEON ____________________

ANAESTHETIST ____________________

DOES PATIENT UNDERSTAND NATURE OF OPERATION?

YES / NO

PROBLEM ORIENTATED RECORD:

SPECIFIC PROBLEM (S)	ACTION TAKEN	BY:

DISCHARGE CRITERIA	**YES**	**NO**
STABLE VITAL SIGNS	______	______
ALERT AND ORIENTATED	______	______
TOLERATING ORAL FLUIDS	______	______
ABLE TO SIT UNAIDED	______	______
RESPONSIBLE ADULT ESCORT ACCOMPANYING THE PATIENT	______	______
WRITTEN AND VERBAL DISCHARGE INSTRUCTIONS GIVEN	______	______
MOBILITY AIDS PROVIDED	______	______

FOLLOW UP APPOINTMENT ....

MEDICATION TO TAKE HOME ....

NURSES SIGNATURE ....

Part 4:
Legal Issues

Chapter 24
Legal Aspects of Day-Case Surgery

N. Davies

In England and Wales most legal actions arising from the professional conduct of a doctor in relation to his or her patient are brought in the civil courts and are founded in negligence.

In order to succeed in an action for medical negligence a patient must establish the following facts:

1 That a duty of care was owed by the doctor to the patient.

2 That the doctor was in breach of the appropriate standard of care imposed by the law.

3 That the breach of duty caused the patient harm or injury recognized by law as meriting compensation.

Duty of care

The duty arises from the fact that the doctor does something to a patient which is likely to cause physical damage unless it is done with proper care and skill. The duty is not reliant on the giving of a representation, undertaking or profession of skill. It exists whether or not there is a contract between the doctor and the patient. If there is a contract between the doctor and the patient, for example private care, a term will be implied into the contract that the doctor will exercise reasonable skill and care in his or her treatment of the patient.

The scope of the doctor's duty will, in general terms, relate to all aspects of patient care including diagnosis [1], treatment [2] and advice [3].

Standard of care

The question which is asked in medical negligence claims is whether the treatment fell below the standard of care reasonably to be expected of an ordinary competent doctor exercising the particular skill in question [4]. In order to answer this question the courts in England and Wales apply the following test: Did the doctor act in accordance with a practice accepted at the time as proper by a responsible body of medical opinion, even though other doctors adopt a different practice? Negligence is tested by the medical practice and knowledge prevalent *at the time* it is alleged to have occurred.

In order to make a decision on the primary question of negligence a judge will hear evidence from practitioners called on behalf of the patient and the doctor or health authority or hospital. In evaluating the evidence of the 'experts' it is not for the judge to prefer one respectable body of professional opinion to another. If there is evidence given by an expert which is honestly held and truthfully given that the doctor acted in accordance with a responsible body of medical opinion, that will be sufficient to defeat a claim in negligence.

Surgery

Surgery is an invasive procedure performed when the patient is anaesthetized or sedated. The patient's ability to take care of himself or herself is compromised by reason of the anaesthesia or sedation. The duty of the doctor performing the surgery is to ensure that the procedure is properly carried out and that the patient is safe throughout the procedure.

This duty is not confined to the performance of the surgery. It also includes the obtaining of consent and following surgery ensuring that the patient is fit to leave hospital. If the doctor carrying out the surgery assumes the responsibility for sedating the patient or allows a second, more junior, member of the staff to carry out this task the surgeon must ensure that the second person has sufficient training and experience not only to sedate the patient but also to deal with resuscitation should it be necessary. Similarly the surgeon must, in these circumstances, be satisfied that the proper equipment for the procedure, the administration of the sedation and adequate facilities for the resuscitation of the patient are readily available.

The duty is one which can be shared. If the patient is to be anaesthetized by an independent anaesthetist then he or she will assume responsibility for providing the correct level of anaesthesia, for monitoring the patient and will be part of the decision to move the patient into the recovery area.

Consent

The issue of consent in the doctor/patient relationship can arise in two areas of the law.

Battery

Battery can be defined as the intentional application of force to the person of another, the force being harmful or offensive and being without the consent of that other and without lawful excuse. Perhaps the best description of the essence of harmfulness and offensiveness is that it lies in the unwanted nature of the touching [5].

In reality what this means is that a doctor acting in good faith with the entirely proper motive of seeking to help the patient is unlikely to be faced with a criminal or civil allegation of battery even though he or she may fail adequately to inform the patient of the nature and extent of the examination, investigation or procedure which he or she is to undergo.

Negligence

It is in this sphere that the issue of consent is most frequently litigated. The question usually raised being whether the patient was adequately informed of the nature, extent and risks of the procedure such as to enable that patient to give real consent.

The courts accept that the decision as to what risks should be disclosed is primarily a question of clinical judgment and require that the doctor acts in accordance with a practice accepted at the time as proper by a responsible body of medical opinion [3]. There is one exception to this rule namely a risk of a substantial nature with grave adverse consequences. If such a risk exists and the patient was not so informed there is authority which would permit a judge to find as a fact that the patient should have been told of the risk even if medical witnesses would not have so advised the patient [3].

Implied or express consent

Consent to treatment may be implied or express. Patients may imply agreement by compliant actions, e.g. by offering an arm for a blood sample to be taken. Express consent is given when the patient confirms his or her agreement to a procedure in clear and explicit terms, verbally or in writing. Written consent should be obtained for any procedure or treatment carrying any substantial risk or side effect.

Surgery is an invasive procedure and written consent should be obtained. A short written form which records the fact that the patient consents to undergo a procedure 'the nature and purpose of which have been explained to me by Dr/Mr...' will not be regarded by the courts as evidence that the patient has been fully and properly informed of the risks of the procedure.

When should the patient be informed of the nature and risks of the procedure?

The time to do this is not immediately before the surgical procedure. A patient has to be given a real opportunity to understand what is being said. Immediately before such a procedure a patient may be agitated, apprehensive or simply worried. The patient will not be in a state of mind which is conducive to listening to and easily understanding what is being said. The patient must have time to understand and appreciate the information and should be given a chance to ask questions or raise any doubts.

The patient should be seen at least 1 day before the procedure and informed of the relevant facts. At this meeting it would be reasonable to ask the patient to sign the consent form. The patient should not be asked to sign the consent form immediately before the procedure because of his or her likely state of mind.

Who should inform the patient of the risks?

The responsibility for ensuring that the patient is adequately informed of the risks ultimately rests with the doctor carrying out the surgery. If this doctor delegates the task to another member of the medical staff then he or she must be satisfied that the second doctor has sufficient knowledge, experience and skill to do the job properly. The fact that the task has been delegated does not absolve the surgeon from this responsibility.

Referred patients

Can a referral from another medical practitioner absolve the surgeon from his or her duty to inform the patient of the risks of the procedure?

Consultant referral

The patient is under the care of another consultant and that consultant has advised that a day-case procedure should take place. The first consultant may have explained the risks of the surgery as part of his or her general advice to and treatment of the patient. In these circumstances the surgeon should ascertain that the risks have been adequately explained.

General practitioner referral

These frequently take place in open access clinics. The surgeon cannot take for granted the fact that the general practitioner has explained the risks. An explanation of the risks must be given by the surgeon or a doctor properly entrusted by him or her with this task.

Referral from another clinic in the same hospital

This patient should be treated in the same manner as the patient referred by a general practitioner.

Consent form

The forms still used in many hospitals in England and Wales are general in their wording and do not specify the risks of the proposed procedure. Given the paucity of information contained in these forms it is in the doctor's interests to record in the medical records the risks of which he or she told the patient and any advice given.*

* In the USA detailed lists of complications and risks are mandatory.

Medical notes

The importance of detailed notes cannot be overemphasized. For many doctors it will provide the sole basis of recalling the advice given or the treatment of a particular patient.

In theory, in any personal injury claim in the UK, patients have 3 years from the date of the alleged act or omission to commence the legal proceedings, section 11(4)(a) Limitation Act 1980. However, section 11(4)(b) of the Limitation Act 1980 permits a patient in a personal injury action to commence proceedings 3 years from the date upon which he or she first had knowledge of facts which are set out in section 14 of the Act. These facts include knowledge that the injury sustained by the patient was significant, that it was attributable in whole or in part to the act or omission which is alleged to constitute negligence and the identity of the defendant or the person against whom the allegation is made.

The Limitation Act also grants the court a discretion to extend the time limits for actions in respect of personal injury or death imposed by the Act (section 33).

The effect of sections 14 and 33 is to permit patients to commence legal proceedings some years after the event. This can create considerable difficulties of recollection for both medical and nursing staff and is one of the reasons why the content of the medical and nursing notes is important. If the notes lack detail defending the case purely on a factual basis can be problematic. Further the content and form of the note can reflect upon the care provided by the treating doctor or nurse. A detailed note may say much about the standard of care. A sloppy and inadequate note can tell its own tale.

Delegation

During the course of day-case surgery it is inevitable that the doctor performing the surgery will delegate certain tasks.

If a task is to be delegated the person so doing must be satisfied that the task given to a delegate is within his or her training, experience and skill. It is essential that the delegate is aware of the nature and extent of the task to be undertaken. It would be appropriate to provide supervision until such time as the person delegating was satisfied that the task was being properly performed. It would be prudent to provide written protocols. The duty on the delegate is to tell the person attempting to delegate if he or she believes the task to be beyond his or her competence.

Conclusion

The doctor who performs the surgery carries the primary responsibility for the safety of the patient and that includes the right of the patient to know and hopefully understand what is involved. The responsibility can be shared with another doctor, e.g. an anaesthetist. The duty commences when the patient is first considered for the surgery and ends when he or she is finally discharged from treatment or follow-up care subsequent to the surgery.

References

1 *Maynard* v. *West Midlands Regional Health Authority* (1985) 1 All ER 635 H.L.
2 *Whitehouse* v. *Jordan* (1981) All ER 261 H.L.
3 *Sidaway* v. *Bethlem Royal Hospital Governors* (1985) 1 All ER 643 H.L.
4 *Bolam* v. *Friern Hospital Management Committee* (1957) 2 All ER 118.
5 Kennedy, Grubb. *Medical Law Text and Materials.*

Chapter 25
The Practitioner, the Anaesthetist and the Law

D. Poswillo

High on the list of medical and dental procedures which are complaint and litigation sensitive is the practice of general anaesthesia and intravenous sedation. Many of the incidents are relatively trivial and simple to redress. For example, damage to mobile teeth or crowns and bridges. Nevertheless some more significant problems relate to procedures which culminate in the loss of limbs, brain death or death outright. When such problems arise they usually lead to many years of anguish for the disadvantaged patient and the unfortunate or allegedly negligent practitioner or his or her assistants.

Those who practice in the healing professions hold a privileged position. The privilege carries with it clear responsibilities. The first principle is to safeguard the patient's physical and mental health and relieve suffering, while respecting human life and dignity. The second is that the practitioner, in the course of professional duty, undertakes to give priority to the medical interests of the patient. Balanced along side these principles are the inalienable rights of the patient and of primary concern, in the eyes of the law, is the principle of consent—the consent of the patient to the procedures used. While society allows the doctor many privileges, the patient, equally in this current era, has what is termed 'rights'. If the privileges of the practitioner are used without the due sense of responsibility it would not be surprising that a climate of public opinion could develop in favour of limiting professional freedom.

Medical and dental intervention of any kind normally requires consent of the patient to the procedures used. Whether or not a patient is sufficiently informed and sufficiently free to consent to medical or dental investigation and treatment is occasionally difficult to resolve. Nevertheless, every effort should be made to ensure that the patient understands the nature and purpose of the clinical procedures involved.

The obtaining of informed consent is an area in which the practitioner must be especially vigilant; familiarity with the diagnosis and treatment of common disorders may promote a paternalistic attitude on the part of the practitioner. This may be seen by some to act to the advantage of the patient but on many occasions we are dealing with sick, frightened and vulnerable people who are out of their usual environment and occasionally in clinical areas where the attention of the patient is not concentrated on the words and warnings of the practitioner.

This, the worst scenario, probably does not lead to problems unless things go wrong; the situation can be worsened by defensive actions of doctors and nurses when problems do arise. By far the largest number of complaints from patients and relatives to health authorities, regulatory bodies or to ligation lawyers stem ultimately from lack of communication. Where errors and mishaps are associated with the allegation of failure to inform, the path to successful litigation becomes more obvious.

To grant or withhold consent to treatment, major or minor, or even a clinical examination is a fundamental right. Without this consent, obtained at a suitable time prior to any intervention on the part of the practitioner and in calm surroundings where communication can be clear and distractions minimal, treatment may be alleged to be assault. Such misunderstandings may result in an action for damages, or in rare circumstances, lead to a criminal trial.

For consent to be valid a number of conditions must be met. The health-care professional, doctor, dentist, nurse or other is required to explain to the patient (or, in the case of a child, a parent or guardian) the nature, purpose and material risks of the planned procedures. Every effort should be made to give this information in clear non-technical language which the patient is capable of understanding. When the patient is of unsound mind or incapable of understanding because of language barriers, informed consent cannot be obtained. If necessary an interpreter should be asked to assist in the explanation. If a close friend or relative can act as an interpreter the task is usually easier. When complex procedures are planned, diagrams and photographs or other visual aids may facilitate the explanation. Without all this effort to obtain true informed consent the signing of a formal consent form is of secondary significance. Even after a thorough explanation and the signing of a consent form a patient may withdraw consent, even up to the moment before undergoing general anaesthesia or sedation, for example. Should this occur it would be most injudicious to proceed unless exceptional circumstances such as a life-threatening emergency presented. In such a situation the opinion of a senior colleague, preferably from a similar discipline but a different professional team, should be requested to advise on whether the planned treatment should proceed. Any information given to the patient with respect to complications known to be reasonably likely to be associated with the procedure should be recorded in the clinical notes. Where difficulties arise either in discussion or in the case of acting in the best interests of the patient without full consent, the records should also be signed by an appropriate witness who has been a party to the discussions on a difficult decision.

While written consent, usually on standard forms, is increasingly common in most significant medical and dental procedures, it is not absolutely necessary to defend an action for assault. Nevertheless, when legal actions can drag on for months or years before they are determined by a court, it is more likely that the verbal evidence of the patient will be considered more reliable by a judge than the recollection of the practitioner if adequate clinical records and a signed consent form cannot be produced. Consent need not always be written. Implied consent is most often used in cases of simple clinical examinations where the patient voluntarily lies on a couch or sits in a dental chair and follows the request of the clinician for a venepuncture, for example.

Express consent, although often oral, should, in the case of anaesthesia or sedation practice, be obtained in writing for any procedure which carries a material risk. Oral consent, if that is all that can be obtained for whatever reason, should be recorded in detail in the clinical records and witnessed by an associate whenever appropriate.

When addressing the element of risk involved in the clinical procedure one must consider the current legal definitions. A procedure which carries with it a risk of temporary 'but recoverable' damage at a level of about 10% should be addressed. Where the risk exists of permanent damage, such as nerve injury perhaps, a risk acknowledged in the literature of the order of 0·5% must be explained. Each practitioner must find his or her own way of addressing the problem of risk in a manner that is fair and understandable but least daunting to the patient. Barring emergency situations consent should be obtained in calm surroundings at least 30 min before a procedure is undertaken and preferably in the outpatient setting reasonably soon before the event. If consent has been obtained weeks or months before the clinical procedure circumstances may have changed and consent should be obtained again. Ideally, consent should be obtained or confirmed about 24 h before a day-case procedure.

Difficulties can arise when the patient says 'just go ahead doctor and do whatever has to be done. I do not wish to know anything about it at all'. When this problem arises the clinician should record the request in the notes, ask the patient to witness the record, and then proceed to provide what is believed to be 'gold standard' treatment for the condition.

There are especial circumstances which create difficult problems with respect to obtaining consent for anaesthesia and sedation. These include the mentally handicapped, the 'battered child or adult' and those who are mentally ill rather than mentally handicapped, and special religious groups. These issues are addressed in Chapters 11, 13, 14 and 19 but they are significant in that the anaesthetist or sedationist may find that he or she is associated with the allegation of negligence if only because consent to the specific procedures for anaesthesia, sedation or postoperative pain control were not adequately addressed.

Negligence and assault, both civil and criminal are the other principal issues which lead to litigation. These problems are inherent in all medical and dental procedures; good communication and preparation of the patient during the consent stage of the consultation reduce the likelihood of many allegations of negligence, but of course not all. Negligence is best avoided by careful preparation and adequate training—preparation for the techniques to be used, preparation of equipment, well-trained and rehearsed staff and preparation for the unanticipated emergency. A trained anaesthetist or sedationist, whether he or she is acting in the hospital or outpatient clinic is unlikely, in law, to be considered negligent if he or she has acted in accordance with the practice accepted as proper by a responsible body of qualified persons skilled in that particular branch of medical science.

Should negligence be alleged, the circumstances of the occurrence will be investigated in depth by experts for both the defendant(s) and the plaintiff. In the event of a collapse or severe adverse outcome associated with anaesthesia or sedation, a series of standard, but difficult questions will have to be answered. In general these may be listed as follows:

1 What went wrong and why?
2 Had an adequate medical history been taken and updated prior to the procedure commencing?
3 Was the anaesthetic or sedative technique justifiable or necessary?
4 Were the agents used correct ones in the circumstances?
5 Were sufficient and properly trained persons present at all times throughout the preparation, the procedure and the full recovery period?
6 Were adequate resuscitation equipment and drugs available?
7 Were those present adequately trained in methods of resuscitation and was each member of the team immediately aware of his or her duties?
8 Was the order of the procedure of resuscitation correct?
9 Was there any failing on anyone's part, during or after the anaesthetic or sedative technique which contributed to the collapse or failure to resuscitate the patient?

The procedures for the use of general anaesthesia, sedation and resuscitation in dentistry have been examined *in extenso*, recently, in the UK and the Report, commissioned by the Standing Dental Advisory Committee and endorsed by the Department of Health have also been enshrined to a large extent in the amendment to the notice for the Guidance of Dentists issued by the General Dental Council in 1992. This report [1] made a number of principal recommendations which have had a considerable impact upon the administration of anaesthesia and inhalation or intravenous sedation in dental practice. Those which are of particular concern cover the training and accreditation of anaesthetists who provide dental anaesthesia and the general standards which must apply equally to hospitals and outpatient clinics. The practice of the operator-anaesthetist is prohibited and there are specific recommendations concerning those who should be available to assist the anaesthetist or sedationist when these procedures are carried out, especially in the dental surgery. All who assist the anaesthetist and the dentist should have received appropriate training and be trained in resuscitation. Every member of the dental team should have their proficiency in cardiopulmonary resuscitation tested and certificated and the relevant procedures should be rehearsed in the dental surgery under simulated conditions at regular intervals.

The drugs and devices required for the safe and effective administration and monitoring of dental anaesthesia and sedation are listed as are other drugs which should be readily available in every dental surgery and which should be equipped to enable resuscitation to be performed. It is specifically recommended that intravenous sedation for the dental outpatient should be limited to one intravenous drug with a single titrated dose with an end-point of administration which falls short of anaesthesia. When combinations of drugs are used the possibility of anaesthesia remains present and such a situation would require the surgery and staff to be trained and equipped to a higher level than that recommended for dental surgeries where only inhalational or intravenous sedation was carried out. It was felt that the benzodiazepine antagonist, flumazenil, should be available in all surgeries where intravenous sedation with benzodiazepines was used but that its use should be reserved for emergencies rather than the convenience of recovering the patient rapidly for faster throughput in the treatment of patients.

The Report makes recommendations for the training and recognition of qualified dental anaesthetists and sedationists and for the additional training of all dental personnel in the handling of an emergency requiring resuscitation. There is little information available, nationally, in the UK of the true incidence of mortality and morbidity in dental anaesthesia and sedation and it is recommended that provision be made for an ongoing national inquiry into such matters so that significant audit statistics can be obtained and lessons learned for the future safety of patients undergoing anaesthesia or sedation in the dental surgery.

The problem of civil assault, or battery, implies the intentional application of force by the practitioner to the patient, which is harmful or offensive, without lawful excuse. Generally, such problems should not arise in the treatment of any dental patient undergoing local or general anaesthesia or sedation for dental treatment. Difficulties can arise, however, when the patient can show that he or she had not been given adequate information on the proposed treatment and any associated hazards. In such a situation, especially coupled with alleged negligent treatment, the patient could insist that consent would have been refused.

Indecent assault is a criminal matter and careful standards of practice should prevent such possibilities ever occurring in dental practice associated with general anaesthesia and sedation. None the less, cases of alleged sexual interference do appear before the courts following dental surgery and the consequences for the practitioner are of the utmost severity when the case is proven. There has, for many years, been anecdotal evidence of sexual fantasies occurring in association with dental surgery under nitrous oxide anaesthesia and latterly sedation with benzodiazepines. The latter situation is particularly worrying when one realizes that the benzodiazepines have the capacity, in almost all cases, to produce considerable amnesia for events. These problems can be avoided entirely by complete preliminary explanation of the practical procedure during the consent phase and the adequate chaperoning of the patients, particularly females and children, at all times from their arrival in the clinic until departure with a responsible accompanying person. In this way allegations of assault or attempts at blackmail can be negated. Particular concern should be given to the propriety of using suppository analgesic drugs inserted rectally prior to recovery from anaesthesia or sedation in patients who are receiving outpatient dental treatment. A full explanation of the procedure and its potential advantages in advance, and gaining consent from the patient is imperative, especially when, accidentally, the suppository is placed in the wrong body orifice of female patients.

In conclusion, the procedure which should be followed after an unfortunate clinical incident should be understood in full. If a mishap has occurred the patient or next of kin should be informed immediately. Failure to do so may not only be negligent but may also negate the original consent. Where a professional colleague has been negligent, simply state the facts as you know them without any accusation of negligence or suggestions of lack of care. After an emergency you may have to recognize that a more competent team of specialists is required for any further intervention. Failure to recognize and act on this may be considered negligent. Last but not least in the handling of the unexpected, beware of the administrative letter requesting information on the incident. Contact your defence organization before you take any action whatsoever.

The outcome of an unfortunate incident associated with dental anaesthesia or sedation depends on the facts. The problems of this nature will involve the setting up of an inquiry to establish the facts. In all jurisdictions the likely procedure would involve the following sequence of events:

1 Interview of the practitioners involved.

2 Interview of the nurses and other members of the practice team.

3 Interview of other practitioners who have treated the patient previously—or other possible witnesses.

4 Inspection of documents—X-rays, study casts/models, treatment cards, appointment books, all contemporaneous records.

5 Inspection and testing of all the equipment used to induce, maintain and monitor anaesthesia or sedation and the facilities available in the recovery area.

6 Reports of independent experts.

The analysis can lead to three possible conclusions if the case becomes the subject of litigation.

1 You will almost certainly lose; in such a situation be prepared to accept advice to achieve a speedy settlement and follow the instructions of your legal advisors.

2 You will almost certainly win; work on the assumption that your legal advisors will convince the plaintiff's advisors that the claim is hopeless. Provide your defence lawyers with all possible information which will assist your case.

3 Your experts are in a quandary. In this situation the defendant is always at risk. Consider the economic factors, the consequences of winning and losing and make a decision based on best advice, to minimize the risk.

Consider most carefully the consequence of losing; publicity, loss of hospital admitting rights and your position amongst your professional peer group. Good communication with your patient prior to any procedure with consent fully understood, preferably at least 24 h before a planned intervention, will remove many of the hazards which can befall a practitioner and which lead to the courts or the disciplinary tribunals. Establish good risk management procedures in your daily practice and strive always to act as would do 'the responsible body of professional men'. Ensure always that any delegated task falls within the competence of the individual who is to perform it.

The object of this section has been to highlight those areas which offer the highest potential for mishap and to suggest remedies which are preventive without being excessively defensive. Remember, however, the wise words of The Rt. Hon. Lord Chief Justice Denning which can be abbreviated as follows: 'All people take risks—but hopefully, not knowingly. Doctors, dentists and the patients must occasionally take risks and a degree of risk continues as long as medical advances continue. If there is no risk there will never be an advance'. If the anaesthetist/sedationist and their team take time occasionally to review safety procedures, particularly the checking of equipment and calibration of monitoring devices on a systematic basis and keeping good records, not only clinical but also of the checking of facilities and the use-by date of drugs, many of the common pitfalls will be avoided. Remember that you have a duty to inform hospital and practice managers of deficiencies in the equipment, the provision of facilities and the availability of trained and competent staff. Advise them of any resultant risks to the well being of your patients before problems arise. Last, but by no means least, do all that you can to minimize risks to yourself and your staff. Establishing current methods of control of cross infection should protect you from the risk of contracting an infectious disease from a patient and equally protect your staff, thus eliminating yet one further medicolegal encounter which you could well do without!

Reference

1 Poswillo D. *General Anaesthesia, Sedation and Resuscitation in Dentistry* (Poswillo Report). London: Department of Health, 1990.

Further reading

Applebaum PS, Lidz IW, Meisel A. *Informed Consent: Legal Theory and Clinical Practice.* Oxford: Oxford University Press, 1987.

Consent to Treatment. London: The Medical Defence Union Ltd, 1992.

Lawton (The Rt. Hon. Lord Justice Lawton). Legal aspects of iatrogenic disorders: a discussion paper. *J Roy Soc Med* 1983; 76: 289–91.

McLoy R, Ed. *Quality Control in Endoscopy. Report of an International Forum.* Berlin: Springer-Verlag, 1991.

Poswillo DE. The benzodiazepine antagonist: medicolegal comment. *Dent Update* 1988; 15: 24–5.

Risk Management in Anaesthesia. London: The Medical Defence Union Ltd, 1991.

Roberts GJ, Rosenbaum NL. *A Colour Atlas of Dental Analgesia and Sedation.* London: Wolfe Publishing, 1991.

Rosenbaum N. *Towards Safer Sedation: Oral Surgery.* London: Meditext, 1992.

Appendices

Appendix 1
Criteria for Day-Cases and Outpatients

Day-case	Outpatient
'Cold' prebooked	Simple prebooked or emergency procedures
Formal admission to day ward or unit	Patient does not usually occupy a bed
Full work-up and documentation with preconsidered consent included in admission statistics, i.e. is part of total booked departmental workload	Documentation simpler. Consent may be urgent without the minimum 24 h requirement for preconsideration
1 Surgery on outpatients previously performed on inpatients.	For children verbal consent by parent or guardian by telephone is allowable, e.g. for procedures in accident and emergency departments
2 Use of modern technology (minimally invasive therapy) to treat patients: (a) surgically, e.g. laparoscopic cholecystectomy; (b) Other disciplines, e.g. interventional radiology, cardiology, gastroenterology, rheumatology departments.	
3 Pain therapy procedures	
Environment	
1 Surgery and endoscopic procedures. Increasing numbers of purpose built day-case operating theatre suites.	
2 Increasing number of patients are being treated in radiology, cardiology and ultrasound departments	
Patients can stay all day i.e. 12 h with the possibility of admission	Short stay, no formal admission

Appendix 2
Malignant Hyperpyrexia

This is a rare condition. Reported incidence varies, e.g. from as high as one in 14 000 in one paediatric report, to an overall incidence from one in 50 000 to one in 200 000 in the UK. A few families can distort the figures in a localized area. Complex multigene inheritance functions as an autosomal dominant. Primary major disorder is in skeletal muscle. Acute, unpredicted increase in oxygen consumption, lactate production, heat production, muscle rigidity (not consistent), sympathetic stimulation and increased cellular permeability. Possibly a spectrum of biochemical conditions. Precise mechanism unknown. Ca^{2+} theory most popular: (a) ionized calcium in unstimulated normal muscle has been found to be lower than normal; and (b) muscle mitochondria in pig models increase their calcium concentration during malignant hyperpyrexia (MH) which is reversed by dantrolene. In many respects MH could be due to regulatory gene activation.

Involvement of the sympathetic nervous system occurs. Sympathomimetic agents (e.g. ketamine) can trigger MH. In a developed case it is not clear whether sympathetic involvement is primary or secondary.

Stress

Wingard, cited by Ellis, regards MH as part of a stress syndrome which can be triggered by excitement, anxiety, exercise or environmental stress, e.g. temperature, hypoxia.

Day-case assessment

Anaesthetic history (patient and family), diathesis of patient and laboratory tests are necessary. Maximal incidence occurs in the second and third decades of life.

Diathesis

Often pronounced muscular development and athletic success. Local hypertrophy of muscles. Muscle cramps. Associations—squint, hernia, laxity of joints, kyphoscoliosis, disc lesions, cartilage tears and pes cavus.

Incidence—risk factors

A squint increases risk factor by approximately 10. The at-risk patients tend to be in the younger age groups because they are undergoing surgery either for associated conditions (see above) or musculoskeletal trauma requiring procedures often in accident and emergency departments as outpatients, or as day-cases. Even susceptible patients may not always trigger on each occasion of an exposure to a trigger agent.

Laboratory tests

May not help. Raised plasma creatine phosphokinase (CPK) can indicate increased membrane permeability. A quadriceps muscle biopsy which includes the motor point may be subjected *in vitro* to static and dynamic halothane tests and a static caffeine test (European MH group). Other tests, e.g. muscle kinases are described by Ellis. More recently, nuclear magnetic resonance imaging and spectroscopy are being investigated for diagnosis.

Anaesthetic triggering agents

Known agents include:

1 Inhalational anaesthetic agents, particularly halothane.
2 Depolarizing muscle relaxants, e.g. suxamethonium.

Agents best avoided include:

1 Ketamine.
2 Phenothiazines.
3 Atropine.
4 Lignocaine.

'Safe' agents include:

1 Thiopentone.
2 Benzodiazepines.
3 Droperidol.
4 Bupivacaine.
5 Nitrous oxide.
6 Opiates.
7 Papaveretum.

Diagnosis

1 Failure to relax after suxamethonium (cf. myotonic and muscular dystrophies which may also show the same phenomena).

2 Tachycardia and rising end tidal carbon dioxide concentration are the earliest indicators of a problem during anaesthesia and intermittent positive pressure ventilation.

3 Cardiac arrhythmias. Ventricular ectopic beats, e.g. ventricular extra systoles.

4 Tachypnoea (if breathing spontaneously).

5 Rising temperature (e.g. up to 43°C).

6 Hot skin, sweating, cyanosis, mottling.

7 Rigidity of some but not all muscle groups in 75% of patients.

8 Severe respiratory and metabolic acidosis $pH < 7{\cdot}0$.

9 Hyperkalaemia. Raised creatine phosphokinase (CPK).

10 Myoglobinuria. Renal failure.

11 Disseminated intravascular coagulation (DIC).

12 Cerebral and pulmonary oedema.

Management

1 Stop potential trigger agents.

2 Arrange to terminate surgery as soon as possible.

3 Increase monitoring level—central venous pressure (CVP) and arterial cannulation, i.e. in addition to blood pressure, ECG, temperature, SaO_2 and $F_{\acute{E}}CO_2$.

4 Simultaneously:

(a) delegate one person to make up dantrolene (dissolves slowly) 1 mg kg^{-1} stat. Further doses—average dose 2·5 mg kg^{-1} and up to 10 mg kg^{-1} has been required;

(b) administer $NaHCO_3$ 100 mmol (may need up to 1500 mmol);

(c) increase ventilation 2–3 times; monitor $F_{\acute{E}}CO_2$ and $PaCO_2$;

(d) blood gases: $PaCO_2$, PaO_2, pHa (other tests if indicated); blood values, Na, K^+, Ca^{2+}, CPK;

(e) urine catheter (save first samples to assess myoglobulinuria);

(f) change anaesthetic tubing and soda–lime; and

(g) fluid balance chart.

5 Hyperkalaemia. Dextrose (50 ml 50%). Insulin (10 U i.v. stat.) regimen.

6 Volume. Saline i.v. (not Hartmanns or Ringer lactate).

7 Cool. Ice cold saline 1–2 l i.v.—follow blood pressure and CVP. Surface cooling (cardiopulmonary bypass or vein to vein perfusion system may be required). Monitor temperature. Can easily overcorrect hypothermia.

8 Frusemide and mannitol + i.v. fluids to maintain urine output.

9 Treat DIC.

10 Monitor and repeat dantrolene, e.g. total dose 4 mg kg^{-1} day^{-1} in divided doses for 2 days.

Prophylaxis

Arguably patients with MH susceptibility should not be managed as day-cases. Avoid anaesthesia with trigger agents. Dantrolene as per data sheet.

Further reading

Ellis FR. Malignant hyperpyrexia. In: Ellis FR, ed. *Monographs in Anaesthesiology*, Vol. 9. *Inherited Disease and Anaesthesia*. Amsterdam: Excerpta Medica, 1981: 163–99.
Gronert GA. Malignant hyperthermia. In: Miller RD, ed. *Anesthesia*, Vol. 3, 2nd edn. New York: Churchill Livingstone, 1986: 1971–94.
Mason RA. *Anaesthesia Databook*. Edinburgh: Churchill Livingstone, 1990: 169–73, 469–70.

Appendix 3
High Frequency Ventilation/ High Frequency Oscillation

Purpose

To reduce V_T:

1 Reduction of intrapulmonary pressures. Decreased barotrauma. Improved circulation until gas trapping occurs at high ventilation frequencies.

2 Ventilation through catheters.

Definitions

HFV	High frequency ventilation
HFPPV	High frequency positive pressure ventilation
HFJV	High frequency jet ventilation
HFO	High frequency oscillation
CFV	Combined HFV and HFO, i.e. twin cycle.

Physiology

1 Effective $\dot{V}_A$ remains 4–6 l min^{-1} $\dot{V}CO_2$ 200 ml min^{-1}. V_D (phys. and anat.) reduced as V_T reduced to minimal values.

2 There is a finite minimum for an effective V_T in adult man around 70–90 ml.

3 Up to 50–80 breaths min^{-1} the inflation pressure is reduced.

4 $>$ 100 breaths min^{-1} lungs cannot empty in the expiratory time available with I:E ratio of 1:1 or 1:2 because of the pulmonary time constant = compliance $\times$ airway resistance (C $\times$ R).

5 Therefore gas trapping occurs with an increase in expiratory lung volume.

6 Above 200–300 breaths min^{-1} at a fixed V_T, CO_2 removal will not improve and may fall due to:

(a) large end expiratory lung volume and anatomical deadspace;

(b) cardiovascular depression.

7 Very high frequencies, e.g. above 400–600 breaths min^{-1}, cause overinflation of the lungs. As a result cardiac output is reduced, O_2 delivery is reduced and non-pulmonary organ damage can occur.

8 Additional monitoring is required (see Table 18.1).

Appendix 4
Semantics of Day-Case Anaesthesia, Analgesia and Sedation

In a booklet of advice for patients, *Anesthesia and Ambulatory Surgery* produced by the American Society of Anesthesiologists (1993) four types of anaesthesia are presented to the patient:

1 General anaesthesia.
2 Regional anaesthesia, i.e. spinal, epidural, limb blocks.
3 Monitored anaesthesia care.
4 Local anaesthesia, local infiltration. (This is the only technique where the anaesthetic drug is administered by the surgeon.)

Monitored anaesthetic care (MAC) is described as a combination of local anaesthetic injection and the use of drugs to produce drowsiness and sedation, while the anaesthesiologist monitors bodily function.

In other health-care groupings, e.g. in the UK, Europe and elsewhere, MAC refers to the presence of an anaesthetist to act as the patient's 'minder' to undertake monitoring and to intervene in ongoing care if necessary. This procedure often occurs when critically ill patients are being investigated in radiology departments, e.g. magnetic resonance imaging and computerized tomography scanners, or undergoing last chance interventions using minimally invasive techniques in a variety of environments, including the operating theatres. Thus MAC is not restricted to day-case anaesthesia as in the USA.

The combination of local anaesthesia and sedation in the UK is termed *sedoanalgesia*. Such patients are monitored with pulse oximetry, ECG and blood pressure; in the USA this technique is referred to as MAC. In many countries, including the UK, it is practised by a variety of specialists who are obliged to employ monitoring, including SaO_2 and a competent 'minder', with training in oxygen therapy, ventilation and for example cardiopulmonary resuscitation. (The current anaesthetic menu in the UK is indicated in Table 10.2.) Much of modern dentistry is an example of this type of practice.

A further point is that sedation is regarded as arguably too deep a state and some practitioners prefer to use the term anxiolysis.

Appendix 5
Bleeding Disorders and Day-Case Surgery

These fall into two categories:
1 Unexpectedly excessive bleeding in the absence of major vessel damage.
2 The patient with a known bleeding diathesis.

Excessive bleeding

Management

1 Immediate replacement of fluids, crystalloid and colloid, $\pm$blood$\pm$blood products.
2 Investigation of coagulation system and immediate correction.
3 Further appropriate management and investigation of the patient.

The clotting system is divided into three phases:
1 Vascular phase (spasm of damaged vessel).
2 Platelet phase. Platelets adhere to wall of injured vessel, with release of adenosine diphosphate and thromboxane A_2 which attract more platelets to the site which aggregate to form a platelet plug.
3 Procoagulant phase. Leads to the formation of fibrin. Either via the extrinsic pathway (activated by thromboplastin released from damaged vessel wall) or the intrinsic pathway. Pathways converge at the stage where factor X is formed. Factor X initiates the final common pathway culminating in the formation of fibrin.

The procoagulant phase contains natural inhibitors of clot formation and a fibrinolytic system which is mediated by plasmin.

Investigations of the clotting system must evaluate platelet and procoagulant phases to facilitate the differential diagnosis of inadequate haemostasis:
1 Tests of platelet phase:
   (a) platelet count estimates only the number and not the function of these cells. Normal count $150–450 \times 10^3$ per mm^3; and
   (b) bleeding time is the best measure of platelet function. The hallmark of a defect in platelet function is a bleeding time longer than 10 min despite a platelet count about 100×10^3 per mm^3.

If the platelet count is inadequate ($< 50 \times 10^3$ per mm^3) or the platelets are defective, platelet transfusion should be given.
2 Tests of procoagulant phase:

(a) prothrombin time (PT) reflects events in the extrinsic coagulation pathway. Normal is 12–14 s. Prolonged with reduction in activity of factors II (prothrombin), V, VII and X;

(b) partial thromboplastin time, e.g. kaolin activated (kPTT), reflects events occurring in the intrinsic and common coagulation pathway. Normal kPTT is 25–35 s. Prolongation occurs in the presence of a plasma deficiency of all procoagulants except VII and XIII. Also prolonged by heparinization; and

(c) thrombin time measures the rate of conversion of fibrinogen to fibrin (i.e. end of common coagulation pathway). Normal is 12–20 s. Prolonged by decreased activity of factors I and II and by heparin.

With diffuse and excessive clotting, fibrinogen levels will fall and levels of fibrin degradation products (FDPs) will rise.

If the tests of the procoagulant phase are prolonged suggesting deficiencies of the various clotting factors, whereas these can be administered in the form of plasma, fresh frozen plasma or cryoprecipitates. The patient should be referred immediately for a haematologist to elucidate the specific defect in the clotting cascade and recommend appropriate therapy.

The patient with a known bleeding diathesis

Either (a) a congenital deficiency of the procoagulant phase; or (b) receiving anticoagulant drug therapy. Most of these patients should be dealt with as inpatients, but mild cases may be admitted as day-stay patients for minor surgery. The haematologist *must* be involved at an early stage.

Congenital disorders of coagulation

Usually due to the absence or decreased presence of a single procoagulant. The three most common disorders are (a) haemophilia A (factor VIII deficiency); (b) haemophilia B (factor IX deficiency, Christmas disease); and (c) von Willebrand's disease.

Haemophilia A

Absence or inadequate activity of factor VIII, a sex (X chromosome) linked recessive gene. Therefore males predominate (but rare cases occur in females). Activity of factor VIII variable. If factor VIII level $> 15\%$ normal, mild cases occur where the bleeding problem may only manifest at time of surgery or major trauma. The kPTT is prolonged in all but very mild cases. Treatment is by administration of factor VIII concentrate.

Preoperatively aim for factor VIII levels approaching 100%. For very mild haemophiliacs for dental extraction or minor surgery, may give an i.v. infusion of desmopressin (DDAVP) 0·3 $\mu g\ kg^{-1}$ over 15 min which causes a three- to fourfold increase in factor VIII activity and may obviate the need for cryoprecipitate or factor

VIII concentrate. Administration of aminocaproic acid or tranexamic acid, which both inhibit fibrinolysis, may also greatly reduce the need for factor VIII by protecting clot which forms from subsequent lysis.

Haemophilia B

Absence or decreased activity of factor IX. Indistinguishable clinically from haemophilia A. Treatment is by specific procoagulant concentrate. Management is as described for haemophilia A.

Von Willebrand's disease

Autosomal dominant disease. Affects both sexes. Due to absence of a protein important for adequate activity of factor VIII and optimal function of platelets. Treatment is with cryoprecipitate. Factor VIII concentrates are ineffective as they lack essential cofactors.

Patients receiving anticoagulant drug therapy

1 Coumarin anticoagulants (e.g. warfarin) interfere with hepatic synthesis of vitamin K dependent procoagulants including factors II, VII, IX and X. Usually administered for long-term prophylaxis against recurrent thrombosis, pulmonary and systolic emboli, patients with arterial, including coronary grafts, valve prostheses, and also those with chronic atrial fibrillation. Therefore most patients will not be suitable for day-stay surgery. Monitored by measurement of the prothrombin time calibrated against an international reference preparation expressed as the international normalized radio (INR). Therapeutic range for INR = 2·0–3·5. Half-life for warfarin is 44 h. Rapid reversal of anticoagulant effect can be achieved by the intravenous infusion of fresh frozen plasma. (Patients who are receiving warfarin, e.g. after valve replacement, carry a card indicating the event and also the last time their coagulation status was checked.)

2 Aspirin and non-steroidal anti-inflammatory drugs (NSAIDs). Inhibition of cyclo-oxygenase by these drugs impairs production of thromboxane A_2 and therefore inhibits secondary platelet aggregation, i.e. they tend to cause drug-induced platelet dysfunction. Bleeding is reduced by the administration of aprotinin (which inhibits the fibrinolytic system) to protect any fibrin clot which forms. It can be argued that patients receiving aspirin or NSAIDs for laparoscopic cholecystectomy should be given 1 million U of aprotonin over 1 h, after a test dose of 5 ml, at time of surgery.

3 Heparin therapy may be administered acutely using long acting low molecular weight heparin (e.g. 5000 u subcutaneously per day, see Chapter 2). Examples are patients with a recent episode of atrial fibrillation, to prevent the formation of clot in the atrial appendices while undergoing restoration of normal rhythm, e.g. with amiodarone or cardioversion. The latter may be a day-case procedure. Arguably, in patients at risk from thrombosis, e.g. deep venous thrombosis, with subsequent

pulmonary embolism, heparin should be administered to some patients undergoing day-case surgery. Low dose heparin is not a contraindication to surgery, and its effects can be rapidly reversed with protamine.

The use of regional anaesthesia (particularly epidural or subarachnoid) in all patients with a known bleeding diathesis (whether congenital or drug induced) is controversial but should probably be avoided in day-stay patients.

Further reading

Lee GR, Bithel TC, Foerster J, Atyens JW, Lukens JN, eds. *Wintrobe's Clinical Hematology*, 9th edn. Philadelphia: Lea & Febiger, 1993.

Macleod J, Edwards C, Bouchier I, eds. *Davidson's Principles and Practice of Medicine*, 15th edn. Edinburgh: Churchill Livingstone, 1987; 541–50.

Mason RA. *Anaesthesia Databook*. Edinburgh: Churchill Livingstone, 1990: 124–7, 307–8, 352–4.

Stoelting RK, Dierdorf SF, McCammon RL, eds. *Anaesthesia and Co-existing Disease*, 2nd edn. New York: Churchill Livingstone, 1988.

Appendix 6
Sickle Disease

The normal forms of haemoglobin are fetal ($\alpha_2\gamma_2$), A($\alpha_2\beta_2$) and A_2($\alpha_2\delta_2$—2–5% of normal Hb in adults).

The basic abnormality in sickle disease is the substitution of valine for glutamic acid in position 6 in the β chain which is inherited as an autosomal dominant. It appears in several forms, e.g. heterozygous SS, homozygous (trait) AS, combinations, e.g. SC disease S thalassaemia. Fetal and haemoglobin A_2 are not affected so that sickling should not occur in infants under 2 months old. Patients with sickle disease produce from 5 to 30% of fetal haemoglobin in adult life.

The homozygous form and some of the combinations manifest as a *severe haemolytic anaemia*. Also the red cells are capable of 'sickling'. This is usually induced by hypoxaemia and the molecules of Hb come out of solution forming tactoids, i.e. chains of Hb, by association of the β chains. This causes distortion of the cells, the *sickle cell phenomenon*, increasing their rigidity so that they will not pass through capillaries and hence they cause microembolization of the tissues. In addition, as in all haemolytic anaemias, the bone marrow shows changes, and episodes of inadequate red cell production are not uncommon so that it is usual to administer folic acid supplements to prevent *aplastic crises*.

The homozygous form is a very serious condition whereas the trait in a pathophysiological sense is rarely serious and should not cause clinical problems, since it is a very late event in a clinical situation with hypoxaemia, unless it is induced by severe local stasis, e.g. the prolonged application of a tourniquet.

The normal PaO_2 (40 mmHg, 5·33 kPa) on the venous side of the circulation is sufficiently low to induce sickling. The principles of sound management include the avoidance of hypoxaemia, circulatory stasis and acidosis. For major surgery or the management of pregnant women near term, in the homozygous condition, it is desirable to replace the patient's endogenous red cells with normal adult haemoglobin A by exchange transfusion.

Sickle haemoglobin has a low affinity for oxygen which means that it is good for oxygen delivery to the tissues. However, it does mean that when old stored blood which has a high oxygen affinity is transfused, oxygen will be taken from the recipient's sickle cells which can cause sickling.

Diagnosis depends on the patient's previous medical and family history. The haemoglobin concentration is very low in the homozygous sickle state, relatively

Table A6.1 Combined abnormalities of sickle disease

Status	Hb	Sickledex test	Film (Heinz bodies)	Electrophoresis
SS	Very low, i.e. > 70–90 G l^{-1}	+	+	Diagnostic
SA	Normal	+	–	Diagnostic
SC	Mild 10–11 G l^{-1}	+	+	Diagnostic

normal in the trait with a modest anaemia in some of the combined abnormalities (Table A6.1). The simplest way of screening if in any doubt is, for example, the sickledex test. A haemoglobin estimation and a blood film will give an indication of the severity of the patient's potential clinical problem.

The disease may cause pigment stones in the biliary system, damage and/or failure of the renal, cardiorespiratory and central nervous system. It often presents with abdominal pain due to involvement of intra-abdominal structures.

In a crisis children may sequestrate their red cells in the spleen, which can be fatal, but in older children, or alternatively for example an acute chest syndrome, the spleen is fibrotic due to repeated infarction. Examples of other associations are von Willebrand's disease, ulcers of the leg and avascular bone necrosis.

The most important aspect of the problem is a correct diagnosis. The genetic predisposition now affects all races.

If there is any doubt about the sickle status of a patient they should be referred to an appropriate haematology unit. Arguably screening should be performed at some stage of the lives of the whole of the coming generation.

The homozygous or active states should not be managed on an outpatient and day-case basis and not without preparation in consultation with a haematologist using blood transfusions.

Patients with the trait can be managed on a day-case basis following three fundamental principles:

1 Avoid hypoxaemia.

2 Avoid local vascular stasis, e.g. tourniquets.

3 Avoid acidosis—which should not apply during day-case procedures. However there is little point in alkalinizing the patient orally preoperatively as this can be unpleasant and induce nausea. Many authorities recommend the administration of sodium bicarbonate, e.g. 1–2 mmol kg^{-1} intraoperatively, but this is not necessary for minor surgery. Clearly monitoring of the SaO_2 and $F_{\acute{E}}CO_2$ are mandatory.

Appendix 7
Summary of Patient Assessment and Process

Phase 1: Preoperative assessment

1 Initial clinic referral.
2 Surgical/medical assessment.
3 History—sources: referring physician, patient, relatives, previous hospital or clinic records. Investigations: referring physician and previous hospital records (specific for current event).
4 Recommendations for day-case procedure:
(a) pathological diagnosis;
(b) suitable diagnostic related group (DRG) for treatment as a day-case;
(c) level of general health—suitability for day-case;
(d) social, domestic and peripheral circumstances; and
(e) Initial consent (implied or documented). Legally the patient is entitled to 24 h to reconsider and the timing of consent often depends on local factors.

Phase 2: day-case assessment unit

Nurses supported by anaesthetist conduct the assessment.
1 History medical/anaesthetic. Nurse with patient: (a) questionnaire (pen and paper); or (b) computerized assessment programme with recommendation for investigations.
2 Examination. Clinic monitor—blood pressure, electrocardiogram (ECG), SaO_2. Anaesthesiologist if required.
3 Investigations. Neither blood tests nor radiology are routine for all patients.
4 Blood values, clotting screen, electrolytes:
(a) referral clinic. Standard profiles may be used in various specialist units during phase 1, i.e. Hb and routine values in patients with anaemia or suspected bleeding (e.g. gastrointestinal, uterine); blood electrolytes (e.g. urological surgery); clotting screen where dissection may cause postoperative haemorrhage (e.g. ear, nose and throat surgery) or where indicated, e.g. known congenital clotting disorder or anticoagulant therapy. These results should be available to the staff of the assessment unit before a date for treatment is booked. Referral to a specialist clinic (e.g. haematology or diabetology) may be indicated.

(b) assessment unit. (i) A single measurement of Hb is still routine in many units. (ii) Blood tests indicated as a result of assessment in questionnaire, programme and physical examination. (iii) Special cases: *Sickle disease*—the sickle gene now affects all ethnic groups, and the incidence for example in Caucasian, Arab or Asian populations clearly depends on local factors, which should be known to the unit. All adults are usually aware of their status, but if the personal or family history at the time of assessment provides a suspicion that they could be sickle positive they should be tested. Sickle testing is not yet routine. *Diabetes*—current control status must be clear. If not, the patient should be referred to the hospital diabetic clinic or a designated physician. (iv) C reactive protein (CRP) (or serum amyloid A protein SAA). This cheap (£0·40 $\approx$ 1\$) investigation is a non-specific but extremely sensitive 'biochemical thermometer' and can be performed with a kit in the unit by nurses. It is elevated in inflammatory, infective, thrombotic and infarctive processes. Its value: firstly to indicate the current level of activity in known intercurrent disease, e.g. rheumatoid arthritis, coronary infarction and angina, and infections, for example in human immunodeficiency virus (HIV) positive patients. Secondly to indicate the presence of unsuspected disease which may not be obvious from the conventional work-up, e.g. active tuberculosis or venous thrombosis (DVT). A high CRP or SAA, unless the reason is known, indicates a need for referral to a medical clinic for further investigation.

5 Chest X-ray. Indications. History and SaO_2.

6 Electrocardiogram. This need not be routine, even in the elderly. Referral for a full ECG evaluation is indicated by history, examination, observation of an abnormal ECG on the portable monitor used for assessment, and possibly an elevated CRP if this measurement is in use.

Choice of anaesthesia

The choice of anaesthesia may be discussed with the patient at this stage, together with any unit policies, i.e. general, regional and local anaesthesia and the use of local anaesthesia combined with sedation with monitoring, referred to as either monitored anaesthetic care in the USA or sedoanalgesia in the UK. The advantages of the use of local anaesthesia or the early introduction of analgesic drugs in the postoperative period, i.e. pre-emptive analgesia will also be discussed with clear instructions for the patient.

The final choice of the type of anaesthesia *must* remain the responsibility of the anaesthesiologist in charge on the day, after discussion with the patient and within the constraints of unit policies.

Ideally a day-case booking should never be cancelled or delayed.

Phase 3: day of procedure

Anaesthesiologist and surgeon

'Good morning'. Review of work-up, consent and current medical status. Diagnostic related group (DRG) and proposed operation site and/or side, e.g. herniorrhaphy, varicose veins, vascular or joint interventions. The anaesthesiologist *must* remain in charge of the choice of anaesthesia at this stage, but should not challenge any opinion previously expressed by a colleague. This approach is part of the discipline of the unit. (Disagreements to be resolved at unit policy meetings.)

Phase 4: postoperative

Recovery from anaesthesia. Pre-emptive analgesia. Management of pain, nausea and vomiting, haemorrhage and complications. Outcome:

1 Retention for observation and further management. Suspected complications, e.g. damage to duct or organ, haemorrhage, severe pain or intractable nausea and vomiting.

2 Discharge. Transport and home arrangements. Contact telephone number, review and readmission procedures.

Phase 5: audit

Short and medium term—morbidity, mortality, admission and/or readmission. Longer term—outcome, e.g. cholecystectomy, skin tumours, endoscopic, prostatic, colonic and laryngeal surgery.

Issues

Responsibility of surgeon or practitioner in charge. Explanation of procedure alternatives and potential complications to the patient. Consent—legally requires a 24 h 'cooling off' period.

Responsibility of anaesthesiologist. Explanation of advantages, disadvantages and complications of different types of anaesthesia, analgesia and sedation, postoperative analgesia and if desirable pre-emptive analgesia. Consent. Recovery and discharge arrangements.

Counselling services. Apart from the core counselling by the surgeons, nurses and anaesthesiologists, specific counselling may be arranged, for example for patients for termination of pregnancy and prostatic surgery. Interventional radiology can be of extended duration and units may arrange counselling sessions with patients usually for about 20 min conducted by interested and trained radiographers or nurses. They are a means of reducing the anxiety in patients by removing fear of the unknown and can be of assistance in their subsequent management.

However, none of this removes the ultimate responsibility of the consultant surgeon, physician, anaesthesiologist or radiologist in charge to explain the procedure to the patient.

Further reading

Whitwam JG. C-reactive and serum amyloid A acute-phase proteins in procedural risk assessment and management. *Curr Op Anaesthesiol* 1993; 6 (suppl 1): S1–S8.

Index

accident and emergency departments, anaesthesia in 359–61
acupuncture in PONV 187
adrenaline
  in cardiopulmonary resuscitation 94, 96
  in infancy and childhood 65
  in management of adverse reactions 80, 81
advanced life support (ALS) 91–6
  in infancy and childhood 98–103
airway pressure measurement 356
alcuronium 322, 325
alfentanil
  adverse reactions to 77
  interaction with benzodiazepines 26
  interaction with propofol 34–5
  perioperative 180, 322
  pharmacology 42–3
  as premedicant 174
alpha-2 agonists 14, 175
ALS *see* advanced life support
amethocaine 65, 333
aminophylline 81
anaesthesia, definition 263
anaesthetic room 175–6
  design 355
anaesthetic technique, choice of 9–13
analgesia
  balanced 180
  in infancy and childhood 308, 326, 342
  postoperative 14–15, 179–83
    after dental procedures 233
  pre-emptive 180
  relative 233–4
anaphylactic/anaphylactoid reactions
  clinical features 71
  diagnostic procedures 72–5
  incidence 70
  management 80–2
  predisposing factors 71–2
  terminology and mechanisms 69–70
  to agents associated with anaesthesia 78–9
  to droperidol 77
  to etomidate 77
  to ketamine 77
  to local anaesthetic agents 79–80
  to muscle relaxants 69–75
  to opioid analgesics 77
  to propofol 76
  to thiopentone 76
angioedema 81
antibiotics
  adverse reactions to 79
  prophylaxis prior to endoscopy 125–7
anticoagulant therapy 408–9
anti-emetics 46–7, 186–8, 310
anxiolysis 9, 174, 405
aortofemoral–popliteal vascular disease, impact of minimally invasive therapy 154–5
aprotinin, adverse reactions to 79
arm–brain time 276
ASA categories 239–40
aspirin in postoperative analgesia 180, 181
asthma, and predisposition to anaphylactic/anaphylactoid reactions 71
asystole 94–6
atopy, and predisposition to anaphylactic/anaphylactoid reactions 71
atracurium
  in infancy and childhood 63, 64, 325
  pharmacology 45, 63, 64
atropine
  in asystole 95
  in infancy and childhood 319
  and PONV 186
audit 188–9, 370, 376, 377, 414–15
Audit Commission, *A Short Cut to Better Services* 348
automated external defibrillator (AED) 93–4

Bain breathing system 291, 292
barbiturates
  interactions with benzodiazepines 25–6
  in sedation 263
basic life support (BLS) 88, 89–91
  in infancy and childhood 98
battery 384–5, 393
Bender Gestalt track tracer 110
benzodiazepines 9, 12, 13, 174
  antagonists 22

chronic use 29
co-induction 10, 35, 38
drug interactions 25–31, 34–5
effect on insulin secretion 134
history 21–2
in infancy and childhood 64, 317–18
in patient controlled sedation 285
pharmacology 22–5, 37, 64
and PONV 185
receptors 22–3
in sedation 47, 264, 265, 267–70
beta-blockers
and predisposition to anaphylactic/anaphylactoid reactions 71
as premedicants 175
Bevan Report 347–8
bleeding disorders 406–9
blood, preoperative biochemical analysis 168–9
blood pressure measurement
in magnetic resonance department 364
preoperative 352
BLS *see* basic life support
body sway measurement 109
bowel damage during laparoscopy 207
brachial plexus block 141, 249–52
Brasslow tape 100, 102
breathing systems 177–8, 289, 290
monitoring 356–7
paediatric 295, 327
semi-closed/closed 293–4
semi-open 289–92
bronchospasm 81
bupivacaine 243
in infancy and childhood 64–5
intra-articular 182
postoperative topical 181
wound infiltration 182, 334
butorphanol 43–4

C-reactive protein, preoperative measurement 168, 352
cancer pain, epidural/subarachnoid opioid administration 145–6
capnography 356
in magnetic resonance department 364
cardiac arrest 87
cardiac arrhythmias during laparoscopy 205
cardiopulmonary resuscitation (CPR)
care after 96–7
ethical aspects 102
in infancy and childhood 98–102
procedures 88–96
cardiovascular collapse 80–1, 87
care plan 375, 379–80
cataract surgery
current practice 212–13
general anaesthesia 220–1
local anaesthesia 221–3
chain of survival 88
chest X-ray, preoperative 169–70, 352
childhood *see* infancy and childhood
chlordiazepoxide 21–2
chloroprocaine 243
choice reaction time test 110
cholecystectomy, impact of minimally invasive therapy 155
cimetidine, interaction with benzodiazepines 27
circle breathing systems 293–4
circuits 177–8, 289–95, 327
monitoring 356–7
civil assault 384–5, 393
clonidine 14, 175
codeine, in infancy and childhood 342
coin counting test 108
co-induction 10, 35, 38
community nurses, involvement in day surgery 377–8
conjunctiva, surface anaesthesia 334
consent 384–5, 389–91
form 386
implied/expressed 385–6, 390–1
and referral 386
continuous quality improvement (CQI) 349
co-ordination assessment 109
corticosteroids, in management of adverse reactions 81
CPR *see* cardiopulmonary resuscitation
cremophor 76
critical flicker fusion threshold 107–8
critical incidents 358
cuirass ventilation 298

day-case surgery
benefits 4, 347
differentiation from outpatient surgery 213, 399
history 3–4
Day Surgery: Making it Happen 348
day surgery unit
administration 370–3
admission to 375
booking visit 171–2
design and management 354–5
facilities 369–70
list organization 376–7
operational policy 370
principles of service provision in 165–95
staffing 352–4, 371–2
deep venous thrombosis (DVT) 47
defibrillation 93–4
delegation 387
dental anaesthesia 226–36

legal aspects 389–95
dentures, preoperative removal 173
desflurane 10
in infancy and childhood 61, 308, 322
in outpatient dental anaesthesia 230
pharmacology 38–40
dexmedetomidine 14, 175
dextran, adverse reactions to 78
diabetes mellitus 133–7
diazepam
bolus injection 25
differentiation from midazolam 24–5
reversal by flumazenil 28
in sedation 264
diclofenac
in infancy and childhood 326, 342
in postoperative analgesia 181
digit span test 108–9
digit symbol substitution test (DSST) 108
digital nerve block 249, 338–9, 340
digital subtraction angiography (DSA) 151
dihydrocodeine, in infancy and childhood 342
Diprivan *see* propofol
discharge 178–9, 364–6
after endoscopy 129
after locoregional anaesthesia 258–9
after pain treatment 149
in infancy and childhood 310–11
dissociative anaesthesia 265
dopamine, in management of adverse reactions 80
dorsal nerve of the penis block 335–7
driving after general anaesthesia 366
driving simulation tests 111
droperidol 46–7
adverse reactions to 77
in PONV 186–7, 310
as premedicant 175
drugs
absorption in infancy and childhood 58
anaphylactic/anaphylactoid reactions to 69–82
distribution in infancy and childhood 59
excretion in infancy and childhood 60
intraosseous administration in infancy and childhood 100
metabolism in infancy and childhood 59–60
side effects 15, 20, 21
see also specific drugs and drug types
duty of care 383

eardrum, surface anaesthesia 333
electrocardiography (ECG) 357
in magnetic resonance department 364
preoperative 169, 351–2
electroencephalography, in postanaesthetic recovery assessment 111
electromechanical dissociation (EMD) 96, 97
emergency anaesthesia 359–61
EMLA 181, 332–3
dosage and indications 244
in infancy and childhood 320
and methaemoglobinaemia 65
end tidal carbon dioxide concentration 356, 364
endoscopy *see* gastrointestinal endoscopy
endotracheal intubation 11
in infancy and childhood 324–5
enflurane 10, 39
in infancy and childhood 60–1, 308
in outpatient dental anaesthesia 229
pharmacology 41, 60–1
and PONV 185
ephedrine, in PONV 187
epicondilitis humeri 140
epidural anaesthesia 182, 254–6
cervical/thoracic 142
in infancy and childhood 340–2
motor loss following 310
etidocaine 243
etomidate 9–10
adverse reactions to 77
in outpatient dental anaesthesia 230
pharmacology 36
in sedation 263
examination under anaesthesia (EUA) in ophthalmic surgery 218–19
external chest compression 90

face masks 11
famotidine 175
fasting, preoperative 8, 173, 314
fentanyl
adverse reactions to 77
interaction with benzodiazepines 26
perioperative 180, 322
pharmacology 42, 43
as premedicant 174
field block 182, 245–6, 247
finger tapping test 109
fluid therapy
intraoperative 187
in management of adverse reactions 80–1
fluids
postoperative intake and PONV 186
preoperative restriction 8, 173, 314
flumazenil 22, 31, 265, 266
and chronic benzodiazepine use 29
pharmacology 27–8
and resedation 28–9
reversal of sedation with 28
therapeutic index 24

and ventilatory response to hypoxaemia and hypercarbia 29–30

gas embolism during laparoscopy 205–6
gasserian ganglion, radiofrequency lesion 147–8
gastric acid aspiration
during laparoscopy 208
prophylaxis 175
gastric suction in PONV 186
gastrointestinal endoscopy
antibiotic prophylaxis 125–7
clinical environment 128–9
complications 119
conscious sedation in 120–2
contraindications to 128
level of monitoring 122–5
patient recovery and discharge 129
risk assessment preceding 125
safety 118–29
training and experience in 127–8
gelatin, adverse reactions to 78, 79
general anaesthesia
comparison with locoregional anaesthesia 238
in diabetes mellitus 135–6
in infancy and childhood 313, 319–27
parental involvement 315–16
preoperative fasting 314
preoperative investigations 314
psychological preparation for 313–14
in ophthalmic day-case surgery 219–21
in outpatient dentistry 226–36
genitofemoral nerve block 141
glaucoma, congenital 218
glycopyrrolate, in infancy and childhood 319
Goldman dental mask 229, 230
golfer's elbow 140
great auricular nerve block 339–40

H_2-receptor antagonists 47, 175
interaction with benzodiazepines 27
haemoglobin, preoperative estimation 168
haemophilia A 407–8
haemophilia B 408
haemorrhage
during laparoscopy 206–7
postoperative in infancy and childhood 310
halothane 10, 39
effect on insulin secretion 134
in infancy and childhood 60–1, 308, 322
in outpatient dental anaesthesia 229–30
pharmacology 41–2, 60–1
and PONV 185
headache, postspinal puncture 257
health-care assistants 371
HealthQuiz 7–8
heart rate measurement, preoperative 352
heparin, prophylactic 47
hepatitis, halothane 41–2, 61
herpes zoster, acute 142
high frequency ventilation 295–8, 404
hospital admission index (HAI) 259
housekeeper 371–2
Humphrey breathing system 177–8, 291, 292
hyoscine 186
hypoglycaemia 134
hypothermia during laparoscopy 206

ibuprofen, in infancy and childhood 342
IgE antibodies, serological tests for 74–5
iliohypogastric nerve block 337–8
ilioinguinal nerve block 141, 337–8
indecent assault 393
indomethacin
in infancy and childhood 326
in postoperative analgesia 181
infancy and childhood
analgesia in 308, 326
anticholinergic agents in 319
cardiopulmonary resuscitation 98–103
day-care facilities 307
discharge criteria 310–11
general anaesthesia 313, 319–27
in outpatient dentistry 226–36
parental involvement 315–16
preoperative fasting 314
preoperative investigations 314
psychological preparation for 313–14
heavy sedation 318
intercurrent and familial medical disorders 305–6
locoregional anaesthesia 332–42
ophthalmic day-case anaesthesia 217–18
pharmacological principles 58–65
postoperative care 309–10
premedication in 308, 316–18
recovery from anaesthesia in 307–9
selection of suitable day-case procedures 303–7
inguinal block 141, 337–8
inhalation agents 10–11
effects on insulin secretion 134
in infancy and childhood 60–1, 308, 322
in outpatient dental anaesthesia 229–30
pharmacology 38–42, 60–1
and PONV 185
inspection time, definition 105, 107
intercostal nerve block 140–1
intestinal perforation during laparoscopy 207
intra-abdominal gas insufflation, complications arising from 203–6

intradermal tests 73–4
intravenous anaesthetic agents 9–10
  in infancy and childhood 61–2, 308, 320–1
  in outpatient dental anaesthesia 230–3
  pharmacology 20–38, 61–2
investigations, preoperative 167–71, 191–4, 314, 412–13
  in ophthalmic day-case surgery 215–16
  procedural issues 351
isoflurane 10, 39
  effect on insulin secretion 134
  in outpatient dental anaesthesia 229
  pharmacology 41, 60–1
  and PONV 185

jet ventilation 295–8, 404

ketamine
  adverse reactions to 77
  in infancy and childhood 318
  in management of adverse reactions 81
  pharmacology 36
  in sedation 264, 265, 271
ketorolac
  in infancy and childhood 326
  interaction with benzodiazepines 27
  pharmacology 44–5
  in postoperative analgesia 181

Lack–Mapleson 'A' breathing system 291–2
Lafayette pursuit rotor 110
laparoscopy 5
  complications 202–9
laparotomy, conversion of laparoscopy to 209
laryngeal mask airway (LMA) 11, 176–7
  in infancy and childhood 303, 323–4
laser surgery, safety issues 361
lateral femoral cutaneous nerve block 141
latex, adverse reactions to 79
legal aspects 383–8, 389–95
lidocaine *see* lignocaine
lignocaine 243
  in infancy and childhood 64, 65
  topical 244, 333
    postoperative 181
Limitation Act 1980 387
LMA *see* laryngeal mask airway
local anaesthesia *see* locoregional anaesthesia
local anaesthetic agents
  adverse reactions to 79–80, 242–3
  in infancy and childhood 64–5
  maximum doses 241
  in postoperative analgesia 181–3
locoregional anaesthesia 14
  in accident and emergency department 360
  central neural blockade 254–8
  comparison with general anaesthesia 238
  conduction anaesthesia 249–54
  in diabetes mellitus 134–5
  discharge criteria and hospitalization 258–9
  extravascular infiltration 244–6
  in infancy and childhood 332–42
  intra-articular infiltration 248–9
  intravascular infiltration 246–8
  in ophthalmic day-case surgery 221–3
  outpatient procedures 241–58
  patient assessment and preparation 238–9
  patient classification 239–40
  premedication 240
  sedation 240–1
  topical 244
lorazepam
  pharmacology 23
  in sedation 271
low back pain 142
low flow to-and-fro breathing system 293, 294
lumbar sympathectomy 144–5
lumbosacral plexus block 252–4

McKesson dental mask 229, 230
Maddox Wing test 111
magnesium sulphate, in management of adverse reactions 81
magnetic resonance department, anaesthesia in 362–4
malignant hyperthermia 217–18, 400–3
Mapleson 'A' breathing system 289–90, 291
mask ventilation 89–90
masseter muscle spasm 218
medical notes 387
memory assessment, longer term 109
meperidine, adverse reactions to 77
mepivacaine 243
mesosalpinx block 182
methaemoglobinaemia 65
methohexitone 9
  in infancy and childhood 61–2, 321
  interaction with benzodiazepines 26
  in outpatient dental anaesthesia 230
  pharmacology 35–6, 61–2
metoclopramide 46, 186, 310
midazolam 9, 12, 13, 22
  adverse effects 24
  bolus injection 25
  co-induction 10, 35, 38
  differentiation from diazepam 24–5
  drug interactions 25–7, 34–5
  effect on insulin secretion 134
  effectiveness 174
  in infancy and childhood 64, 317–18

in patient controlled sedation 285
pharmacology 23, 37, 64
plasma half-life 25
resedation after reversal 28–9
reversal by flumazenil 28
in sedation 47, 264, 265, 267–70
therapeutic index 24
minimal access surgery 151–3
implications for anaesthesia 153–9
minimally invasive therapy (MIT) 151–3
implications for anaesthesia 153–9
mivacurium
in infancy and childhood 64, 325
pharmacology 46, 64
monitored anaesthetic care (MAC) 405
monitoring 178, 355–8
in outpatient dentistry 234
in gastrointestinal endoscopy 122–5
in infancy and childhood 326
in locoregional anaesthesia 243
patient controlled sedation 285
performance indicators 348–9
morphine 42, 43
adverse reactions to 77
in infancy and childhood 322, 342
interaction with benzodiazepines 26
intra-articular 182
intraoperative 322
mortality in outpatient dentistry 235
mouth-to-mouth ventilation 89–90
muscle relaxants
anaphylactic/anaphylactoid reactions to 69–75
in infancy and childhood 63–4, 325
monitoring effects 357
pharmacology 45–6, 63–4
myofascial pain syndrome 139
myringotomy 333

nalbuphine 26, 43–4
naloxone 31, 266
naproxen 181
nasal intubation 232
nausea *see* postoperative nausea and vomiting
neck pain 142
negligence 383–5, 391–2
neonates
pharmacological principles 58–65
suitability for day-case procedures 304–5
neostigmine 186
nerve blockade 138–9
in cancer pain 145–6
central 142, 254–8
destructive
with neurolytic solution 146–7
with radiofrequency lesions 147–9
discharge criteria and hospitalization 149
in pain treatment 138–49
peripheral 140–1, 249
in accident and emergency department 360
in infancy and childhood 335–40
plexus 141, 249–54
in postoperative analgesia 181–3
regional intravenous sympathetic 145
sympathetic 143–5
therapeutic reversible 139–45
nerve injury during laparoscopy 208
neuralgia, postherpetic 142
neurolytic blocks 146–7
neuromuscular blocking agents *see* muscle relaxants
nitrous oxide 39
pharmacology 42
and PONV 185
non-steroidal anti-inflammatory drugs (NSAIDs) 14
in infancy and childhood 326, 342
pharmacology 44–5
in postoperative analgesia 180–1
noradrenaline, in management of adverse reactions 80
NSAIDs *see* non-steroidal anti-inflammatory drugs
nursing staff 353, 371
role in patient assessment 374–5
stress and burn out 372
training and education 373

Oakley chart 100, 101
occipital nerve block 140
oculocardiac reflex 217
omeprazole 47, 175
ondansetron 15, 47, 187, 310
operating theatre
design 355
staff 353
ophthalmic day-case surgery 212–13
anaesthesia for 216–23
patient selection 213–16
opioid analgesics 14
adverse reactions to 77
in combination with patient controlled sedation 286–7
epidural/subarachnoid administration 145–6
in infancy and childhood 322, 342
interactions with benzodiazepines 25–6
in perioperative analgesia 180, 322
pharmacology 42–4
and PONV 185
as premedicants 174–5
in sedation 263, 265
oral airways 11
outpatient surgery, differentiation from day-case

surgery 213, 399
oxazepam pharmacology 23
oxycodone 174
oxygen, supplemental in gastrointestinal endoscopy 122
oxymorphone 174

p-deletion test 107
pacemakers in magnetic resonance 364
pain
chronic 139
following laparoscopy 209
and PONV 185
postoperative 309, 366
therapy of 138–49
painful shoulder injection 139–40
pancuronium 325
paracetamol
in infancy and childhood 326, 342
in postoperative analgesia 180
patient controlled sedation (PCS) 223, 267, 269–70, 275, 288
choice of drug 285
choice of procedure 286
in combination with opioid analgesics 286–7
efficacy 282
equipment 277–9, 284–5, 287–8
maximum mean infusion rate 279–81
monitoring 285
patient selection 286
pharmacokinetic principles 276–7
principles 279–84
safety 282–4
patient hotels 378
patients
age of 7
classification by ASA categories 239–40
information for 172, 195, 376
preparation 8–9
selection 5–6, 166–7, 191–4, 373–5, 412
in infancy and childhood 305–6
for locoregional anaesthesia 238–9
for ophthalmic day-case surgery 213–16
for patient controlled sedation 286
procedural issues 350–1
PCS *see* patient controlled sedation
pegboard test 109
penicillin, adverse reactions to 79
penile block 335–7
perceptive accuracy test (PAT) 107
perceptual speed test 107
performance indicators 348–9
peribulbar anaesthesia 222
perioperative complications, factors influencing 6
pethidine 42, 43, 322
pharmacodynamics 20
pharmacokinetics 20
in infancy and childhood 58–60
pharmacology 20–48
in infancy and childhood 58–65
plasma proteins
adverse reactions to 78
in infancy and childhood 59
pneumomediastinum during laparoscopy 205
pneumopericardium during laparoscopy 205
pneumoperitoneum, induced, complications arising from 203–6
pneumothorax
after brachial plexus block 252
during intercostal nerve block 140–1
pollution by anaesthetic gases 235
PONV *see* postoperative nausea and vomiting
posterior facet syndrome 148
postherpetic neuralgia 142
postoperative nausea and vomiting (PONV) 183–8, 365–6
after ophthalmic surgery 218
in infancy and childhood 309–10
Poswillo Report 227, 234
Prausnitz–Kuestner test 74
precordial thump 92
premedication 173–5
drugs 47
in infancy and childhood 308, 316–18
in locoregional anaesthesia 240
preoperative assessment 7–8, 166–71, 191–4, 373–5, 412–13
in infancy and childhood 315
in locoregional anaesthesia 238–9
in ophthalmic day-case surgery 215–16
procedural issues 351
preoperative management 172–6
in infancy and childhood 313–18
prepuce, surface anaesthesia 334
prilocaine 243
in infancy and childhood 65
ototoxicity 333
procaine 81, 243
professional organizations 158–9
propofol 10, 31, 176
adverse effects 34
anaphylaxis 76
drug interactions 34–5
in infancy and childhood 62, 308, 320–1
interaction with benzodiazepines 26
metabolism 32
in outpatient dental anaesthesia 230
in patient controlled sedation 285
pharmacokinetics 31–2
and PONV 185
recovery characteristics 32–4
in sedation 263, 264–5, 266, 267–70

therapeutic index 24
propranolol 175
prostatectomy, impact of minimally invasive therapy 155
psoas block 252–3
psychomotor tests of postanaesthetic recovery 105–14
pulmonary oedema 81
pulse oximetry 358
in magnetic resonance department 364

quality control/assurance 358–9, 376, 377

radio-allergosorbent test 74–5
radiofrequency nerve lesions 147–9
radiology department, anaesthesia in 362
ranitidine 27, 47, 175
RAST 74–5
reception area 355
staff 371
recovery 364–6
after endoscopy 129
after propofol induction 32–4
assessment of 104–14, 309
in infancy and childhood 307–9
recovery area 178, 307
design 355
staffing 353
recovery position 91
rectus sheath block 182
referral and consent 386
reflex sympathetic dystrophy 144
regional anaesthesia *see* locoregional anaesthesia
regional intravenous sympathetic block 145
relative analgesia 233–4
respiratory arrest 90
retinoblastoma 218
retrobulbar anaesthesia 221–2
rhizotomy, percutaneous radiofrequency 148–9
rocuronium 46

saccadic eye movements 111
safe practice, issues in 347–66
salbutamol, in management of adverse reactions 81
sciatic nerve block 253
scopolamine 186
secretarial staff 354
sedation
in accident and emergency department 360–1
complications 271–2
conduct of 266
deep 120
definition 263
dissociation 234
drugs available for 263–6
end-point 271
in gastrointestinal endoscopy 120–2
grades 263
heavy in infancy and childhood 318
inhalational 233
in locoregional anaesthesia 240–1
and minimally invasive therapy 156
objectives 263
for ophthalmic local anaesthesia 223
in outpatient dentistry 233–4
patient controlled *see* patient controlled sedation
techniques 267–71
sedoanalgesia 262–3, 267, 405
conduct of 266–7
semantics of anaesthetic technique 405
serological tests for IgE antibodies 74–5
serum amyloid A protein, preoperative measurement 168
sevoflurane 11, 39
in infancy and childhood 61, 308
pharmacology 40
short-term memory assessment 108–9
sickle disease 228, 231, 410–11
silver nitrite dressings, and methaemoglobinaemia 65
simple reaction time test 110
skin prick test 72–3
Society for Minimally Invasive Therapy (SMIT) 158–9
spasmophilia, and predisposition to anaphylactic/anaphylactoid reactions 71–2
spinal anaesthesia 142, 182, 256–8
spinal facets, radiofrequency denervation 148
standard of care 383–4
stellate ganglion
radiofrequency lesion 148
therapeutic reversible block 143–4
step-down unit 365
Steward simplified postanaesthetic recovery score 105, 309
strabismus correction 217–18, 219–20
street fitness 114
Stroop phenomenon 108
subarachnoid block 142, 182, 256–8
subconjunctival anaesthesia 222
sub-Tenon's infiltration 222
sufentanil
interaction with propofol 34
pharmacology 43
surgical day-case, definition 347
suxamethonium
in infancy and childhood 63, 64, 325
pharmacology 45, 63, 64
synergism 10

triple 34–5, 38
syringe drivers 277–9, 284–5, 287–8

temazepam 9, 23
temperature monitoring 358
tennis elbow 140
thiopentone 9
anaphylaxis 76
effect on insulin secretion 134
in infancy and childhood 51, 308, 320
interaction with benzodiazepines 26
in outpatient dental anaesthesia 230
pharmacology 35–6, 51
therapeutic index 24
three in one block 253
timolol 175
to-and-fro breathing system 293, 294
topical anaesthesia 244, 332–4
tracking tests 110–11
training 157–8
Trieger dot test 110
trigeminal neuralgia 147–8
trigger point injections 139

unconsciousness 91
urinary tract injury during laparoscopy 207
urine, preoperative testing 168–9

vecuronium
in infancy and childhood 63, 64, 325
pharmacology 45, 63, 64
venous access 94
in infancy and childhood 99–100
ventilation systems 157, 295–8
ventricular fibrillation (VF) 91–4
visualization tests 107
vomiting *see* postoperative nausea and vomiting
Von Willebrand's disease 408

Waters breathing system 293, 294
wisdom teeth, surgical removal 231–3
wound infiltration by local anaesthetic agents 181–2, 334